Cardiopulmonary
Physical Therapy

Cardiopulmonary Physical Therapy

A Clinical Manual

Joanne Watchie, MA, PT, CCS

W.B. SAUNDERS COMPANY

A Division of Harcourt Brace & Company

Philadelphia   London   Toronto   Montreal   Sydney   Tokyo

W.B. SAUNDERS COMPANY

A Division of Harcourt Brace & Company

The Curtis Center
Independence Square West
Philadelphia, PA 19106

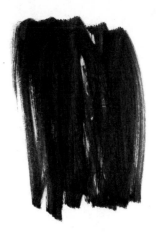

Library of Congress Cataloging-in-Publication Data

Watchie, Joanne.
    Cardiopulmonary physical therapy: a clinical manual / Joanne
Watchie. — 1st ed.
        p.   cm.
  ISBN 0-7216-6709-0
    1. Cardiopulmonary system—Diseases—Physical therapy—Handbooks,
manuals, etc.   I. Title.
    [DNLM: 1. Cardiovascular Diseases—rehabilitation—handbooks.
2. Lung Diseases—rehabilitation—handbooks.   3. Physical Therapy—
methods—handbooks.   WG 39 1995]
  RC702.W38   1995
  616.1'2062—dc20
  DNLM/DLC   95-3949

CARDIOPULMONARY PHYSICAL THERAPY: A CLINICAL MANUAL   ISBN 0-7216-6709-0

Printed in the United States of America

Last digit is the print number: 9 8 7 6 5 4 3 2 1

To Andrew
for his support and patience
through the long years it took to complete this book
and especially for his help
in keeping the computer operational.

To Tony
for his love, patience, and acceptance
of all the time I spent on this book
and unavailable to him.
I promise to take you to a movie!

PREFACE

Cardiopulmonary Physical Therapy: A Clinical Manual is intended to be a ready reference for physical therapists working in the acute care setting, particularly the intensive care unit, cardiac care unit, cardiac step-down unit, or general medical wards. In addition, it will be valuable for clinicians working in a number of other acute, home care, and rehabilitation settings, such as orthopedics, oncology, and neurology, where patients frequently have secondary medical diagnoses of hypertension, cardiovascular disease, diabetes, and/or pulmonary disease. Finally, students of physical therapy will enjoy the wide variety of practical information contained in this book.

The idea for this clinical manual developed during an Executive Committee meeting of the Cardiopulmonary Section of the American Physical Therapy Association in 1988, during which several members expressed frustration over the amount of time and effort required to find appropriate materials to use in the orientation and instruction of staff and students who rotate through the various physical therapy services that provide treatment to patients with cardiopulmonary diseases or dysfunction. In addition, some members receive frequent requests for reference materials and bibliographies from practicing therapists who are interested in developing more expertise in cardiopulmonary physical therapy. *Cardiopulmonary Physical Therapy: A Clinical Manual* was created in response to these needs.

The purpose of this book is to provide a quick convenient source for a wide variety of information relating to the physical therapy management of patients with cardiopulmonary problems. This information is typically obtainable only by consulting numerous other textbooks dealing with cardiology, pulmonology, exercise physiology, cardiac and pulmonary rehabilitation, and cardiopulmonary physical therapy. This manual is not intended to obviate the need for these more detailed and complete reference materials in the physical therapy department, for their information is often vital to a true understanding of a specific patient's problems and appropriate management.

Included are basic cardiopulmonary anatomy and physiology, pathophysiology of commonly encountered cardiac and pulmonary disorders, diagnostic tests and procedures, therapeutic interventions, pharmacology, physical therapy evaluation and treatment of cardiopulmonary dysfunction, pediatric cardiopulmonary topics, and clinical laboratory values and profiles. In addition, there is an extensive list of cardiopulmonary abbreviations and a glossary. Finally, an attempt was made to facilitate the location of related materials within the book by noting cross-reference page numbers and making the index as complete as possible.

Joanne Watchie

CONTRIBUTOR

Coreen Woodford, PharmD, is a former assistant professor of clinical pharmacy at the University of Southern California School of Pharmacy. She is currently a preceptor for Level IV USC pharmacy students in the community pharmacy clerkship at the San Marino Pharmacy, San Marino, California.

ACKNOWLEDGMENTS

My creation of this book is partially an accident; one of our Cardiopulmonary Section members, Kate Grimes, had pulled together some materials for a simple pocket-sized handbook containing lab values and other useful information, and I merely volunteered to finish putting it together. Thanks, Kate, for your start, but I kept finding other bits of information I thought would be nice to have at my fingertips.... Unfortunately, the book is no longer pocket-size, but I hope it is useful nonetheless.

The most important people to thank for their patience, support, and understanding during the long years it took to complete this project are my husband and son. I know they are at least as happy as I am that this is finally done!

However, there are a few others who directly contributed to the production of the book whom I would like to include. First and foremost is my colleague and friend, Ellen Hillegass, who provided constant encouragement and frequent advise. Next, Joy Moore at Cracom Corporation was always helpful and reassuring as the book went through publication. My illustrator, Jeanne Robertson, was incredibly patient and persistent as we tried to create a number of figures for this book. David Prout provided guidance throughout the editorial phase and helped me know when it was time to call it quits. And finally, Margaret Biblis from W.B. Saunders kept me going when I grew tired of all the demands and then learned to back down a bit with the endless deadlines. I extend my sincerest thanks to all of you.

CONTENTS

1

CARDIOLOGY

This chapter begins with a review of basic cardiovascular anatomy and physiology, with emphasis on the factors that influence cardiac function. The remainder of the chapter presents the various diagnostic tests and procedures and therapeutic interventions available for the management of cardiac disease. In many instances the implications for physical therapy treatments for important findings from the most common diagnostic tests, as well as for some treatment interventions, are included. The cardiac diseases and disorders frequently encountered in rehabilitation patients are described in Chapter 3.

1.1 THE HEART AND CIRCULATION

A brief review of cardiac anatomy and some of the physiologic principles essential for understanding cardiac function are offered in this section.

ANATOMY

THE HEART

- The heart chambers and valves are shown in Figure 1–1.
- Terminology used to describe the regions of the heart:
  - Basal: top, superior
  - Apical: bottom, inferior
  - Lateral: lateral left ventricle
- Layers of cardiac tissue:
  - Endocardium: innermost layer (endothelium and subendothelial connective tissue)
  - Myocardium: middle layer (muscle tissue)
  - Epicardium: inner layer of the serous pericardium lying directly on the heart
  - Pericardium: fibrous sac around the heart

THE CONDUCTION SYSTEM OF THE HEART

Conduction of the spontaneous electrical activity of the heart normally occurs along the pathway illustrated in Figure 1–2:

- Cells in the sinoatrial (SA) node depolarize fastest, at a rate of 60 to 100 beats per minute (bpm), and a wave of depolarization is sent through the atria along the internodal pathways, causing atrial contraction.
- After a brief delay in the atrioventricular (AV) node, the impulse is conducted through the AV bundle (bundle of His), the right and left bundle branches, and the Purkinje fibers to the ventricular muscle cells, which then contract, initiating systole.
- During diastole, the ventricles repolarize and refill with blood.

If the SA node does not function, the role of pacemaker is taken over by the next functioning portion of the conduction system, according to its intrinsic rate of depolarization: the AV node at 40 to 60 bpm and the ventricular pacemaker cells at 25 to 40 bpm.

INNERVATION OF THE HEART

- The heart is innervated by the autonomic nervous system, consisting of two antagonistic parts, the sympathetic and parasympathetic nervous systems (SNS and PNS, respectively), which are illustrated in Figure 1–3.
- The PNS, via the vagus nerves, is dominant during basal conditions, when the SNS is inhibited. However, during any form of stress the SNS becomes dominant and effects many complex changes involving most systems of the body.
- The effects of the autonomic nervous system on the heart are listed below:
  - *PNS:* decreases heart rate (negative chronotropic effect), decreases strength of atrial

1

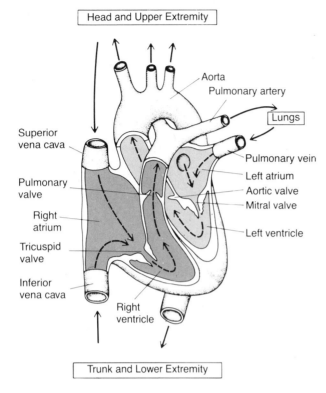

Head and Upper Extremity

Aorta
Pulmonary artery

Lungs

Superior vena cava

Pulmonary vein
Left atrium
Aortic valve
Mitral valve

Pulmonary valve

Right atrium

Tricuspid valve

Left ventricle

Inferior vena cava

Right ventricle

Trunk and Lower Extremity

FIGURE 1-1. The heart chambers and valves. Blood flows into the right atrium from the superior and inferior vena cavae, then through the tricuspid valve to the right ventricle and out through the pulmonic valve and pulmonary arteries to the lungs; blood returns to the left atrium via the pulmonary veins, then passes through the mitral valve to the left ventricle, and is finally ejected through the aortic valve into the aorta and the coronary arteries to supply all tissues of the body. (From Guyton AC: *Textbook of Medical Physiology,* 8th Ed. Philadelphia, W.B. Saunders Co., 1991. Used with permission.)

FIGURE 1-2. The conduction system of the heart. Impulses travel from the SA node through the atria to the AV node, then through the bundle of His, right and left bundle branches, and Purkinje fibers to the ventricular muscle. (From Guyton AC: *Textbook of Medical Physiology,* 8th Ed. Philadelphia, W.B. Saunders Co., 1991. Used with permission.)

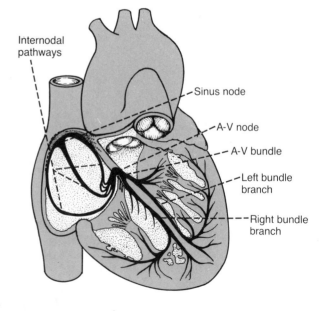

Internodal pathways

Sinus node
A-V node
A-V bundle
Left bundle branch
Right bundle branch

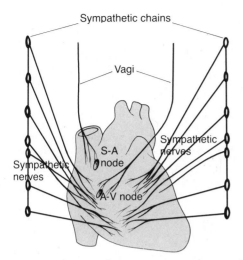

FIGURE 1-3. Autonomic nervous system innervation of the heart. SNS stimulation reaches the heart via the sympathetic chain while the PNS acts through the vagus nerves. (From Guyton AC: *Textbook of Medical Physiology,* 8th Ed. Philadelphia, W.B. Saunders Co., 1991. Used with permission.)

contraction (negative inotropic effect), and slows conduction through the AV node.
- *SNS:* increases heart rate (positive chronotropic effect), increases contractility (positive inotropic effect), and increases conduction velocity throughout the atria, AV node, and ventricles.

BLOOD SUPPLY TO THE HEART: THE CORONARY ARTERIES

- The heart muscle receives its blood supply via the coronary arteries, which are shown in the common angiographic views in Figure 1–4:
  - Right coronary artery (RCA)
  - Left main coronary artery (LMCA)
  - Left anterior descending (LAD)
  - Circumflex (Cx)
- The most common distribution of blood supply is described in Table 1–1.
- Coronary blood flow occurs almost exclusively during the diastolic phase of the cardiac cycle, when the ventricles are filling.

PHYSIOLOGY

BASIC FUNCTIONS OF THE CARDIOVASCULAR SYSTEM

- Circulation of blood
- Delivery of oxygen, nutrients, and water
- Circulation of hormones
- Temperature regulation
- Removal of metabolites
- Maintenance of acid-base balance (pH)

IMPORTANT RELATIONSHIPS

- Cardiac output (CO, or $\dot{Q}$) is the product of heart rate (HR) and stroke volume (SV): CO = HR × SV.
  - Factors that influence heart rate and stroke volume are listed in Table 1–2.

TABLE 1-1. Common Distribution of the Coronary Arteries

CORONARY ARTERY	DISTRIBUTION
Right coronary artery (RCA)	Right atrium, SA node, posterior right ventricle, AV node, bundle of His, and usually serves as origin of the posterior descending artery (~80–90% of people)
Left main	Bifurcates within 2–10 mm into the left anterior descending and circumflex arteries
Left anterior descending (LAD)	Anterior left ventricle, anterior intraventricular septum and adjacent right ventricle, portions of both bundle branches, and often the proximal inferior portion of both ventricles and apex
Circumflex (Cx)	Left atrium, lateral and inferior walls of the left ventricle, and sometimes serves as origin of the posterior descending artery (~10–20% of people)
Posterior descending artery (PDA)	Posterior intraventricular septum, plus at least half of the inferior left ventricle

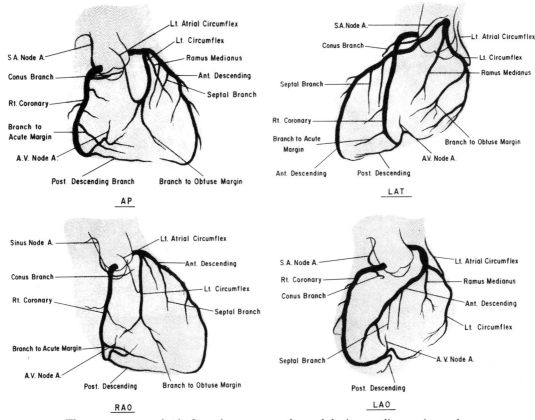

FIGURE 1–4. The coronary arteries in four views commonly used during cardiac angiography: anteroposterior, AP; lateral, LAT; right anterior oblique, RAO; and left anterior oblique, LAO. (From Abrams H, Adams DF: *N. Engl. J. Med.* 281:1277, 1969. Used with permission.)

- Cardiac function is affected by a number of factors:
  - Preload, which is the resting tension or stretch on the myocardial cells and is considered to be the volume of blood in the ventricle at the completion of filling (i.e., the end-diastolic volume, EDV)
    — An increase in preload results in an increase in stroke volume.
    — Because end-diastolic pressure (EDP) is directly related to end-diastolic volume, either of them can be used as indicators of preload.
  - Afterload, or the load or pressure against which the ventricle must work in order to eject blood, which corresponds to the diastolic pressure initially (e.g., of the aorta for the left ventricle) and then rises with the systolic pressure as blood is ejected
    — An increase in afterload results in a decrease in stroke volume.
  - Contractility, or inotropic state, which refers to the innate rate and intensity of force development during contraction
    — An increase in the inotropic state results in faster myocardial shortening at any given preload and afterload, as well as a greater degree of shortening and force development, so a greater stroke volume of blood is ejected.

TABLE 1–2. **Factors That Influence Heart Rate and Stroke Volume**

FACTOR	INFLUENCED BY
Heart rate	The intrinsic rate of spontaneous pacemaker function.
	The balance of SNS and PNS stimulation.
	Levels of circulating catecholamines and other substances.
Stroke volume	*Preload,* which is affected by:
	Active atrial contraction(results in ↑ EDV by 10–20%)
	Heart rate (↑ HR results in ↓ diastolic filling time)
	Venous blood return
	Total blood volume, state of hydration
	Ventricular compliance (the ease with which the ventricle distends when it is filled with blood)
	Afterload, which is affected by:
	Total peripheral resistance
	Stroke volume
	EDV
	Impedance (blood viscosity, aortic compliance)
	Presence of outflow obstruction
	Contractility, which is affected positively and negatively by multiple factors (see Table 1–3)

SNS = sympathetic nervous system, PNS = parasympathetic nervous system, EDV = end-diastolic volume, HR = heart rate, ↑ = increased, ↓ = decreased.

— Inotropism is affected by numerous factors, as listed in Table 1–3.
- Ventricular compliance, or the ease with which the ventricle distends when it is filled with blood (i.e., its degree of stiffness)
  — If compliance is decreased (i.e., the ventricle is stiffer, as in left ventricular hypertrophy), a given volume of filling will result in a higher end-diastolic pressure.
  — If compliance is increased (i.e., left ventricular dilatation), a given volume of filling will result in a lower end-diastolic pressure.
- The amount of energy the heart requires to produce cardiac output is related to the *wall tension or stress* the ventricles must develop in order to eject the stroke volume against the afterload and the frequency with which it contracts (i.e., the heart rate).
- As ventricular pressure rises during systole, wall tension is directly related to the intraventricular pressure and the radius and in-

TABLE 1–3. **Factors That Influence Contractility/Inotropism**

POSITIVE INOTROPIC INFLUENCE	NEGATIVE INOTROPIC INFLUENCE
↑ Sympathetic tone	Beta blockers
↑ Endogenous catecholamines	Calcium antagonists
Digitalis	Barbiturates
Sympathetic amines	Acidosis
↑ Heart rate	Hypoxia
Glucagon	General anesthesia
Angiotensin	Antiarrhythmic agents
Aldactone	Heart failure
Corticosteroids	↓ Functional ventricular muscle mass
Hyperthyroidism	↓ Myocardial oxygen supply:demand
Serotonin	Circulating myocardial depressant factors

↑ = increased, ↓ = decreased.

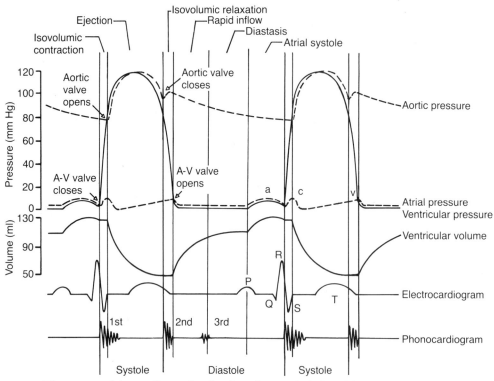

FIGURE 1-5. The events of the cardiac cycle, showing changes in left atrial pressure, left ventricular pressure, aortic pressure, ventricular volume, the electrocardiogram, and the heart sounds via a phonocardiogram. (From Guyton AC: *Textbook of Medical Physiology,* 8th Ed. Philadelphia, W.B. Saunders Co., p. 102, 1991. Used with permission.)

versely related to the ventricular wall thickness (i.e., T = P × R/h).

• A commonly used indirect index of myocardial energy cost (i.e., myocardial oxygen consumption) is the rate-pressure product (RPP), or double product, which is equal to the product of heart rate and systolic blood pressure (SBP): RPP = HR × SBP, which is usually expressed as the three-digit number × 10^2. For example, in an individual with a HR of 145 and a blood pressure of 160/80 during running, the RPP would equal 145 × 160, or 232 × 10^2.

CARDIAC CYCLE

The cardiac cycle includes all the events that occur within the heart during the filling phase, or diastole, and the pressure-development and ejection phase, or systole. These events are illustrated in Figure 1–5 and occur as follows:

• During *diastole,* blood flows continuously into the right atrium (RA) and left atrium (LA) via the vena cavae and pulmonary veins, respectively, and continues its flow across the atrioventricular (AV) valves (tricuspid [TV] on the right and mitral [MV] on the left) into the right ventricle (RV) and left ventricle (LV), respectively.

• Spontaneously, the SA node initiates a wave of *depolarization* that travels through the atria and is depicted as the P wave on the electrocardiogram (ECG).

• Depolarization is followed by *atrial contraction,* the final event of diastole (the *a* wave), which forces a last increment of blood into the ventricles and results in RV and LV end-diastolic pressure.

- The wave of depolarization traverses the AV node, bundle of His, bundle branches, and Purkinje fibers to excite the right and left ventricular muscle fibers, causing *left then right ventricular contraction* (normally 20 to 30 mseconds apart).
- With the onset of contraction, the respective *ventricular pressures* begin to *rise* so that they exceed the pressures in the atria and force *MV and TV closure.*
- Now all the heart valves are closed and there is a fixed volume of blood in each ventricle. Ventricular contraction continues against this volume (the *isovolumic phase)* until the pressures within the ventricles exceed that in the aorta on the left and pulmonary artery (PA) on the right.
- At this point, the *ejection valves* (aortic valve on the left and pulmonic valve on the right) *open* and the *ejection* phase begins. Additional ventricular contraction results in ejection of the final *stroke volume* for that heart beat.
- Ventricular contraction is followed by *relaxation* with *repolarization* of the myocardial cells and diminution of ventricular pressures. When the *ventricular pressures fall* below that in the aorta and PA, the *ejection valves close.*
- Further decline in ventricular pressures results in *MV and TV opening* so that the *diastolic filling phase* begins again.
- The atria, which have been filling with blood throughout the ejection phase, initially empty rapidly into the ventricles (y descent). Continued slower ventricular filling occurs until the next atrial contraction occurs.

HEART SOUNDS

Most commonly, only two heart sounds can be auscultated, but on occasion a third and/or fourth heart sound may be present.

- S_1: first heart sound, which is associated with MV and TV closure and corresponds with the onset of ventricular systole.
- S_2: second heart sound, which is associated with aortic and pulmonary valve closure and corresponds with the start of ventricular diastole.
- S_3: third heart sound, which is associated with early rapid diastolic filling of the ventricles and is called a "ventricular gallop";

most frequently associated with heart failure though may occur normally in the young or very old.
- S_4: fourth heart sound, which is associated with active ventricular filling due to atrial contraction and is called an "atrial gallop"; often heard following acute myocardial infarction.

1.2 EVALUATION OF CARDIAC FUNCTION

Although physical therapists rarely participate in or read the data of most of the diagnostic tests and procedures described in this section, we are frequently challenged to interpret the results of these investigations and their implications for our patients. By comprehending the information presented in a patient's chart, we can have a fairly accurate perception of the patient's status and probable or possible physiologic responses to our interventions even before we begin our assessment. At the least, we should be able to determine when caution is particularly warranted.

SIGNS AND SYMPTOMS OF CARDIOVASCULAR DISEASE

Generally, the first information that is presented in a patient's medical history is the patient's complaints. Table 1–4 tabulates the most common patient complaints and their cardiovascular causes. There may be other possible explanations for some of these complaints, and these are presented on pages 42 and 153.

PHYSICAL EXAMINATION

The history and physical examination section of a patient's chart is a valuable source of important information relating to the patient's status and level of function. The relevant data and their implications are discussed in Chapter 5 (see Table 5–3, page 150).

ELECTROCARDIOGRAPHY

An electrocardiogram (ECG) records the electrical activity of the heart on a graph of voltage versus time. It can be obtained using a single lead, as in a rhythm strip, or multiple leads, as in the standard 12-lead ECG.

TABLE 1–4. **Signs and Symptoms of Cardiovascular Diseases**

SIGN OR SYMPTOM	CARDIOVASCULAR CAUSES
Chest pain or discomfort	Mismatch between myocardial oxygen supply and demand (due to coronary disease, LV hypertrophy, LV outflow obstruction, coronary spasm, microvascular angina), autonomic dysfunction, MV prolapse
Claudication	Peripheral arterial disease with mismatch between peripheral O_2 supply and demand
Clubbing of digits	Right-to-left shunting in congenital heart disease
Cough, hemoptysis	Acute pulmonary edema, MS
Cyanosis	Right-to-left shunting in congenital heart disease, significant ↓ cardiac output
Dizziness, syncope	Inadequate cardiac output resulting in ↓ perfusion of the brain (due to ↓ LV function, LV outlet obstruction, arrhythmias, blood pooling in lower extremities)
Dyspnea, shortness of breath	↑ Pulmonary venous pressure caused by LV diastolic or systolic dysfunction (due to coronary ischemia, valvular disease, ↓ myocardial function), peripheral arterial disease with lactic acidosis
Edema	↑ Systemic venous pressure due to ↑ RA pressure (e.g., LV failure, MS, cor pulmonale, TS, TR, constrictive pericarditis)
Fatigue, weakness	Depressed cardiac output (due to ↓ LV function, LV outlet obstruction, arrhythmias), drugs
Abnormal funduscopic examination	Hypertension, diabetes mellitus, sometimes infective endocarditis
Hemoptysis	Acute pulmonary edema, MS
Hypotension	↓ Cardiac output, vasodilation
Jugular venous distension (JVD)	↑ Systemic venous pressure caused by ↑ RA pressure (see "Edema," above)
Nocturia	CHF with some peripheral edema
Orthopnea	In CHF, SOB when lying flat due to ↑ pulmonary venous pressure caused by ↑ venous return to heart that is not able to handle ↑ workload
Palpitations	Arrhythmias
Paroxysmal Nocturnal Dyspnea (PND)	In CHF, sudden onset of SOB that awakens patient at night because of ↑ pulmonary pressures caused by the gradual reabsorption of edema fluid from the LEs (which are no longer dependent), which results in ↑ venous return to heart that is not able to handle ↑ workload
Pulmonary rales	CHF, exercise-induced ↑ pulmonary pressures
Abnormal pulse rate or rhythm	Arrhythmias
S_3, S_4	See "Heart Sounds" (page 163)
Shortness of breath (SOB)	See "Dyspnea" entry above
Syncope	Profoundly ↓ cardiac output (see "Dizziness" entry above)
Weakness	See "Fatigue" entry above

LE = lower extremity, LV = left ventricle, MV = mitral valve, O_2 = oxygen, MS = mitral stenosis, RA = right atrium, TS = tricuspid stenosis, TR = tricuspid regurgitation, CHF = congestive heart failure, SOB = shortness of breath, S_3 = third heart sound, S_4 = fourth heart sound, ↑ = increased, ↓ = decreased.

RHYTHM STRIPS

An ECG recording obtained from one to three leads, which can be acquired via "hard" wiring (where wires connect the patient to the monitor) or via telemetry (where a radiotelemeter sends the ECG signal to the monitor), produces a rhythm strip.

- Rhythm strips are used mainly to monitor heart rate and rhythm and are commonly seen in intensive care units, step-down or transi-

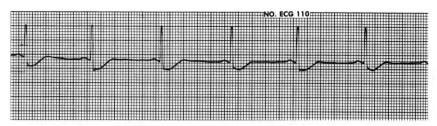

FIGURE 1-6. Rhythm strip showing normal sinus rhythm. Abnormal ST–T changes are also present.

tional care units, and cardiac and pulmonary rehabilitation programs.

- A rhythm strip showing normal sinus rhythm is depicted in Figure 1–6.
- Information related to ECG lead setups and basic interpretation of rhythm strips is presented in Chapter 5 (see pages 176 to 186).

12-LEAD ECG

The electrical activity of the heart can be recorded from 12 specific leads, as shown in Figure 1–7, to provide a "map" of the electrical voltages created by the different areas of the heart.

- Lead placement for a 12-lead ECG is depicted in Figure 1–8.
- Information that can be obtained from a 12-lead ECG includes:
  - Rate and rhythm
  - Electrical axis of the heart
  - Presence of specific abnormalities, such as chamber enlargement and hypertrophy, conduction defects, myocardial ischemia and infarction and their location, and drug effects
- Some specific abnormalities that can be identified using a 12-lead ECG include:
  - Left ventricular hypertrophy (LVH)
    — Characterized by tall R waves in V_{5-6} (>27

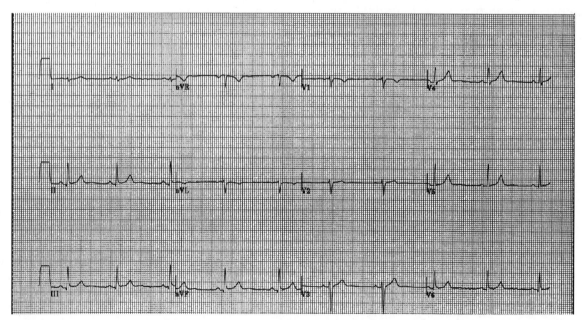

FIGURE 1-7. A normal 12-lead electrocardiogram. Note the progression of the QRS waves across the precordium (leads V_{1-6}) as the deflections transition from predominantly negative to very positive. (Courtesy of Ellen Hillegass.)

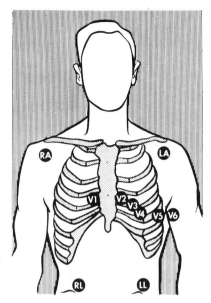

FIGURE 1-8. Location of electrodes for the standard 12-lead ECG, in this case for exercise testing. For a standard 12-lead ECG, the RA electrode would be attached to the right arm, the LA on the left arm, the RL on the right leg, and the LL on the left leg. (From Wilson PK, et. al.: *Cardiac Rehabilitation, Adult Fitness, and Exercise Testing.* Philadelphia, Lea & Febiger, p. 261, 1981. Copyright © Williams & Wilkins 1981. Used with permission.)

mm), total of S wave voltage in V_1 plus R wave voltage in V_{5-6} >35 mm, possible ST depression and T wave inversion in V_{5-6}
— Caused by increased pressure load on the LV (e.g., hypertension, aortic stenosis) or hypertrophic cardiomyopathy
— ECG changes occur late in progression of LVH so that there is already significant diastolic and possibly systolic dysfunction by the time of their appearance
— May mask ischemic changes
• Right ventricular hypertrophy (RVH)
— Characterized by prominent R waves in aVR and precordial V_{1-2} leads; secondary ST-T wave changes, as described above
— Caused by increased pressure load on the RV (e.g., pulmonary hypertension, mitral stenosis, LV failure) or hypertrophic cardiomyopathy
— ECG changes occur late in progression of RVH so that there is already significant di-

astolic and possibly systolic dysfunction by the time of their appearance
— May mask ischemic changes
• Left bundle-branch block (LBBB)
— Characterized by QRS >0.12 seconds, broad notched R in V_{5-6} plus wide, slurred S in V_1, and abnormal T waves, often in the opposite direction of the predominant QRS voltage
— Seen in coronary disease, any cause of LVH, congenital heart disease; or may be idiopathic
— May be transient (e.g., acute myocardial infarction, congestive heart failure, myocarditis, drug toxicity), or rate related
— May mask ischemic changes
• Right bundle-branch block (RBBB)
— QRS >0.12 seconds, rSR′ or notched R in V_{1-2} plus wide, slurred S in V_{5-6}
— Seen in coronary disease, hypertensive heart disease, any cause of RVH, congenital heart disease; or may be idiopathic
— May be transient (e.g., pulmonary embolism, exacerbation of chronic obstructive pulmonary disease (COPD), or rate related
— Occurs in up to 10% of normal individuals
• Myocardial ischemia
— Characterized by ST depression ≥1.0 to 1.5 mm at 0.08 seconds after the J point (see page 177), possible T wave inversion (see pages 12 and 22)
— Usually develops during activity or mental stress and resolves within minutes of rest or taking a nitroglycerin tablet
• Myocardial infarction (MI)
— Acute transmural MI is characterized by abnormal Q or QS with ST elevation in the area of infarct and reciprocal ST depression in the area opposite to infarct (Fig. 1–9)
— Acute subendocardial MI is characterized by ST depression and inverted T wave in the area of infarct ("non-Q wave" infarct)
— ECG pattern evolves over days to months (see Chapter 3, page 71)
• In addition, localization of acute MI is possible using 12-lead ECG, as described in Table 1–5 and demonstrated in Figure 1–9. By appreciating the location of infarcted tissue, the ther-

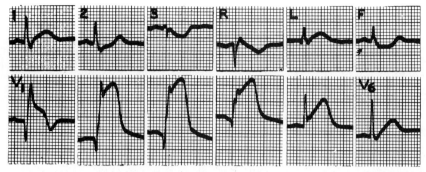

FIGURE 1-9. Acute anterior myocardial infarction with ST elevation in V_{1-5}, and abnormal ST segments in other leads. (From Marriott HJL: *Practical Electrocardiography*, 5th Ed. Baltimore, Williams & Wilkins, 1972. Used with permission.)

apist is better able to understand what impact the loss of myocardium will have on cardiac function.

AMBULATORY/HOLTER MONITORING

Ambulatory monitoring creates a 12- to 24-hour continuous recording of one or more ECG leads, which is useful for the diagnosis of cardiac arrhythmias, evaluation of symptoms and correlation with arrhythmias, diagnosis of myocardial ischemia (Fig. 1–10), evaluation of efficacy of antiarrhythmic drug therapy, and evaluation of artificial pacemaker function.

By knowing what kind of arrhythmias a patient demonstrated on holter monitoring and how often and whether any therapeutic interventions have been instituted by the physician,

the therapist may have an idea of what kind of rhythm changes might be expected and can inform the physician about the patient's current status and effectiveness of any therapeutic modifications.

VECTORCARDIOGRAPHY

A modified ECG that records the electrical activity of the heart from three-dimensional views creates a vectorcardiogram (VCG).

- Using a special camera and instant film, VCG produces vector loops instead of a simple graph of voltage versus time.
- VCG is particularly informative in patients with right ventricular hypertrophy (RVH) and myocardial infarction involving the inferior or posterior wall of the left ventricle.

TABLE 1-5. Localization of Myocardial Infarction by ECG

AREA OF INFARCTION	ECG CHANGES
Inferior	II, III, aVF: Q waves, ST elevation, T wave inversion (primary changes)
Inferolateral	II, III, aVF + V_{4-6}: primary changes as above
Inferoposterior	II, III, aVF: primary changes as above + V_{1-2}: broad initial R wave, ST depression, tall upright T wave
Anteroseptal	V_{1-3}: primary changes as above
Anterior (apical)	V_{2-4}: primary changes as above
Anterolateral	I, II aVL + V_{4-6}: primary changes as above
Extensive anterior	V_{1-6}, I, aVL: primary changes as above
Posterior (posterobasal)	V_{1-2}: broad initial R wave, ST depression, tall upright T wave (reciprocal changes)
Posterolateral	V_1 + V_{4-6}: reciprocal changes V_1 + primary changes V_{4-6}
Right ventricular	V_1 and V_4: primary changes; usually occurs in association with inferior myocardial infarction

FIGURE 1-10. Myocardial ischemia induced by an exercise stress test: 4 mm ST segment depression at stage 2 of a Bruce protocol treadmill test. Ambulatory ECGs from lead V_5 also show ischemic changes during a number of activities, especially playing tennis during which he was asymptomatic. Coronary angiography revealed severe left anterior descending stenosis (see arrow). (From Nabel EG, et al.: Characteristics and significance of ischemia detected by ambulatory monitoring. *Circulation* 75[Suppl V]:74, 1987. Used with permission of the American Heart Association, Inc.)

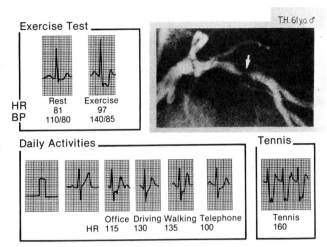

STRESS TESTING

Stress testing involves the use of exercise or other interventions to increase the workload of the heart in order to document the cardiovascular, and sometimes respiratory, responses to physiologic stress.

EXERCISE TESTING

Static or, more commonly, progressive dynamic exercise (e.g., using a treadmill or bicycle ergometer) can be performed in order to assess the physiologic responses to increasing demands on the body.

- The parameters most commonly monitored during exercise testing include:
  - Heart rate
  - Blood pressure
  - ECG
  - Signs and symptoms
- The purpose of exercise testing may be to assess any of the following:
  - Functional capacity
  - Possible presence and extent of coronary disease (as shown in Fig. 1–10)
  - Prognosis
  - Effects of therapeutic interventions
- In addition, ancillary techniques such as radionuclide imaging and echocardiography can provide supplementary information and augment the value of exercise testing in selected patients.
- The energy expenditure associated with the different stages of some common exercise test protocols are depicted in Figure 1–11.

- The information obtained from exercise testing is very valuable to the therapist, as it documents the patient's exercise tolerance and physiologic responses to exercise and gives a good indication how well the patient will tolerate vigorous rehabilitation activities (for norms, see page 194). Testing also reveals what factor(s) limited exercise tolerance.

CARDIOPULMONARY EXERCISE TESTING

- Cardiopulmonary exercise testing incorporates metabolic gas analysis, including the measurement of oxygen uptake ($\dot{V}O_2$), carbon dioxide production ($\dot{V}CO_2$), and other ventilatory parameters, during exercise testing (see above).
- During testing the patient usually breathes through a one-way nonrebreathing valve with nose plugged so that expired air can be analyzed and air flow can be measured, as demonstrated in Figure 1–12.
- Among the data that can be provided, in addition to that from a standard exercise test, are:
  - Maximal oxygen uptake ($\dot{V}O_{2\,max}$)
  - Anaerobic threshold (AT)
  - Respiratory rate (f)
  - Tidal volume (V_T)
  - Expired ventilation ($\dot{V}E$)
  - Heart rate (HR)
  - Oxygen pulse ($\dot{V}O_2$/heart beat)
  - Maximal MET (metabolic equivalent of energy expenditure) capacity
  - Cardiac output ($\dot{Q}$)

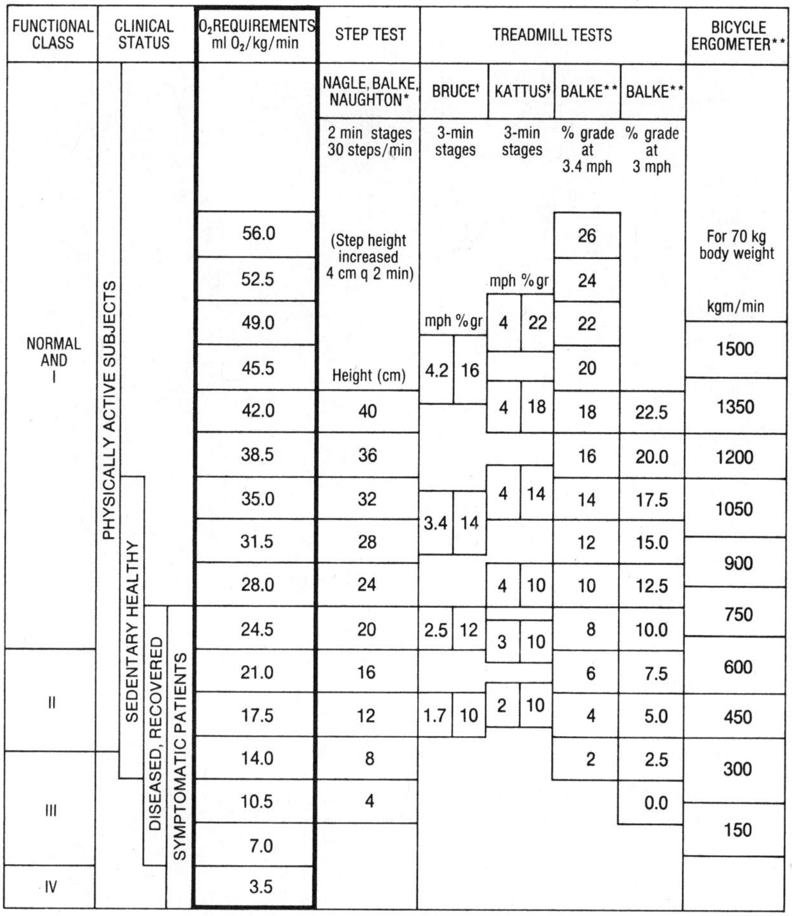

FUNCTIONAL CLASS	CLINICAL STATUS	O₂ REQUIREMENTS ml O₂/kg/min	STEP TEST — NAGLE, BALKE, NAUGHTON* (2 min stages 30 steps/min)	BRUCE† (3-min stages) mph	BRUCE† %gr	KATTUS‡ (3-min stages) mph	KATTUS‡ %gr	BALKE** % grade at 3.4 mph	BALKE** % grade at 3 mph	BICYCLE ERGOMETER** (For 70 kg body weight) kgm/min
NORMAL AND I	PHYSICALLY ACTIVE SUBJECTS	56.0	(Step height increased 4 cm q 2 min)					26		
		52.5						24		
		49.0				4	22	22		1500
		45.5	Height (cm)	4.2	16			20		
		42.0	40			4	18	18	22.5	1350
		38.5	36					16	20.0	1200
	SEDENTARY HEALTHY	35.0	32			4	14	14	17.5	1050
		31.5	28	3.4	14			12	15.0	900
		28.0	24			4	10	10	12.5	
		24.5	20	2.5	12	3	10	8	10.0	750
II		21.0	16					6	7.5	600
	DISEASED, RECOVERED	17.5	12	1.7	10	2	10	4	5.0	450
	SYMPTOMATIC PATIENTS	14.0	8					2	2.5	300
III		10.5	4						0.0	150
		7.0								
IV		3.5								

FIGURE 1-11. The energy expenditure, or oxygen requirements, associated with different stages of some common exercise test protocols. Lowest workloads are at the bottom of the chart and then progress upward. *Nagle FS, Balke B, Naughton JP: Gradational step tests for assessing work capacity. *J. Appl. Physiol.* 20:745–748, 1965. †Bruce RA: Multi-stage treadmill test of submaximal and maximal exercise. Appendix B, source publication. ‡Kattus AA, Jorgensen CR, Worden RE, Alvaro AB: S-T-segment depression with near-maximal exercise in detection of preclinical coronary heart disease. *Circulation* 41:585–595, 1971. **Fox SM, Naughton JP, Haskell WL: Physical activity and the prevention of coronary heart disease. *Ann. Clin. Res.* 3:404, 1971. (From the American Heart Association Committee on Exercise: *Exercise Testing and Training of Apparently Healthy Individuals: A Handbook for Physicians.* American Heart Association, p. 13, 1972. Used with permission.)

- This data allows for the differentiation of either cardiovascular or pulmonary causes limiting exercise tolerance (see Chapter 2, page 54).

PHARMACOLOGIC STRESS TESTING

When patients are unable to perform a standard exercise test (e.g., because of peripheral vascular, neurologic, chronic respiratory, orthopedic, or other disease), pharmacologic agents can be used as an alternative form of stress.

- The agents currently used include dipyridamole, adenosine, and dobutamine.
- Usually, pharmacologic stress testing is combined with echocardiography or radionuclide studies (e.g., thallium-201 scanning), or it may be used during cardiac catheterization.

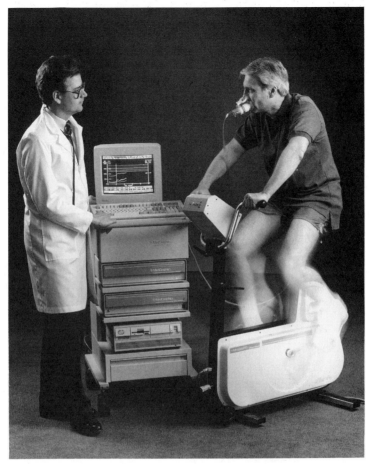

FIGURE 1-12. An individual performing a cardiopulmonary exercise test with analysis of respiratory gases. (Courtesy of Medical Graphics Corp., St. Paul, MN.)

CHEST RADIOGRAPHY

Using roentgen rays passed through the body to a film plate, various structures in the chest can be imaged.

- Because of the excellent contrast between the air-filled lungs and soft tissue structures, the pulmonary vasculature is distinctly visualized and the cardiac silhouette is clearly outlined on a routine chest radiograph.
- Prominence of particular parts of the cardiac silhouette suggests structural enlargement.
- The diameter of the heart can be measured to denote heart size using the standard posteroanterior inspiration view (Fig. 1–13).

ECHOCARDIOGRAPHY

Echocardiography uses inaudible, variable-frequency sound waves to depict cardiac structures and function.

M-MODE ECHOCARDIOGRAPHY

The ultrasonic beam produces a one-dimensional view of the heart showing time on the x-axis, distance on the y-axis, and intensity of echocardiography on the z-axis, as depicted in Figure 1–14. The ECG is recorded for timing of events.

- It is particularly useful for the evaluation of pericardial effusions, mitral valve disease, and hypertrophic obstructive cardiomyopathy.

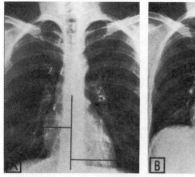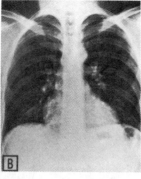

FIGURE 1-13. Measurement of the transverse cardiac diameter on a posteroanterior inspiration chest radiograph using the spinous processes to draw the vertical reference point and the longest distances to the right and left heart borders. The normal value of 50% is not valid in an expiration film *(B)*. (From Kloner RA: *The Guide to Cardiology*, 2nd Ed. New York, Le Jacq Communications, 1990. Used with permission.)

- The normal adult ranges for echocardiographic measurements are listed in Table 1–6. Larger chamber values indicate some degree of dilatation due to a higher volume load, whereas higher wall thicknesses indicate hypertrophy and thus decreased compliance.

TWO-DIMENSIONAL ECHOCARDIOGRAPHY/ SECTOR SCANNING

A B-mode echocardiographic tracing is rapidly and sequentially scanned across a sector field at a rate sufficiently fast enough to provide a continuous picture, as shown in Figure 1–15.

- Common clinical uses of two-dimensional (2-D) echocardiography include evaluation of LV function: end-systolic volume (ESV), end-diastolic volume (EDV), and ejection fraction (EF); calculation of LV mass; assessment of wall motion; detection of complications following acute MI; evaluation of valve structure and motion; identification of vegetations in infective endocarditis; detection of intracavitary masses; and assessment of congenital heart disease.
- Many abnormalities noted on echocardiography carry direct implications regarding possi-

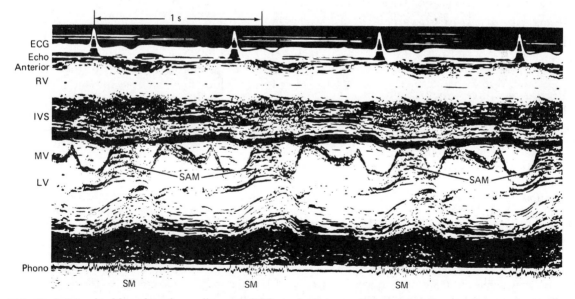

FIGURE 1-14. An M-mode echocardiogram, ECG, and phonocardiogram showing systolic anterior motion (SAM) of the mitral valve (MV) in a patient with hypertrophic obstructive cardiomyopathy. IVS = interventricular septum, LV = left ventricular chamber, RV = right ventricular chamber, SM = systolic murmur. (From Sokolow M, McIlroy MB: *Clinical Cardiology*, 4th Ed. Los Altos, CA, Lange Medical Publications, p. 91, 1986. Used with permission.)

TABLE 1–6. Normal Adult Ranges for Echocardiographic Measurements

STRUCTURE	RANGE
Intraventricular septum thickness	8–12 mm
Posterior LV wall thickness	8–12 mm
Left atrial dimension	15–35 mm
Aortic root dimension	20–35 mm
RV dimension	10–26 mm
LV dimension: diastolic/systolic	40–52/25–35 mm
LV volume: diastolic/systolic	64–141/16–43 ml
Stroke volume	50–100 ml
Ejection fraction	65–85%

From the Warren G. Magnuson Clinical Center, The National Institutes of Health, Bethesda, MD.
LV = left ventricular, RV = right ventricular.

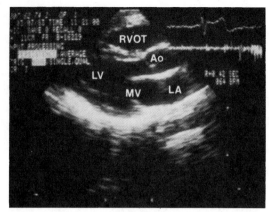

FIGURE 1–15. A normal two-dimensional echocardiogram, long-axis view. LV = left ventricle, MV = mitral valve, LA = left atrium, RVOT = right ventricle outflow tract, Ao = aorta. (From Cheitlin MD, Sokolow M, McIlroy MB: *Clinical Cardiology*, 6th Ed. Los Altos, CA, Lange Medical Publications, 1993. Used with permission.)

ble problems during exercise. For example, patients with an EF <40%, large areas of abnormal wall motion, significant valvular abnormalities, and increased LV mass are likely to exhibit abnormal responses to activity.

DOPPLER ECHOCARDIOGRAPHY

Doppler echocardiography uses ultrasound to record blood flow within the cardiovascular system.

- There are three types: continuous, pulsed, and multiple-pulsed or high-pulsed repetition frequency (high PRF).
- Doppler echocardiography can be used to measure cardiac output from the aorta and pulmonary artery, blood flow through heart valves, and peak velocity of blood flow across a stenosed valve allowing for calculation of pressure gradient.
- In addition, Doppler echocardiography with color flow mapping depicts the direction of blood flow and therefore provides documentation of valvular incompetence with regurgitant flow, as shown in Figure 1–16, and is often used intraoperatively to assess the adequacy of surgical reconstruction.
- Patients with significant valve disease usually exhibit abnormal responses to activity and have diminished exercise tolerance. Those

with severe aortic stenosis and obstructive hypertrophic cardiomyopathy (>75 mm Hg gradient) across the aortic valve are usually restricted to only mild exertion because of the increased risk of syncope and sudden death.

TRANSESOPHAGEAL ECHOCARDIOGRAPHY

High-quality 2-D and Doppler images are obtained by placing a transducer at the end of a flexible endoscope and inserting it in the esophagus. Transesophageal echocardiography (TEE) is particularly useful in assessing prosthetic valve function, vegetations, and aortic dissections. It is also used to monitor cardiac function during cardiac surgery.

INTRACARDIAC ULTRASOUND

A tiny echocardiography transducer can now be inserted into the coronary arteries via an arterial catheter, which allows for the documentation of atherosclerotic lesions and their composition. This technique is particularly useful in identifying diffuse disease without focal lesions, an inherently problematic condition for coronary angiography. By distinguishing the composition of various lesions, the most appropriate interventional technique can be selected (e.g., angioplasty for intimal/medial hypertrophy versus atherectomy for calcified lesions).

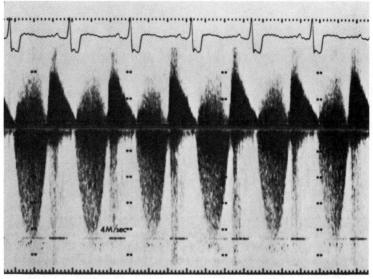

FIGURE 1-16. Continuous wave Doppler recording of a patient with pulmonic stenosis and regurgitation. In systole (downward reflection) the velocity is very high and exceeds 4 m/s. The diastolic reverse flow signifies the presence of regurgitation. (From Feigenbaum H: Echocardiography. In Braunwald E (ed.): *Heart Disease— A Textbook of Cardiovascular Medicine.* Philadelphia, W.B. Saunders Co., 1992. Used with permission.)

EXERCISE ECHOCARDIOGRAPHY

Many centers now perform ultrasonic examination during or immediately following some form of stress, most commonly exercise, in order to detect stress-induced regional wall motion abnormalities in patients with ischemic heart disease and to assess global changes in LV function during stress and hemodynamic changes in patients with valvular heart disease.

- These studies have used supine or upright bicycle exercise, immediate posttreadmill exercise, pharmacologic stress (i.e., dipyridamole, adenosine, or dobutamine), and atrial pacing.
- Results revealing increased ventricular end-diastolic volume, wall motion abnormalities, or valvular dysfunction during or immediately following exercise may indicate significant exercise intolerance and the need for careful monitoring during activity of limited intensity.

PHONOCARDIOGRAPHY

Using a special device capable of magnifying the heart sounds, a graphic recording of the timing, duration, and intensity of the various sounds is provided. Phonocardiography is most valuable as a means of timing the events of the cardiac cycle and demonstrating their relationship with simultaneous recordings of arterial and venous pulse wave forms, the ECG, respiration, and/or the echocardiogram. A phonographic recording is included in Figure 1–14 on page 15.

CARDIAC IMAGING TECHNIQUES

Various diagnostic tests involving sophisticated methods of imaging the cardiac structures are becoming increasingly more popular. Some of them include the injection of specially prepared radiopharmaceuticals that can be detected either in the blood stream or in the tissues and imaged by nuclear scanning devices.

COMPUTED TOMOGRAPHY

Computed tomography (CT) uses highly sensitive detectors around the body to measure attenuation of an x-ray beam that has passed through a body part in multiple projections; several million attenuation values are fed into a computer, which constructs a matrix of a cross-sectional slice of the body part and processes it to create a clear image with excellent contrast resolution of tissues.

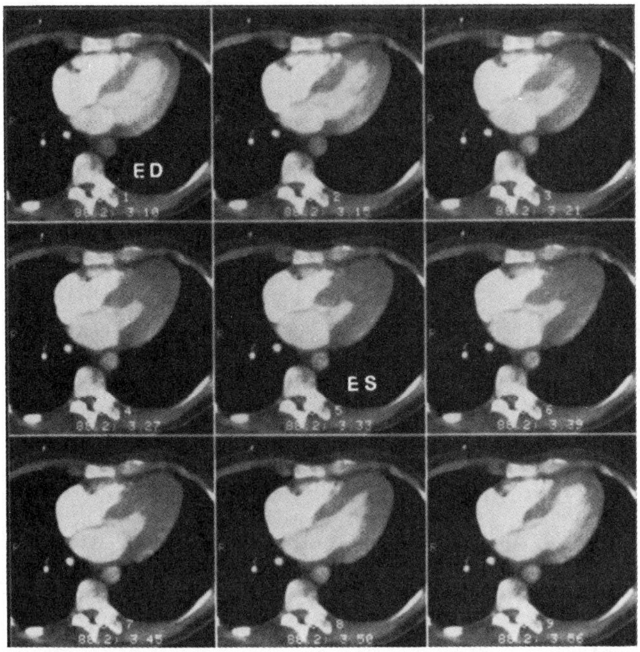

FIGURE 1-17. Series of CT scans of the heart at the same anatomic level acquired every 50 mseconds during a single cardiac cycle in a patient with hypertrophic cardiomyopathy. These are 9 of 17 scans acquired in approximately one cardiac cycle. Frame at upper left is near end-diastole (ED) and middle frame is near end-systole (ES). Note the change in ventricular volumes during the cardiac cycle and wall thickening during systole. (From Braunwald E (ed.): *Heart Disease—A Textbook of Cardiovascular Medicine.* Philadelphia, W.B. Saunders Co., 1992. Scan courtesy of J. Rumberger, Ph.D., M.D., Mayo Clinic. Used with permission.)

- CT images documenting thoracic aorta disease, pericardial disease, paracardiac and intracardiac masses, and patency of coronary arterial bypass grafts can be obtained by using newer standard CT scanners with exposure times of less than 2 seconds.
- Precise definition of intracardiac anatomy and assessment of cardiac function require either ECG gating of a standard CT scanner or the use of an ultrafast (cine) CT scanner, as in Figure 1–17.

MAGNETIC RESONANCE IMAGING

In magnetic resonance imaging (MRI), radiofrequency pulse sequences, with the patient positioned in a strong magnetic field to stimulate aligned protons, are used to generate signals that can be amplified and converted into images of body tissues. Two techniques, ECG-gated spin echocardiography and fast gradient echocardiographic imaging (cine MRI), produce high-contrast images that are useful for defining cardiac anatomy, including wall thickness, chamber volumes, valve areas, and vessel cross sections and lesion sizes (Fig. 1–18); identifying pericardiac and intracardiac masses; evaluating regional and global function of the ventricles; and determining the severity of valvular insufficiency.

MYOCARDIAL PERFUSION IMAGING

Radioisotopes that accumulate in the myocardium according to regional blood flow can be used to determine relative myocardial perfusion. Imaging can be performed either at rest or immediately following peak exercise or pharmacologic stress.

- During maximal exercise, coronary vascular reserve is recruited in order to meet the demand for increased flow. Coronary flow will be maximal in myocardium supplied by normal coronary arteries so that there will be excellent deposition of radioisotope in these regions; however, zones supplied by stenotic coronaries will show substantially less radionu-

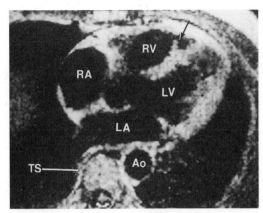

FIGURE 1-18. MRI of a normal heart. LV = left ventricle, RV = right ventricle, LA = left atrium, RA = right atrium, Ao = aorta, TS = thoracic spine. The black arrow points to the moderator band in the right ventricle. (From Herfkens RJ, et al.: Nuclear magnetic resonance imaging of the cardiovascular system: Normal and pathologic findings. *Radiology* 147:749, 1983. Used with permission.)

clide deposition because of the limited ability to augment blood flow. Thus, the relative distribution of radioisotope indicates the relative perfusion in various portions of the myocardium.

- A repeat scan can be performed 3 to 24 hours after the stress scan to distinguish between reversible defects resulting from stress-induced ischemia (Fig. 1–19) and permanent defects resulting from myocardial infarction.
  - Patients with reversible defects require careful monitoring during activity in order to prevent ischemia.
- The most common radioisotope in use is thallium-201 (^{201}Tl), but other isotopes are being studied, including technetium-99m (^{99m}Tc) labeled SestaMlBl and teboroxime.
- In addition, computer processing and analysis (i.e., single-photon emission tomography (SPECT) imaging) can be used to acquire multiple planar images around an object in order to reconstruct the three-dimensional object by "back projection," and thus allows the identification of disease in specific coronary artery distributions.
- The major uses for myocardial perfusion imaging, aside from diagnosing myocardial ischemia, include documenting acute myocardial infarction, indicating the size of infarction and thus providing prognostic information, and demonstrating reversible defects and thus viable myocardium in unstable angina and postinfarction chest pain.

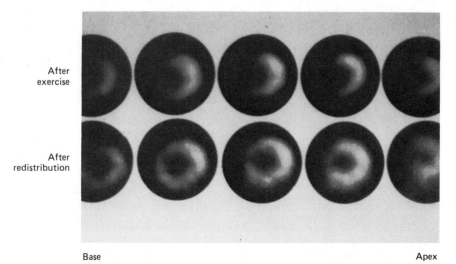

After exercise

After redistribution

Base

Apex

FIGURE 1-19. Tomographic thallium-201 images in the left anterior oblique position immediately after exercise *(A)* and after recovery and reperfusion *(B)*. The septal area is ischemic during exercise and well perfused after recovery. (From Cheitlin MD, Sokolow M, McIlroy MB: *Clinical Cardiology,* 6th Ed. Los Altos, CA, Lange Medical Publications, 1993. Used with permission.)

INFARCT-AVID IMAGING

Using radiotracers, such as technetium-labeled pyrophosphate or radiolabeled antimyosin antibody, which bind selectively to necrotic myocardial cells, it is possible to establish a diagnosis of acute MI, as shown in Figure 1–20.

- These scans are most valuable in patients who are first seen several days after the onset of symptoms when other studies are equivocal or when a perioperative MI is suspected.
- The intensity of the image is greatest at approximately 72 hours after infarct and lasts up to 7 to 10 days.

RADIONUCLIDE ANGIOGRAPHY OR VENTRICULOGRAPHY (RNA, RNV)

Assessment of cardiac performance using radionuclides is possible using two different techniques:

First Pass Technique

- A bolus of ^{99m}Tc is injected intravenously and followed through the heart chambers; then the ratio of the number of counts at end-systole and end-diastole is used to determine

these two volumes, as well as ejection fraction.

- With data acquisition time of <30 seconds, it is possible to define rapidly changing physiologic states. The first pass technique is particularly useful for evaluating RV function and intracardiac shunts, acutely ill patients who cannot remain in a stable position for long periods of time, and patients performing upright exercise.

Gated Equilibrium Technique

- Following injection of ^{99m}Tc, which is allowed to equilibrate with the blood volume for 5 to 10 minutes, images "gated" to the ECG can be obtained that define specific events within the cardiac cycle, as demonstrated in Figure 1–21. Data from several hundred beats are stored in a computer to obtain signals of adequate intensity; thus, it is sometimes called a MUGA (multiunit gated acquisition) scan.
- The equilibrium technique allows for multiple studies following a single radionuclide injection so that regional assessment can be performed in as many views as are relevant for analysis, and sequential and serial data can be

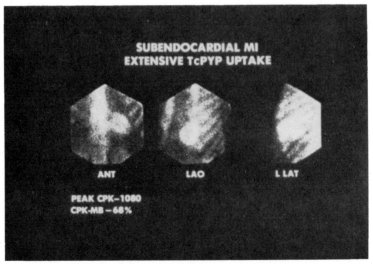

FIGURE 1–20. A ^{99m}Tc-labeled pyrophosphate scan showing uptake in the anterior (ANT), left anterior oblique (LAO), and left lateral (LLAT) views by infarcted tissue in a patient with extensive subendocardial infarction. (From Sokolow M, McIlroy MB: *Clinical Cardiology*, 6th Ed. Los Altos, CA, Lange Medical Publications, 1993. Used with permission. Scan courtesy of EH Blotrinick.)

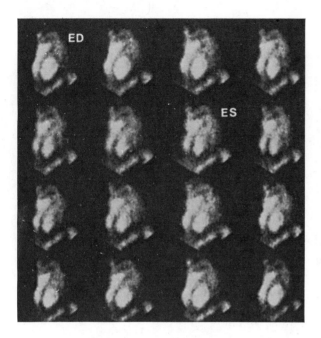

FIGURE 1–21. Serial images from a multigated equilibrium blood pool study with 16 frames in a single cardiac cycle (left anterior oblique position). End-diastole (ED) is shown in the first image and end-systole (ES) in the seventh image. The temporal sequence is read from left to right. This study shows normal uniform ventricular contraction throughout the cardiac cycle. (From Berger HJ, Gottschalk A, Zaret BL: Radionuclide assessment of left and right ventricular performance. *Radiol. Clin. North Am.* 18:441, 1980. Used with permission.)

obtained during a variety of control, physiologic, and/or pharmacologic states. However, to obtain meaningful data, cardiac performance must be relatively stable and the patient must remain fairly still beneath the detector for up to 10 minutes of data acquisition per position.

- Patients with an ejection fraction (EF) <40% are more likely to exhibit abnormal physiologic responses to exertion.
- The normal response to activity is an increase in EF. If a patient exhibits a rise in EF during activity, that patient will usually exhibit reasonably normal responses to exertion and will tolerate exercise better, even if the initial EF was very low.
- A significant drop in EF with activity is abnormal regardless of the initial EF; the lower the EF and the more pronounced the drop, the lower will be the individual's exercise tolerance and the greater will be the need for careful monitoring.
- Further application of this technique to ambulatory monitoring for several hours after blood pool labeling is now possible using an ambulatory ventricular function monitor called the VEST.

POSITRON EMISSION TOMOGRAPHY

Positron emission tomography (PET) is an imaging technique that uses biologically active positron emission radiopharmaceuticals (e.g., ^{18}F deoxyglucose or ^{11}C acetate) to display and quantify metabolic processes, receptor occupancy, and blood flow. In cardiology, it is being used to assess coronary blood flow, quantify coronary reserve, measure regional myocardial oxygen consumption, and demonstrate ischemic but viable myocardium that would benefit from revascularization surgery (Fig. 1–22).

INVASIVE MONITORING

Monitoring of cardiovascular status can be performed using specially designed intravascular catheters capable of measuring temperature, pressure, and volume.

INTRAARTERIAL CATHETERIZATION

Catheters, placed usually within the brachial or femoral artery, are commonly used in intensive care units for obtaining repeated arterial blood gas samples and directly recording arterial pressures (often displayed on the monitoring equipment).

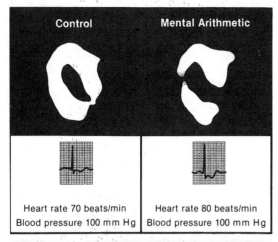

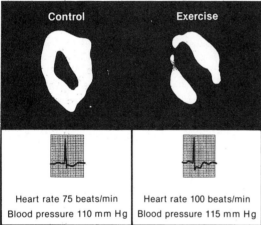

Control	Mental Arithmetic
Heart rate 70 beats/min	Heart rate 80 beats/min
Blood pressure 100 mm Hg	Blood pressure 100 mm Hg

Control	Exercise
Heart rate 75 beats/min	Heart rate 100 beats/min
Blood pressure 110 mm Hg	Blood pressure 115 mm Hg

FIGURE 1–22. PET scan of the heart showing regional myocardial uptake of rubidium-82 in a patient with chronic stable angina, a positive exercise test, and proven coronary disease. The two control images show uniform perfusion to the posterior wall, free wall, anterior wall, and septum of the left ventricle. However, regional perfusion abnormalities and ST segment depression on ECG are evident during both mental arithmetic and exercise. Notably, the patient evidenced no symptoms during the mental arithmetic. (From Deanfield JE, et al.: Silent myocardial ischemia due to mental stress. *Lancet* 2:1001, 1984. © by the Lancet Ltd. 1984. Used with permission.)

PULMONARY ARTERY CATHETER

A balloon-tip catheter (often referred to as a Swan-Ganz catheter, after the original brand) can be placed into the pulmonary artery (PA) via a large central vein, usually the subclavian or internal jugular, to obtain the PA wedge pressure (PAWP, formerly referred to as the pulmonary capillary wedge, PCW, pressure) and indirectly the left atrial pressure (LAP).

- Patients with pulmonary pressures >20 mm Hg are likely to become symptomatic during exertion.
- A pulmonary artery pressure of 35 mm Hg is often considered to be a contraindication to exercise training.

THERMODILUTION CATHETER

A thermodilution catheter, a special catheter placed like a pulmonary artery catheter, is used to measure cardiac output. Cold saline is injected through the proximal lumen lying in the right atrium and the resulting temperature change, recorded at the tip of the catheter in the PA by means of a thermistor bead embedded in the catheter wall, is used to calculate cardiac output.

COMBINATION CATHETERS

A combination of catheters, including those described above, with two or more lumens and ports serving different purposes, can be contained within one device. An example of a triple-lumen catheter is depicted in Figure 1–23.

CENTRAL VENOUS PRESSURE LINE

An intravenous line in the subclavian, basilic, jugular, or femoral vein and passed to the right atrium (RA) can be used to measure the pressure in the vena cavae or RA. The central venous pressure (CVP) line provides information about the adequacy of right heart function, including effective circulating blood volume, effectiveness of pump function, vascular tone, and venous return.

- A CVP line is especially useful in assessing fluid volume and replacement needs.
- However, if the patient has chronic obstructive pulmonary disease or myocardial ischemia or infarction, CVP measurements may reflect pathologic changes rather than fluid volume.

CARDIAC CATHETERIZATION

Using one or more catheters inserted into the heart through the venous and/or arterial systems, cardiac anatomy and function can be eval-

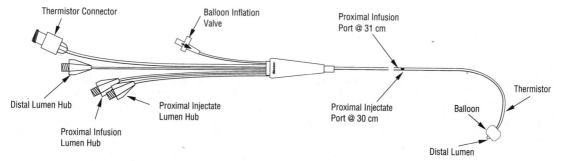

FIGURE 1–23. A typical triple-lumen pulmonary artery catheter. (VIP-831 catheter courtesy of Baxter Healthcare Corporation, Edwards Critical-Care Division, Santa Ana, CA.)

uated. Through these catheters, intracardiac pressures can be measured to define the hemodynamic function of the heart (Table 1–7) and dye can be injected to study ventricular performance and intracardiac and coronary arterial anatomy (see Fig. 1–10, page 12).

- Because of the improved sensitivity and specificity of newer noninvasive cardiac tests, standard diagnostic cardiac catheterization is often reserved for patients who need further quantification of the severity of their disease or determination of the appropriateness of surgical intervention.
- However, in recent years, the use of cardiac catheterization has been expanded to include bedside hemodynamic monitoring, intracardiac electrophysiologic testing, endomyocardial biopsy, percutaneous transluminal angioplasty and atherectomy, and percutaneous balloon valvotomy.

RIGHT HEART CATHETERIZATION

Right heart catheterization is commonly used for:

- Determination of RA, RV, PAW, and PA pressures
- Blood sampling from the RV to evaluate shunts
- Measurement of cardiac output
- Measurement of LV function if an atrial septal defect (ASD) or ventricular septal defect (VSD) is present

LEFT HEART CATHETERIZATION

Left heart catheterization is used for:

- Evaluation of mitral and aortic valve disease
- Evaluation of regional and global LV function
- Measurement of LV and aortic pressures
- Assessment of pressure gradients across aortic and mitral valves
- Performing coronary angiography

TABLE 1–7. Normal Resting Hemodynamic Values

VALUE	RANGE	MEAN
Right atrium (mm Hg)	2–10	0–8
Right ventricle: systolic/end-diastolic (mm Hg)	15–30/0-8	—
Pulmonary artery: systolic/end-diastolic (mm Hg)	15–30/3–12	9–16
Pulmonary artery wedge and left atrium (mm Hg)	3–15	1–10
Left ventricle: systolic/end diastolic (mm Hg)	90–140/3–12	—
Systemic arteries: systolic/end-diastolic (mm Hg)	90–140/60–90	70–105
Cardiac index (L/min/m²)	2.6–4.2	3.4
Stroke index (ml/beat)	30–65	47
Oxygen consumption (ml/min/m²)	110–150	—
Arteriovenous oxygen difference (ml/L)	30–50	—
Pulmonary vascular resistance (mm Hg/L/min)	20–130	70
Systemic vascular resistance (mm Hg/L/min)	700–1600	1150
Arterial saturation (%)	94–100	98

Patients with coronary occlusions >70–75% usually exhibit symptoms during activity but often benefit from exercise training, evidencing increased exercise tolerance and decreased symptoms.

ELECTROPHYSIOLOGIC STUDIES

Electrophysiologic studies (EPS) involve the use of electrode catheters to assess the electrical activity and responses of the heart. EPS involve the introduction of electrode catheters into the right and/or left sides of the heart, which are then positioned at various intracardiac sites to stimulate and record electrical activity from portions of the atria or ventricles, His bundle region, bundle branches, or accessory pathways, depending on the purpose of the study. EPS may be performed in patients with symptomatic, recurrent, or drug-resistant supraventricular or ventricular tachyarrhythmias (particularly when they produce serious hemodynamic consequences) and in those patients with unexplained syncope.

1.3 THERAPEUTIC INTERVENTIONS

As in most areas of medicine, the types of therapeutic interventions in cardiology continue to expand. Some of the more common ones, as well as some newer procedures currently under investigation, are described briefly in this section.

MEDICAL MANAGEMENT

Generally speaking, most types of cardiac dysfunction are treated medically for as long as possible. Medical management may include pharmacologic agents, diet modification, risk factor reduction, and rehabilitation. When symptoms become disabling, surgery may be warranted.

PHARMACOLOGIC THERAPY

The various medications used to treat cardiovascular dysfunction are described in Chapter 4.

DIET MODIFICATION

Specific diet modifications that may be advised for cardiac patients include the following:

- A low cholesterol, low saturated fat diet is commonly recommended for patients with atherosclerotic cardiovascular disease. In addition, the general public is encouraged to follow such a diet for the prevention of atherosclerotic heart disease (ASHD).
- High-fiber intake is often recommended for the prevention of ASHD (as well as colon cancer).
- Sodium restriction is often used to decrease preload in heart failure and is sometimes used in the management of hypertension.
- Caloric restriction may be recommended to achieve weight loss in obese individuals and thus reduce the workload of the heart for those with heart failure and decrease blood pressure in hypertensive individuals.
- Because of the extended contact we have with patients, physical therapists are in an ideal role to reinforce the importance of diet modification and share the findings of current literature or, better yet, great low fat, low cholesterol recipes with patients.

RISK FACTOR REDUCTION

Since the atherosclerotic process has been linked to specific risk factors, their reduction is often recommended for patients with atherosclerotic coronary, cerebrovascular, and peripheral vascular disease.

- Risk factor reduction commonly includes cessation of smoking, treatment of hypertension, exercise training, diet modification (see above), weight control, stress reduction training, and control of blood glucose levels.
- There is scientific data to support risk factor reduction both for primary prevention of atherosclerotic diseases as well as for secondary prevention of recurrent events.
- As physical therapists practice more independently, we have an increasing responsibility to assess the overall health status of the patients we treat and make appropriate recommendations for their general health and well-being. Risk factor reduction for cardiovascular disease is a critical element because it is the leading cause of death in the United States.

CARDIAC REHABILITATION

Cardiac rehabilitation is a multidisciplinary program aimed at restoring the cardiac patient to optimal physiologic, social, vocational, and emotional status. It usually includes patient assessment and development of an individualized treatment plan, patient and family education, risk factor modification, exercise training, psychologic counseling, and patient reassessments to document progress. Physical therapists have unequaled expertise in prescribing exercise, especially for patients with chronic medical problems (see pages 197 to 203), and in the prevention and treatment of exercise-related injuries; therefore physical therapists are assets to the cardiac rehabilitation team.

SURGICAL INTERVENTIONS

A variety of surgical interventions are used in the treatment of patients with heart disease. Most are described briefly in the following pages.

PERCUTANEOUS TRANSLUMINAL CORONARY ANGIOPLASTY

During percutaneous transluminal coronary angioplasty (PTCA) a balloon-tip catheter is inserted into a coronary artery narrowed by atherosclerotic plaque, and the balloon is inflated. The goal is to increase the intraluminal diameter, which is probably accomplished via plaque splitting and mural stretching, as illustrated in Figure 1–24. Percutaneous transluminal angioplasty can also be applied to the renal, mesenteric, and peripheral arteries.

CORONARY ARTERY BYPASS GRAFT

Coronary artery bypass graft (CABG) surgery uses autogenous saphenous vein or internal mammary arterial grafts to bypass stenotic lesion(s) of the coronary arteries. Figure 1–25 shows both types of CABG. Multiple lesions in the same coronary artery can be bypassed using sequential grafting, especially when an internal mammary artery graft is used.

- CABG is performed via a median sternotomy, and at closing, the sternum is wired back together again. Reasonable healing takes approximately 6 to 8 weeks.
  - During the interim period, patients are usually restricted as to the amount of weight they can lift without unduly stressing the sternotomy site; the amount of restriction and the time period vary tremendously from surgeon to surgeon but often fall in the range of not more than 10 to 20 pounds for 6 to 12 weeks.
  - Patients are also restricted from doing pushups and other resisted exercises that involve the pectoralis muscles.
- Immediately after surgery, the patient usually has two chest tubes in place, one to drain the mediastinum and one to reinflate the left lung, which was collapsed during surgery. The second, or intrapleural, chest tube requires water seal and often gentle suction to evacuate air from the pleural space and create the desired negative pressure.
  - At first there is marked bubbling from the water chamber if it is set to suction; however, the amount of bubbling diminishes as the air leak seals off.
  - If the water seal is set to suction, there should always be some bubbling. If the bubbling ceases, the tube has become kinked or blocked. If a change of position and release

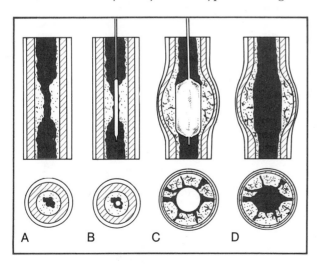

FIGURE 1–24. Current concept of the mechanism of balloon dilatation in PTCA. Serial panels show the baseline stenosis *(A)*, passage of the deflated balloon catheter *(B)*, balloon inflation *(C)*, and the postdilatation appearance *(D)*, as drawn in longitudinal and transverse cross-sectional views. Note fracture and outward displacement of atherosclerotic plaque and stretching of the media and adventitia (panels *C* and *D*). (From Castaneda-Zuniga WR, et al.: The mechanism of balloon angioplasty. *Radiology* 135:565, 1980. Used with permission.)

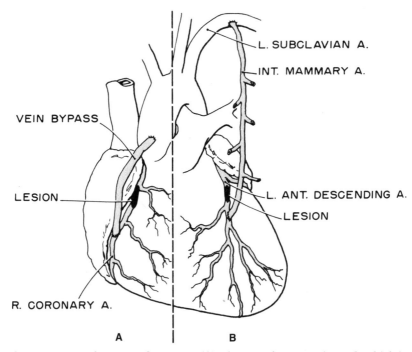

FIGURE 1-25. Coronary artery bypass graft surgery: *(A)* using a saphenous vein graft, which is sutured from the ascending aorta to a coronary artery (the right coronary artery in this example) distal to stenosis, and *(B)* using an internal mammary artery anastamosed to a coronary artery (the left anterior descending coronary artery) distal to the site of occlusion. (From Price SA, Wilson LM: *Pathophysiology: Clinical Concepts of Disease Processes,* 4th Ed. St. Louis: Mosby–Year Book, 1992. Used with permission.)

of the chest tube does not result in resumption of the bubbling, the nurse or physician should be notified. Likewise, a sudden increase in the amount of bubbling should be reported.

• During healing of the sternotomy, patients should be encouraged to maintain full range of motion of their shoulders, trunk, and neck and to practice good posture.

• In addition, patients should be discouraged from crossing their legs when they sit, especially if saphenous vein grafts were harvested.

• Exercise training is important in these patients, both as a means of increasing exercise tolerance and as a way of reducing the rate of atherogenesis.

INVESTIGATIONAL TECHNIQUES FOR TREATING CORONARY STENOSIS

Currently, a number of new techniques for treating coronary stenosis are under investigation. Three of them are introduced here.

Intracoronary Stents

Coronary stents are intraluminal prostheses made of polished metal wires or tubes (Fig. 1–26), which are inserted via an intracoronary catheter in order to scaffold a segment of vessel that does not maintain patency following percutaneous transluminal coronary angioplasty (PTCA).

Atherectomy

Atherectomy involves the insertion of a special-tipped intracoronary catheter to cut away and remove atherosclerotic plaque within a vessel, somewhat like a "Roto-Rooter" or a little "Pac Man" with suction. It is usually combined with PTCA in order to achieve adequate lumen size.

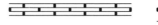 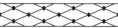

Unexpanded stent   Expanded stent

FIGURE 1-26. An intracoronary stent before inflation and in its expanded configuration used to maintain the patency of a vessel following PTCA.

TABLE 1–8. Intersociety Commission for Heart Disease (ICHD) Code for Pacemaker Modes

CHAMBER PACED	CHAMBER SENSED	RESPONSE TO SENSING
V = ventricle A = atrium D = dual (A + V)	V = ventricle A = atrium D = dual (A + V) O = none	I = inhibited T = triggered D = dual (atrium triggered and ventricle inhibited) O = none

PACEMAKER'S PROGRAMMABILITY	TACHYARRHYTHMIA FUNCTIONS
P = programmable rate and/or output M = multiprogrammability O = none	B = burst N = normal rate competition S = scanning E = externally activated

The top three features are most commonly used to identify pacemaker modes (e.g., a VVI pacemaker); the lower two features are also included on occasion.

Laser Angioplasty

Thermal heating of a vessel or direct ablation of plaque material using laser energy can be performed during PTCA in order to overcome the vessel's elasticity and provide a smooth luminal surface despite preexisting dissections or flaps.

PACEMAKER INSERTION

Pacemakers are electronic devices that use an external energy source to stimulate the heart when disorders of impulse formation and/or transmission create significant hemodynamic problems. They are surgically implanted usually in the left infraclavicular area, a subxiphoid pocket, or the left chest wall (and therefore full range of motion in the shoulders and trunk should be encouraged once the pacemaker is stable).

• Modern pacemakers have a variety of func-

tions, which can be programmed according to patient need.

• Pacemaker modes are most commonly described using the three- to five-letter notation proposed by the Intersociety Commission for Heart Disease Resources (ICHD), which are described in Table 1–8.

• There are several types of pacemakers, as listed in Table 1–9. They are briefly described below:

  • *Asynchronous, or fixed-rate pacemakers* (AOO, VOO) have no sensing function and therefore stimulate the designated chambers at a constant rate regardless of the underlying rhythm. They are rarely used today because of the potential risk of initiating fibrillation.

  • *Demand pacemakers* (AAI, AAT, VVI, VVT) sense spontaneous activity of the designated

TABLE 1–9. Types of Pacemakers and Their Modes

PACEMAKER TYPE	ICHD CODE*	SENSES	PACES
Atrial asynchronous	AOO	O	A
Ventricular asynchronous	VOO	O	V
Atrial demand	AAI, AAT	A	A
Ventricular demand	VVI, VVT	V	V
Atrial synchronous	VAT	A	V
Atrial synchronous ventricular inhibited	VDD	A + V	V
AV sequential	DVI	V	A + V
Optimal sequential	DDD	A + V	A + V

*Refer to Table 1–8 for explanation of pacemaker codes.
A = atria, V = ventricles, O = none, D = dual, I = inhibited, T = triggered.

chamber and respond by either inhibiting or triggering a stimulus to that chamber.

— For example, an AAI pacer provides fixed-rate atrial pacing unless inhibited by sensed atrial activity.

— In contrast, a VVT pacer delivers a ventricular stimulus every time it senses ventricular depolarization.

- *Atrial synchronous ventricular pacemakers* (VAT, VDD) act as dual chamber "physiologic pacemakers," which more closely approximate normal cardiac function.

— The VAT pacer, which senses atrial activity and after a suitable delay stimulates the ventricles, is used in patients with normal sinus function but impaired atrioventricular (AV) conduction. It allows for the preservation of the atrial contribution to ventricular filling and maintenance of sinus node control over ventricular rate within the upper and lower limits programmed into the pacer.

— In order to avoid the potential risk of delivering a ventricular stimulus on the T wave of a premature ventricular complex, which would not be sensed, the *atrial synchronous ventricular inhibited pacemaker* (ASVIP) was developed. Using the VDD mode, both the atria and ventricles are sensed and a ventricular stimulus can be either inhibited or triggered.

- *AV sequential pacemakers* (DVI) are designed for patients who have bradycardia and impaired AV conduction and allow preservation of the atrial contribution to ventricular filling.

— Sensing only the ventricles but able to pace both the atria and the ventricles, this pacemaker stimulates the atria if ventricular activity is not detected within a prescribed escape interval; in addition, it then waits long enough to allow normal AV conduction, and if no ventricular activity is sensed, it paces the ventricles.

— However, if ventricular activity is sensed, the ventricular stimulus is inhibited and all pacemaker timing is reset.

- *Optimal sequential pacemakers* (DDD) sense and pace both the atria and ventricles and adapt to the underlying rhythm automatically, according to a specific scheme.

— If the pacemaker senses normally conduc-

ted sinus rhythm, it is totally inhibited.

— If the pacemaker senses normally conducted atrial bradycardia, it provides atrial pacing.

— If the pacemaker senses atrial bradycardia and prolonged or blocked AV conduction, it provides AV sequential pacing.

— If the pacemaker senses sinus rhythm with prolonged or blocked AV conduction, it functions as an atrial synchronous ventricular pacemaker.

- Finally, pacemakers may also be used to control certain tachyarrhythmias.
  - Maintaining normal rate through pacing helps prevent bradycardia-dependent tachycardias (e.g., ventricular tachycardia associated with complete AV block).
  - Some tachyarrhythmias can be terminated using overdrive suppression (i.e., short bursts at high-stimulus rates) or underdrive termination (i.e., delivering an appropriately timed stimulus during a particular part of the tachycardia cycle).
  - Pacemakers can be programmed to pace with short AV intervals for patients who have accessory bypass tracts (e.g., Wolff-Parkinson-White [WPW] syndrome) for the prevention of tachycardia.

AUTOMATIC IMPLANTABLE CARDIOVERTER/ DEFIBRILLATOR

An automatic implantable cardioverter/defibrillator (AICD) is a self-contained diagnostic-therapeutic system, which is surgically implanted via left thoracotomy, median sternotomy, or subxiphoid or subcostal incision in patients with documented lethal ventricular arrhythmias not associated with acute MI.

- Its functions include continuous monitoring of the ECG, identification of ventricular tachycardia or fibrillation, and delivery of therapeutic pacing or cardioversion/defibrillation.
- The purpose is to provide arrhythmia prevention or termination, low-energy synchronized cardioversion for termination of ventricular tachycardia, and/or high-energy defibrillation for resuscitation of ventricular fibrillation.
- Refer to comments regarding sternotomy (page 25), thoracotomy (page 63), and pacemaker insertion (page 27) for important recommendations for physical therapy management.

VALVE REPAIRS AND REPLACEMENT

Percutaneous Balloon Valvuloplasty

Percutaneous balloon valvuloplasty uses a balloon-tip catheter, which is inserted into the orifice of a stenotic valve and inflated, in order to increase the area of the valve orifice. Percutaneous balloon valvuloplasty is most successful in mobile, minimally calcified, minimally thickened valves without severe subvalvular fibrosis.

Valvotomy and Commissurotomy

Valvotomy and commissurotomy involve an incision into the chest (either median sternotomy or left thoracotomy) followed by surgical cutting or digital manipulation of a valve or its adherent diseased commissures in order to relieve stenosis.

- Closed valvotomy/commissurotomy can be performed either by simple transatrial finger fracture of the valve commissures (where a small incision is made in the appropriate atrium through which an index finger is inserted into the stenotic valve orifice to expand it) or with the aid of a transventricular dilator (which works with one finger to expand the valve orifice).
- Open commissurotomy involves the use of cardiopulmonary bypass and direct visualization of the stenotic valve and is the preferred technique in the United States. It allows for removal of atrial thrombi, incision of commissures, separation of fused chordae, splitting of underlying papillary muscle, and debridement of valvular calcium.

Physical therapy recommendations for patients with sternotomy incisions can be found on page 25, whereas those for thoracotomy are located on page 63. Because patients requiring surgical management of valve disease have generally experienced a long period of progressive physiologic deterioration, they tend to be fairly deconditioned and also benefit greatly from exercise training (see Chapter 6, page 223).

Valvectomy

Complete excision of right-sided heart valves may be performed for some congenital defects or for infective endocarditis in drug abusers where reinfection is likely.

Annuloplasty

Annuloplasty consists of the surgical repair or reconstruction of a defective valve.

- Annuloplasty may be possible in patients with mitral or tricuspid valvular incompetence caused by myxomatous degeneration, rupture of chordae tendinae or papillary muscle, or dilation of the valve annulus.
- Valve reconstruction offers the advantages of avoiding the problems associated with chronic anticoagulation and thromboembolism, as well as eventual valve failure (see below).

Valve Replacement

When other interventions have failed or are not possible, excision of a heart valve and replacement with a prosthetic valve is performed, usually through a median sternotomy or left thoracotomy incision.

- Valve replacement is commonly performed for severe mitral and aortic disease and sometimes for pulmonic or tricuspid valve disease.
- Prosthetic valves can be either mechanical or tissue (Fig. 1–27), with each having its own advantages and disadvantages.
  - The major advantage of mechanical prostheses is their durability; however, they require chronic anticoagulation because of the risk of thromboembolic complications.

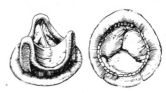

Tissue valve

Caged ball

Tilting disk

FIGURE 1–27. Examples of artificial heart valves. (From Way LW (ed.): *Current Surgical Diagnosis and Treatment*, 7th Ed. Los Altos, CA, Lange Medical Publications, 1985. Used with permission.)

- Conversely, tissue prostheses have a very low risk of thromboembolic complications without anticoagulation but tend to degenerate over time, especially in younger patients. Newer cryopreserved allografts may offer improved durability.
- Timing of valve replacement is a crucial aspect in managing patients with valve disease.
  - Because all prosthetic valves are fairly stenotic when placed within the valve orifice, surgical replacement for valvular stenosis offers benefits only when the original valve is more stenotic than the prosthesis.
  - Chronic valvular regurgitation is often tolerated for decades with few complaints.
  - Yet, patients respond to valve replacement better if surgery is performed before the development of significant ventricular dysfunction.

Refer to comments under valvotomy and commissurotomy (page 29) for physical therapy recommendations.

SURGICAL TREATMENT OF THE FAILED HEART

A limited number of surgical procedures are used to treat the failed heart. Some are still considered investigational and thus are not widely available.

Intraaortic Balloon Pump

Intraaortic balloon counterpulsation (or pump, IABP) uses inflation and deflation of a balloon in the aorta to provide mechanical circulatory assistance for patients with certain types of cardiogenic shock.

- Inflation of the balloon with carbon dioxide or helium during diastole boosts intraaortic pressure and thus restores arterial pressure and improves coronary perfusion.
- Rapid deflation of the balloon during ventricular systole decreases afterload and therefore assists the emptying of the LV, resulting in enhanced stroke volume and reduced myocardial oxygen consumption.

Physical therapists must be careful not to interfere with the tubes running between the patient and the IABP when they are providing any type of treatment for these patients. When a femoral vessel is used as part of the circuit, hip flexion is usually prohibited.

Cardiac Assist Devices and Artificial Hearts

Devices that assist or virtually take over the pumping action of the left, right, or both ventricles are being used to support patients in post-cardiotomy and acute MI shock and to bridge patients to cardiac transplantation.

- Among these devices are right and left ventricular assist devices (RVAD and LVAD, respectively), biventricular assist devices (BVAD), extracorporeal membrane oxygenation (ECMO) systems, and orthotopic biventricular replacement prostheses (artificial hearts).
- Most are powered externally; some are implantable.

Patients are often referred to physical therapy for general strengthening and endurance training (to increase peripheral efficiency) while they are using one of these devices and awaiting transplantation. Usually they tolerate gradual, low-level exercise very well; their progress is limited by peripheral deconditioning. The physician should be consulted regarding any specific precautions or guidelines that might be indicated.

Heart and Heart-Lung Transplantation

The surgical implantation of a donor heart or heart and lungs within a patient with end-stage cardiac disease offers the opportunity for return to an active lifestyle.

- Heart transplantation may be performed for patients with cardiomyopathy, coronary artery disease, valvular disease, and congenital heart disease.
  - Heart transplantation is usually orthotopic, where the recipient's heart is removed and replaced with a donor heart. The recipient's heart is excised leaving part of both atria, including the entrances of the vena cavae and pulmonary veins and the SA node. The donor's heart is removed in total and incisions are made to anastamose each atria, then the aorta and the pulmonary artery trunk. Care is taken during anastamosis of the RA to avoid injury to the donor SA node.
  - Less common is heterotopic transplantation, where the donor heart is placed in the right lower thorax in series with the retained native heart.

- For cardiac patients with fixed elevated pulmonary vascular resistance, either heterotropic heart transplantation or heart-lung transplantation can be used.
- Combined heart-lung transplantation has been successful in patients with primary or secondary pulmonary hypertension, as well as diffuse pulmonary diseases with right heart failure, such as emphysema, diffuse pulmonary arteriovenous fistulas, and cystic fibrosis.
- Immunosuppression using multiple agents, including cyclosporine, steroids, azathioprine, and OKT3, is required to avoid organ rejection. Moderate doses are prescribed initially, but doses of some drugs can be tapered to lower maintenance levels by the time of discharge at 2 to 3 weeks after transplantation. Newer immunosuppressive agents are currently under investigation. Refer to Chapter 4.

Because patients are extremely debilitated by the time they qualify for transplantation, they are often referred to physical therapy for general strengthening and physical conditioning exercise during the waiting period. The goal is to increase peripheral efficiency (which is achieved by a very gradual, low-level aerobic exercise program) and thus aid the patient in returning more quickly to a more functional lifestyle following transplantation.

Following transplantation, physical therapy is typically initiated within a few days after surgery and consists of breathing exercises, coughing, progressive mobility, light range of motion, calisthenic and postural exercises, and progressive aerobic exercise, usually walking and/or stationary cycling.

- Postoperative sternotomy precautions are followed (see page 25).
- Physiologic monitoring is extremely important in this patient group because of the denervated status of the donor heart and the hypertensive side effects of cyclosporine.
  - The denervated heart usually has a higher resting heart rate (HR) than normal because of the lack of vagal stimulation, and there is no HR response to the Valsalva maneuver or changes in position from supine to sitting to standing.
- ECG monitoring reveals two independent P waves (one from the native heart remnant and one from the donor heart); only the P wave from the donor heart will be associated with QRS complexes.
- Warm up must be prolonged to allow HR increases via rising levels of circulating catecholamines rather than direct sympathetic nervous system stimulation of the heart.
- Maximal HR is lower than normally expected for age, but stroke volume is greater so that peak cardiac output is only slightly lower than normal. Blood pressure responses are fairly normal initially, but many patients develop hypertension as a side effect of the immunosuppressive drugs. Exercise ventilation is higher in transplant patients during submaximal exercise, but maximal oxygen consumption and anaerobic threshold are decreased. All these respiratory parameters improve with physical training.
- Recovery HRs decrease more gradually in denervated hearts because of the slow reuptake of the circulating catecholamines.
- The blood pressure responses to isometric exercise show an increase similar to normal ranges because of a greater increase in total peripheral resistance; however the HR response remains flat, as would be expected in a denervated heart.
- With denervation, patients are also unable to perceive the pain associated with myocardial ischemia.
- Other medication side effects that should be addressed include hypercholesterolemia and increased atherogenesis, as well as musculoskeletal problems due to glucocorticosteroids.

Cardiomyoplasty

A newer experimental procedure involves the use of a latissimus dorsi muscle (LDM) flap with its neurovascular bundle still attached to reconstruct the LV wall in order to augment and support ventricular function.

- For successful function, the procedure also requires:
  - Insertion of an AV sequential pacemaker with the atrial electrodes attached to the LV wall and the ventricular electrodes attached

to the LDM flap so that synchronized function can be achieved
- A 6- to 8-week muscle training program to condition the fast-twitch Type IIA skeletal muscle fibers to gradually take on the oxidative characteristics of slow-twitch Type I fibers

OTHER SURGICAL INTERVENTIONS

Aneurysectomy/Myectomy

Aneurysectomy/myectomy involves the surgical resection of a dyskinetic region of the myocardium (i.e., a LV aneurysm) or another segment of cardiac muscle. The primary indications for aneurysectomy are angina pectoris associated with prior myocardial infarction and multivessel coronary artery disease and recurrent hemodynamically significant ventricular arrhythmias; the indications for myectomy are recurrent arrhythmias and outflow tract obstruction.

Myotomy and Myectomy

When patients with hypertrophic cardiomyopathy (HCM) experience obstruction to ventricular ejection of blood due to contact of the anterior mitral valve leaflet during systole, some centers perform an experimental procedure, called a left ventricular myotomy and myectomy (LVMM), to relieve the outflow obstruction. In LVMM, a surgical incision is made through the LV and a small amount of muscle tissue is excised from the interventricular septum at the point where the mitral valve leaflet makes contact. Alternatively, the procedure may be performed via cardiac catheterization using a bioptome or laser. In both cases there is risk of creating a ventricular septal defect if too much tissue is excised.

Surgical Treatment of Tachyarrhythmias

Surgical treatment of tachyarrhythmias include excision, isolation, or interruption of cardiac tissue critical for the initiation, maintenance, or propagation of tachycardia.

- Surgical treatment for tachyarrhythmias may be employed for patients with symptomatic, drug-resistant, recurrent tachyarrhythmias, such as supraventricular tachycardias (e.g., Wolff-Parkinson-White syndrome; AV nodal reentry rhythms, atrial tachycardia, atrial flutter) or ventricular tachycardia.

- Usually, patients are required to undergo preoperative electrophysiologic studies, as well as intraoperative intracardiac recordings and programmed stimulation, in order to achieve successful results.

- In addition, indirect surgical approaches including aneurysectomy, coronary artery bypass grafting, and valve surgeries, may provide relief from tachyarrhythmias by improving cardiac hemodynamics and myocardial blood flow.

REFERENCES

1. Andreoli TE, Bennett JC, Carpenter CCJ, Plum F, Smith LH, Jr.: *Cecil Essentials of Medicine*, 3rd Ed. Philadelphia, W.B. Saunders Co., 1993.
2. Arthur EK: Rehabilitation of potential and cardiac transplant recipients. *Cardiopulmonary Record* 1(3):11–13, 1986.
3. Braunwald E (ed.): *Heart Disease—A Textbook of Cardiovascular Medicine*. Philadelphia, W.B. Saunders Co., 1992.
4. Cahalin LP: Cardiac muscle dysfunction. *In* Hillegass EA, Sadowsky HS (eds.): *Essentials of Cardiopulmonary Physical Therapy*. Philadelphia, W.B. Saunders Co., 1994.
5. Chung EK (ed.): *Quick Reference to Cardiovascular Diseases*, 3rd Ed. Baltimore, Williams & Wilkins, 1987.
6. Fink AW: Exercise responses in the transplant population. *Cardiopulmonary Record* 1(3): 7–10, 1986.
7. Guyton AC: *Textbook of Medical Physiology*, 8th Ed. Philadelphia, W.B. Saunders Co., 1991.
8. Hurst JW, Schlant RC, Rackley CE, Sonnenblick EH, Wenger NK (eds.): *The Heart, Arteries and Veins*, 7th Ed. New York, McGraw-Hill Information Services Co., 1990.
9. Kelley WN (ed-in-chief): *Textbook of Internal Medicine*, 2nd Ed. Philadelphia, J.B. Lippincott Co., 1992.
10. Kloner RA (ed.): *The Guide to Cardiology*, 2nd Ed. New York, Le Jacq Communications, 1990.
11. Marriott HJL: *Practical Electrocardiography*, 5th Ed. Baltimore, Williams & Wilkins, 1972.
12. Phillips RE, Feeney MK: *The Cardiac Rhythms— A Systematic Approach to Interpretation*, 3rd Ed. Philadelphia, W.B. Saunders Co., 1990.
13. Sadowsky HS: Anatomy of the cardiovascular and respiratory systems. *In* Hillegass EA, Sadowsky HS (eds.): *Essentials of Cardiopulmonary*

Physical Therapy. Philadelphia, W.B. Saunders Co., 1994.

14. Sadowsky HS: Cardiovascular and respiratory physiology. *In* Hillegass EA, Sadowsky HS (eds.): *Essentials of Cardiopulmonary Physical Therapy.* Philadelphia, W.B. Saunders Co., 1994.

15. Sokolow M, McIlroy MB: *Clinical Cardiology,* 4th Ed. Los Altos, CA, Lange Medical Publications, 1986.

16. Tilkian AG, Daily EK: *Cardiovascular Procedures—Diagnostic Techniques and Therapeutic Procedures.* St. Louis, The C.V. Mosby Co., 1986.

17. Underhill SL, Woods SL, Sivarajan ES, Halpenny CJ: *Cardiac Nursing.* Philadelphia, J.B. Lippincott Co., 1982.

18. Wyngaarden JB, Smith LH Jr, Bennett JC (eds.): *Cecil Textbook of Medicine,* 19th Ed. Philadelphia, W.B. Saunders Co., 1992.

2

PULMONOLOGY

The first part of this chapter offers a review of basic pulmonary anatomy and physiology, with emphasis on the factors that influence lung function. The remainder of the chapter presents the various diagnostic tests and procedures and therapeutic interventions available for the management of pulmonary disease. The implications for physical therapy treatments of important findings from the most common diagnostic tests, as well as for some treatment interventions, are included. The pulmonary diseases and disorders frequently encountered in rehabilitation patients are described in Chapter 3.

2.1 RESPIRATORY SYSTEM AND ITS FUNCTION

ANATOMY OF THE RESPIRATORY SYSTEM

The thorax consists of 12 thoracic vertebrae, 12 ribs, sternum, and costal cartilage. The upper airways consist of the nose, pharynx, and larynx. The lower airways, the tracheobronchial tree, are depicted in Figure 2–1. The two lungs with their various lobes and segments are illustrated in Figure 2–2.

MUSCLES OF RESPIRATION

The respiratory muscles, their innervations, and their functions are listed in Table 2–1. The primary muscles of inspiration are the diaphragm and the intercostal muscles, especially the external intercostal muscles. During deep or labored breathing, the accessory muscles of inspiration are recruited. At rest, expiration is a passive process, occurring as the inspiratory muscles relax. During forced expiration and coughing, the abdominal and internal intercostal muscles become active.

INNERVATION

The lungs and airways are innervated by the pulmonary plexus (located at the root of each lung), which is formed from branches of the sympathetic trunk and vagus nerve. SNS stimulation results in bronchodilation and slight vasoconstriction, whereas PNS stimulation causes bronchoconstriction and indirect vasodilation.

The function of the lungs is controlled through a complex system that integrates information from a number of specialized receptors, as illustrated in Figure 2–3.

BLOOD SUPPLY TO THE LUNGS

The bronchial arteries supply the airways, pleura, and connective tissue. The pulmonary arteries supply the alveoli and participate in gas exchange.

RESPIRATORY PHYSIOLOGY

BASIC FUNCTIONS OF THE RESPIRATORY SYSTEM

The basic functions of the respiratory system include oxygenation of the blood, removal of carbon dioxide, control of acid-base balance, and production of vocalization.

PHYSIOLOGY OF RESPIRATION

The physiology of respiration involves:

- Inspiration:
  - Active muscle contraction results in expansion of the thorax and a fall in alveolar pressure, which causes air to flow into lungs.
- Expiration:
  - The passive return of the respiratory muscles to their resting positions causes alveolar pressure to rise, and air flows out of the lungs.
  - During forced expiration and coughing, active contraction of the expiratory muscles (plus closure of the glottis during coughing)

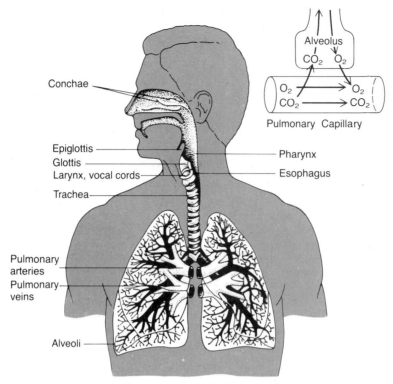

FIGURE 2-1. The respiratory passages. (From Guyton AC: *Textbook of Medical Physiology*, 8th Ed. Philadelphia, W.B. Saunders Co., p. 410, 1991. Used with permission.)

TABLE 2-1. **Muscles of Respiration, Their Innervations, and Functions**

MUSCLE (INNERVATION)	FUNCTIONS
Inspiratory Muscles	
Diaphragm (C_{3-5})	Expands thorax vertically and horizontally; essential for normal vital capacity and effective cough
Intercostals (T_{1-12})	Anterior and lateral expansion of upper and lower chest
Sternocleidomastoid (cranial nerve XI and C_{1-4})	When head is fixed, elevates sternum to expand chest superiorly and anteriorly
Scalenes (C_{3-8})	When neck is fixed, elevate first two ribs to expand chest superiorly
Serratus anterior (C_{5-7})	When scapulae are fixed, elevates first 8–9 ribs to provide posterior expansion of thorax
Pectoralis major (C_5–T_1)	When arms are fixed, elevates true ribs to expand the chest anteriorly
Pectoralis minor (C_{6-8})	When scapulae are fixed, elevates third, fourth, and fifth ribs to expand the chest laterally
Trapezius (cranial nerve and XI C_{3-4})	Stabilizes scapulae to assist the serratus anterior and pectoralis minor in elevating the ribs
Erector spinae (C_1 down)	Extend the vertebral column to allow further rib elevation
Expiratory Muscles	
Abdominals (T_{5-12})	Help force diaphragm back to resting position and depress and compress lower thorax leading to $\uparrow$ intrathoracic pressure, which is essential for effective cough
Internal intercostals (T_{1-12})	Depress third, fourth, and fifth ribs to aid in forceful expiration

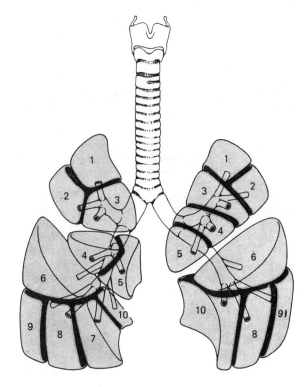

FIGURE 2-2. The bronchopulmonary segments. *Left and right upper lobes:* (1) apical, (2) posterior, and (3) anterior segments. *Left upper lobe:* (4) superior lingular, and (5) inferior lingular segments. *Right middle lobe:* (4) lateral and (5) medial segments. *Lower lobes:* (6) superior, (7) medial basal (no medial basal segment in the left lung), (8) anterior basal, (9) lateral basal, and (10) posterior basal segments. (From Weibel ER: Design and structure of the human lung. *In* Fishman AP (Ed.): *Pulmonary Diseases and Disorders,* vol. 1. New York, McGraw-Hill, 1980. Reproduced with permission of McGraw-Hill, Inc.)

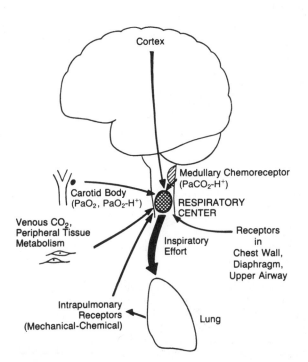

FIGURE 2-3. The complex system involved in the integration and control of respiratory function. (From Zwillich CW: Control of ventilation. *In* Kelly WN (ed.): *Textbook of Internal Medicine,* 2nd Ed. Philadelphia, J.B. Lippincott Co., p. 1690, 1992. Used with permission.)

causes a marked rise in intrathoracic pressure so that expiration occurs more rapidly and completely.

A number of factors determine respiratory function (Table 2–2):

- Pulmonary compliance, which is the ease with which the lungs inflate during inspiration
- Airway resistance, or the resistance to air flow through the airways
- Ventilation, which is the process by which air moves into and out of the lungs
- Diffusion, which involves the movement of gases into and out of the blood

TABLE 2–2. Factors Affecting Respiratory Function

FACTOR	INFLUENCED BY

Compliance (C)	Lung compliance
	    The elastic properties of the lungs tend to collapse the lungs if they are
	        not acted on by external forces.
	Chest wall compliance
	    The elastic forces of the chest wall cause it to expand if unopposed by the
	        elastic recoil of the lungs.

Airway resistance (R_{aw})	Upper airways
	    Provide ~ 45% of total airway resistance
	Lower airways, which are affected by:
	    External pressure
	    Bronchial smooth muscle contraction/relaxation
	    Mucosal congestion, edema, mucous
	    Inspiration versus expiration ($\uparrow$ versus $\downarrow$, respectively)
	    Loss of structural support (e.g., emphysema)

Ventilation ($\dot{V}$)	Regional differences
	    Greatest ventilation in lower lung fields
	    Least in upper lung fields
	Body position
	    Greatest ventilation in dependent regions

Diffusion	Interference at the alveolar capillary membrane (i.e., thickening, fibrosis, fluid, edema, etc.) Surface area available for gas exchange
Perfusion ($\dot{Q}$)	Body position/gravity Dependent/lower lung regions > upper Interaction of alveolar, arterial, and venous pressures down the lungs Vasoconstriction (triggered by hypoxia, acidemia, etc.)

Ventilation-perfusion ($\dot{V}/\dot{Q}$) Matching	Uneven ventilation, which can result from:
	    Uneven compliance
	    Uneven airway resistance
	Uneven perfusion, which can result from:
	    Obstruction of part of the pulmonary circulation
	    Compression of blood vessels

Oxygen-hemoglobin (O_2-Hb) binding	Arterial oxygen concentration (PO_2)
	    If $PO_2 > 60 \rightarrow O_2$ saturation will be > 90%
	    A decrease in PO_2 results in $\downarrow$ association + $\uparrow$ dissociation of O_2-Hb (so
	        less O_2 is bound to Hb but what is bound is more easily given off to the
	        tissues)
	    A number of factors result in shift of the oxyhemoglobin curve:
	        $\uparrow$ pH, $\downarrow$ PCO_2, $\downarrow$ temperature, and others cause a shift to the left so
	            there is $\uparrow$ association + $\downarrow$ dissociation of O_2-Hb
	        $\downarrow$ pH, $\uparrow$ PCO_2, $\uparrow$ temperature, and others cause a shift to the right so
	            there is $\downarrow$ association + $\uparrow$ dissociation of O_2-Hb

ARTERIAL OXYGENATION

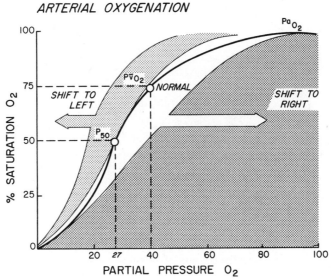

FIGURE 2-4. The oxyhemoglobin (O_2-Hb) dissociation curve. Factors that cause a shift of the curve to the left (e.g., acute alkalosis, hypocapnia, hypothermia) result in increased association and decreased dissociation of O_2-Hb, whereas factors that cause a shift of the curve to the right (e.g., acute acidosis, hypercapnia, fever) lead to reduced association and enhanced dissociation of O_2-Hb. (From Hobson L, Dean E: Review of respiratory physiology. *In* Frownfelter DL: *Chest Physical Therapy and Pulmonary Rehabilitation,* 2nd Ed. Chicago, Year Book Medical Publishers, Inc., p. 55, 1987. Used with permission.)

- Perfusion, or the blood flow through the pulmonary circulation that is available for gas exchange
- Ventilation-perfusion matching, or the degree of physical correspondence between ventilated and perfused areas of the lungs
- Oxygen-hemoglobin binding, or the level of oxygen saturation of the arterial blood, as shown in Figure 2–4.

LUNG VOLUMES AND CAPACITIES

As illustrated in Figure 2–5, it is possible to measure various lung volumes and capacities. The lung volumes and capacities are described in Table 2–3.

- Tidal volume (V_T) represents the most efficient breathing pattern and volume.
- Functional reserve capacity (FRC) reflects the balance of the elastic forces exerted by the chest wall and the lungs and is the resting volume of the respiratory system after a normal expiration.
- At total lung capacity (TLC), the elastic forces of the lungs are balanced by the maximal inspiratory muscle forces.
- At residual volume (RV), the elastic forces of

the chest wall are balanced by the maximal expiratory muscle forces.
- RV includes the amount of air in the nonrespiratory conducting airways, or the *anatomic dead space,* as well as that remaining in the pulmonary acini following a maximal forced expiration; it is normally $\sim$ 20% to 30% of V_T.

2.2 EVALUATION OF THE PULMONARY SYSTEM

Although physical therapists seldom participate in or read the raw data of most of the diagnostic tests and procedures described in this section, we are frequently challenged to interpret the results of these investigations and their implications for the patients we treat. Through better comprehension of the information in a patient's chart, we can grasp more completely the patient's status and the possible physiologic effects of our treatment interventions.

SIGNS AND SYMPTOMS OF PULMONARY DISEASE

Generally, the first information presented in the admission note in a patient's chart relates to the

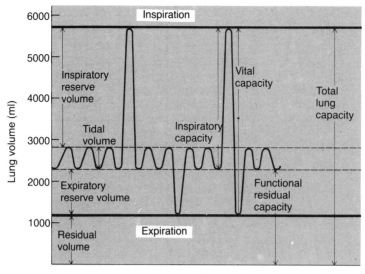

FIGURE 2-5. A spirogram showing the lung volumes and capacities. (From Guyton AC: *Textbook of Medical Physiology*, 8th Ed. Philadelphia, W.B. Saunders Co., p. 407, 1991. Used with permission.)

patient's subjective complaints. Table 2–4 describes the most common signs and symptoms and their pulmonary causes. There may be other possible explanations for some of these symptoms; the cardiovascular causes are listed in Table 1–4 on page 8, and other causes are presented in Table 5–5 on page 153.

PHYSICAL EXAMINATION

The history and physical examination section of a patient's chart is a valuable source of impor-

tant information relating to patient status and level of function. The data relevant to physical therapy evaluation and their implications for treatment are discussed in Chapter 5.

CYTOLOGIC AND HEMATOLOGIC TESTS

A variety of cytologic and hematologic tests are used to identify disease-causing organisms and to monitor the body's responses to them.

TABLE 2-3. The Lung Volumes and Capacities

VOLUME OR CAPACITY	DESCRIPTION
Tidal volume (VT)	Amount of air inspired or expired during normal breathing
Inspiratory reserve volume (IRV)	Extra volume inspired over and above the tidal volume
Expiratory reserve volume (ERV)	Extra amount of air forcefully expired after the end of a normal tidal expiration
Residual volume (RV)	Volume of air still remaining in the lungs after a complete forceful expiration
Inspiratory capacity (IC)	Maximal volume of air that can be inspired after a normal tidal expiration = TV + IRV
Functional residual capacity (FRC)	Amount of air remaining in the lungs after a normal tidal expiration = RV + ERV
Vital capacity (VC)	Maximal volume of air that a person can forcefully expire after taking in a maximal inspiration = IRV + TV + ERV
Total lung capacity (TLC)	Maximal volume of air that the lungs can contain following a maximal inspiration = RV + ERV + TV + IRV

TABLE 2-4. **Signs and Symptoms of Pulmonary Disease**

SIGN OR SYMPTOM	COMMON PULMONARY CAUSES
Anorexia, weakness, fatigue, weight loss	Chronic respiratory disease (probably caused by ↑ work of breathing), pulmonary infection
↓ Breath sounds	Pneumothorax, emphysema, pleural effusion, local bronchial occlusion, atelectasis, hypoventilation of any cause, diaphragmatic paralysis, obesity
Bradycardia	Profound hypoxemia
Bronchial breath sounds	Consolidation, tumor, alveolar collapse, or fibrosis in close approximation to a patent bronchus
↓ Chest expansion (focal, generalized)	Pulmonary consolidation, fibrosis, atelectasis, pleural effusion, pneumothorax, obesity, kyphoscoliosis, obstructive lung disease, respiratory muscle weakness
Chest pain	Pleurisy, pneumonia, cancer, tuberculosis, pulmonary emboli or infarction, pneumothorax, violent coughing, rib fracture or other trauma, tracheobronchial infection, inhalation of noxious fumes, intercostal neuritis, pulmonary hypertension
Coma, convulsions	Rapid ↑ P_{CO_2}
Confusion, ↓ concentration, restlessness, irritability	Hypoxemia, hypercapnia
Cough	Stimulation of airway mucosal irritant receptors by inflammation, secretions, foreign bodies, chemical substances, and intrabronchial masses
Crackles, or rales	Interstitial fibrosis, pulmonary edema, COPD
Cyanosis	Hypoxemia
Diaphoresis	Infection (fever), ↑ sympathetic nervous system (SNS) activity (e.g., anxiety re: SOB), night sweats (unknown mechanism)
Digital clubbing	Unknown; seen in bronchial carcinoma, certain forms of pulmonary fibrosis (e.g., asbestosis, cryptogenic fibrosing alveolitis), chronic sepsis (empyema, lung abscess, bronchiectasis, cystic fibrosis)
Dullness to percussion	Pleural effusion, lobar consolidation, lobar or whole lung atelectasis
Dyspnea, shortness of breath (SOB) (air hunger)	*Acute onset:* pulmonary embolism, pneumothorax, acute asthma, pulmonary congestion caused by congestive heart failure (CHF), pneumonia, upper airway obstruction.
	Subacute or chronic: airflow limitation/COPD, ↓ lung volume, impaired gas exchange, ↓ lung compliance (e.g., pneumonia, congestion, atelectasis, pleural effusion, pulmonary fibrosis), ↓ chest wall compliance (e.g., kyphoscoliosis, obesity, neuromuscular impairment), ↑ demand
Fever	Pulmonary infection, tissue degeneration, trauma
Hemoptysis (expectoration of bloody or blood-streaked secretions)	Acute exacerbation of chronic bronchitis, bronchial carcinoma, tuberculosis, bronchiectasis, pulmonary hypertension, pulmonary infarction, pneumonia (especially *pneumococcal*)
Hypercapnia (↑ P_{CO_2})	↑ Ventilation-perfusion mismatching, alveolar hypoventilation, pulmonary arteriovenous malformations
Hypoxemia (↓ P_{O_2})	↑ Ventilation-perfusion mismatching, diffusion defect, alveolar hypoventilation, pulmonary arteriovenous malformations, ↓ F_{IO_2} (e.g., altitude)
Mediastinal shift	Pulmonary fibrosis, atelectasis (toward affected side); pneumothorax, pleural effusion, hyperinflation of one lung caused by check-valve obstruction of a bronchus (away from affected side); severe kyphoscoliosis (toward side of compressed lung)

Continued on following page

TABLE 2–4. **Signs and Symptoms of Pulmonary Disease** *Continued*

SIGN OR SYMPTOM	COMMON PULMONARY CAUSES
↑ Nasal secretions	Infection, irritants, allergens
Orthopnea (SOB when recumbent)	Paralysis of both hemidiaphragms, CHF
Paroxysmal nocturnal dyspnea (PND) (awakening with SOB in the middle of the night)	Pooling of secretions, gravity-induced ↓ lung volumes, sleep-induced ↑ airflow resistance, CHF
Pleural friction rub	Irritation of the pleura (e.g., pneumonia, pleurisy)
↑ Resonance to percussion	Emphysema, pneumothorax
Rhonchi, wheezes	↑ Secretions in airway(s)
Sputum production	Pulmonary suppuration, lung abscess, chronic bronchitis, bronchiectasis, neoplasm, pulmonary edema, pneumonia
Stridor	Narrowing of the glottis, trachea, or major bronchi, as by foreign body aspiration, external compression by tumor, or tumor within the airways
Tachycardia	Hypoxemia
Tachypnea	Pneumonia, pulmonary edema, pulmonary infarction, diffuse pulmonary fibrosis, anxiety, exertion
↑ Vocal fremitus	Consolidation
↓ Vocal fremitus	Pleural effusion, pneumothorax, obesity, ↑ chest musculature
Wheezes	Narrowing of a bronchus (e.g., bronchoconstriction, stenosis, ↑ secretions, edema, inflammation, tumor, foreign body aspiration)

Sputum Analysis

Collection and examination of expectorated sputum is the most common method of obtaining a sample for cytologic evaluation. Other methods, such as bronchoscopy and needle aspiration are presented later.

Hematologic Tests

Blood tests that may aid in the assessment of pulmonary disease include arterial blood gases, complete blood counts, and coagulation studies (see Chapter 8).

CHEST RADIOGRAPHY

Despite the technologic advances yielding a number of new imaging modalities in recent years, the standard chest radiograph remains a critical element of the clinical examination.

- The various projections that can be used during chest radiography are described in Table 2–5.
- The structures that can be identified in a normal posteroanterior chest radiogram are shown in Figure 2–6.
- The difference between an inspiratory versus an expiratory radiogram is illustrated in Figure 1–13 (see page 15).
- Physical therapists working in cardiopulmonary care often become familiar with the basic principles of chest x-ray interpretation and use the results to anatomically locate the patient's pathologic condition and direct treatment interventions.

DIGITAL IMAGING

Acquired directly from a fluoroscopic image or latent image on a plate or via digitization of an x-ray film, digital imaging uses a computer processing system to replace conventional radiography.

- The image created is opposite in contrast to that normally seen on radiographs.
- The main advantages are the ability to manipulate and process the images in innumerable

TABLE 2–5. **Various Projections Used for Chest Radiography**

PROJECTION	DESCRIPTION
Posteroanterior (PA)	The x-ray beam passes back to front with the subject standing or sitting with the chest against the film plate, usually with the breath held following a deep inspiration.
Anteroposterior (AP)	The x-ray beam passes front to back with the patient's back against the film; most often obtained with a portable x-ray machine when patients are too ill or unable to travel to the radiology department.
Lateral (Lat.)	The beam passes side to side, usually right to left, with the side of the chest against the film plate in an upright position; commonly obtained along with a PA film.
Oblique	The beam passes PA or AP with one of the patient's sides in contact with the film plate and the chest rotated 10–45 degrees.
Decubitus	The beam travels PA or AP with the patient lying on one side. Used to confirm presence of pleural fluid or suspected foreign body in small children.
Lordotic	The x-ray is taken in the PA position with the patient tilted backward. Because structures change their relative positions, this view allows better visualization of subapical, posterior, middle lobe, and lingular lesions.
Expiratory	The x-ray is obtained following expiration or forced expiration to document focal air trapping or delayed emptying.

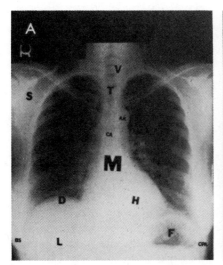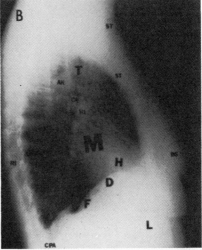

FIGURE 2–6. Posteroanterior *(A)* and lateral *(B)* chest radiographs of a young woman showing all the structures that are reviewed during chest xray evaluation. Soft tissues and extrathoracic structures: soft tissues (ST), breast shadow (BS), diaphragm (D), liver (L), and fundus of stomach (F). Bony thorax: ribs (RI), vertebrae (V), scapulae (S), clavicles (CL), and sternum (ST). Mediastinal structures: mediastinum (M), trachea (T), carina (CA), aortic knob (AK), heart (H), anterior clear space (ACS), and hilum of lungs (HI). Lung fields: hilum of lungs (HI), pulmonary vessels, costophrenic angle (CPA), and lung apices (LA). (From Johnson T: Principles of chest x-ray interpretation. *In* Frownfelter DL: *Chest Physical Therapy and Pulmonary Rehabilitation, An Interdisciplinary Approach,* 2nd Ed. Chicago, Year Book Medical Publishers, Inc., p. 769, 1987. Used with permission.)

ways allowing improved diagnostic value and the ability to store images and transmit them from one location to another.

- Digital imaging is often useful for imaging diaphragmatic function, which is valuable information to therapists who must interpret the patient's physiologic response to exertion and devise appropriate treatment goals and plans.

ELECTROCARDIOGRAPHY

A 12-lead electrocardiogram is commonly obtained to ascertain the presence of right ventricular hypertrophy (RVH) and/or strain in patients with chronic lung disease, acute asthma, and pulmonary embolism.

- Specific indicators of RVH and/or strain include:
  - Right-axis deviation (axis $> +100°$)
  - P-pulmonale (a tall, peaked P wave taller than 2.5 mm in leads II, III, and aVF)
  - A dominant R wave in aVR and V_1.
- In addition, hypoxemia and acidosis are often associated with atrial and ventricular arrhythmias.

PULMONARY IMAGING STUDIES

FLUOROSCOPY

Flouroscopy is a technique of radiographic imaging with intensification, producing a real time display of a patient's breathing that may be highlighted with a radioopaque contrast agent.

- Flouroscopy offers two advantages over standard radiograph:
  - Offers a quick and inexpensive method of detecting lesions that can be seen clearly only in an unusual oblique projection (e.g., some pleural plaques, retrocardiac nodules)
  - Demonstrates lesions in real time, allowing identification of small pulmonary nodules obscured by ribs as they move relative to the ribs with respiration and detection of pulsation of nodules and masses
- Another important use is documenting diaphragmatic function, as shown in Figure 2–7, which is valuable information to physical therapists.
- Fluoroscopy is also used to diagnose air trapping in small children with suspected foreign body aspiration and to guide needle biopsies.

CONVENTIONAL TOMOGRAPHY

Mechanically linked movement of an x-ray tube and film cassette holder in opposite curvilinear directions allows structures overlapping the area of interest to blur out so the area can be more clearly visualized. Chest tomography is most commonly used to differentiate between benign versus malignant processes when a solitary opacity is found on a chest radiograph, evaluate suspicious hilar findings, demonstrate suspected intrabronchial masses, and document tracheal structure when stricture or tumors are suspected.

COMPUTED TOMOGRAPHY

With computed tomography (CT), highly sensitive detectors around the body measure attenuation of an x-ray beam that has passed through a body part in multiple projections; several million attenuation values are fed into a computer, which constructs a matrix of a cross-sectional slice of the body part and processes it. The result is a clear image with excellent contrast resolution of tissues (see Fig. 1–17 on page 18).

- Chest CT is valuable in evaluating mediastinal masses, hilar abnormalities, diffuse lung disease, pleural abnormalities, presence of metastatic lesions, and resectability of bronchial carcinoma.
- CT is also widely used to detect and localize mediastinal lymph nodes for mediastinoscopy and transbronchial biopsy, focal bronchial abnormalities for bronchoscopic biopsy, and lung lesions for percutaneous needle biopsy.

MAGNETIC RESONANCE IMAGING

Magnetic resonance imaging (MRI) uses radiofrequency pulse sequences with the patient positioned in a strong magnetic field to stimulate aligned protons, which generate signals that can be amplified and converted into images of body tissues, as shown in Figure 1–18 (see page 19). Thoracic MRI is most useful for imaging mediastinal masses, thrombosis of the superior vena cava and great vessels, central pulmonary emboli, vascular stenoses, aneurysms, and dissections, and soft tissues of the chest wall. Notably, expanded lungs have insufficient density of protons to generate adequate images for the evaluation of pathologic processes involving the parenchyma.

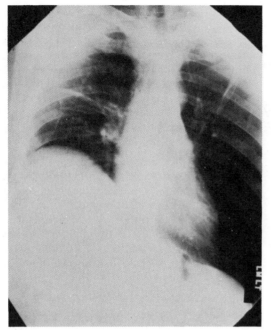 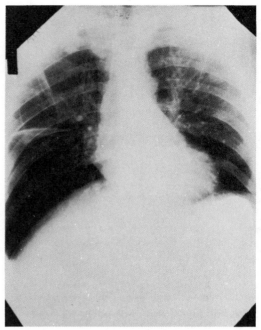

A   B

FIGURE 2–7. Fluoroscopic image showing diaphragmatic function in a patient with right hemidiaphragm paralysis: *(A)* Paradoxic upward motion of the paralyzed right hemidiaphragm during sudden inspiration. *(B)* Paradoxical downward motion during expiration. (From Prakash UBS: Neurologic diseases. *In* Baum GL, Wolinsky E (eds.): *Textbook of Pulmonary Diseases,* 4th Ed. © 1989. Published by Little, Brown and Company, Boston, p. 1418. Used with permission.)

POSITRON EMISSION TOMOGRAPHY

Positron emission tomography (PET) scanning is an imaging technique that uses biologically active positron emission radiopharmaceuticals (i.e., ^{18}F deoxyglucose or ^{11}C acetate) to display and quantify metabolic processes, receptor occupancy, and blood flow (see Fig 1–22 on page 22). In pulmonary medicine, PET is being used to study regional expansion and oxygen concentration, ventilation-perfusion relationships, glucose metabolism, and central chemical control of ventilation.

ULTRASONOGRAPHY

Although ultrasound is not useful for evaluating aerated lung and any structures lying immediately beneath bone or air, it can be valuable for differentiating pleural fluid from pleural thickening.

VENTILATION-PERFUSION ($\dot{V}/\dot{Q}$) SCANNING

The use of radionuclides in the gaseous form or dissolved in liquid and a gamma counter provides information on the distribution of ventilation and perfusion within the lungs.

- Perfusion and ventilation studies are obtained separately and then the images are compared, as shown in Figure 2–8.
- The most common uses of $\dot{V}/\dot{Q}$ scanning include the diagnosis of pulmonary embolism, prediction of postoperative lung function following pneumonectomy, diagnosis of early airflow obstruction (as indicated by delayed washout), and assessment of appropriateness of surgical excision of emphysematous bulla.
- Unfortunately, $\dot{V}/\dot{Q}$ scanning is not very sensitive at identifying smaller areas of mismatch,

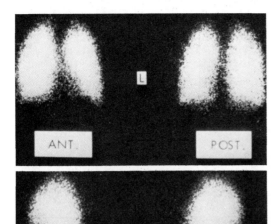

FIGURE 2–8. Ventilation and perfusion scans in a 37-year-old female with sudden onset of dyspnea. Note the lack of perfusion in the right lower lobe (upper left image). (From Gamsu F, Rozenman J: Diagnostic imaging. *In* Baum GL, Wolinsky E (eds.): *Textbook of Pulmonary Diseases,* 4th Ed. © 1989. Published by Little, Brown and Company, Boston, p. 307. Used with permission.)

so that results are stated in terms of the probability of pulmonary embolism, as described in Table 2–6.

- Abnormal findings inform the therapist that significant mismatch between ventilation and perfusion exists and the patient will have limited tolerance for activity.

OTHER SCINTIGRAPHIC IMAGING STUDIES

Scintigraphy can also be used for other pulmonary diagnostic purposes including localization of tumor, assessment of interstitial lung disease, and detection of opportunistic infections (via gallium-67 scanning); measurement of mucociliary clearance (via radiolabeled aerosol studies); evaluation of lung epithelial permeability (via ^{99m}Tc-DPTA clearance studies); and assessment of cardiac function in cor pulmonale (via gated blood pool imaging).

PULMONARY FUNCTION TESTS

Pulmonary function tests (PFTs) consist of a series of tests designed to assess the integrity and function of the respiratory system. They include measurements of the lung volumes and capacities, ventilation, pulmonary mechanics, and dif-

TABLE 2–6. Interpretation of Ventilation-Perfusion ($\dot{V}/\dot{Q}$) Scans

CATEGORY	$\dot{V}/\dot{Q}$ SCAN PATTERN*	APPROXIMATE INCIDENCE OF PULMONARY EMBOLISM†
Normal	No perfusion defects	0
Low probability	Small $\dot{V}/\dot{Q}$ mismatches	10
	$\dot{V}/\dot{Q}$ mismatches without corresponding roentgenographic changes	
	Perfusion defect substantially smaller than roentgenographic density.	
Intermediate probability	Severe, diffuse COPD with perfusion defects	30
	Perfusion defect of same size as roentgenographic changes	
	Single medium or large $\dot{V}/\dot{Q}$ mismatches‡	
High probability	Two or more medium or large $\dot{V}/\dot{Q}$ mismatches	90
	Perfusion defect substantially larger than roentgenographic density.	

Reprinted with permission from Biello DR: Radiological (scintigraphic) evaluation of patients with suspected pulmonary thromboembolism. *JAMA* 257(23):3257–3259, 1987. Copyright © 1987, American Medical Association.
*A small perfusion defect involves <25% of the expected volume of a pulmonary segment; medium, 25% to 90%; and large, ≥90%.
†Detected by pulmonary angiography.
‡Controversy exists regarding whether single large $\dot{V}/\dot{Q}$ mismatches are categorized as high or intermediate probability. The more conservative interpretation has been used in this table.

fusion. The information provided by PFTs is helpful to the therapist in establishing realistic treatment goals and an appropriate treatment plan according to the patient's current pulmonary problems and any permanent impairment.

DATA AVAILABLE FROM PFTS

Lung Volumes and Capacities

- The various lung volumes and capacities are described in Table 2–3 (see page 40).
  - Total lung capacity may be decreased in disease processes with space-occupying lesions (such as edema, atelectasis, tumors, and fibrosis) and in pleural effusion, pneumothorax, or thoracic deformity. It may be normal or increased in obstructive lung diseases.
  - Examples of proportional changes typically seen in obstructive and restrictive lung disease compared with normal function are illustrated in Figure 2–9.

Ventilation

- The parameters that describe ventilatory function include:
  - Tidal volume (VT)

— Values should always be assessed within the context of respiratory rate and minute ventilation.

— Values of 400 to 700 ml are typical, although there is considerable variation. Values may be decreased in restrictive lung dysfunction.

- Respiratory rate (*f*, RR)
  — Normally, f = 12 to 20 breaths per minute (bpm) in adults. Values are increased with exercise, hypoxia, hypercapnia, acidosis, increased dead space volume, and other causes, and may be decreased in central nervous system depression, carbon dioxide narcosis, and obstructive lung disease.
  — f is often considered to be a good indicator of the stimulus to breathe and of normal versus abnormal ventilatory status.

- Minute ventilation (expired) ($\dot{V}E$)
  — $\dot{V}E$ = VT × f and is usually between 5 to 10 L/min. $\dot{V}E$ will be increased in hypoxia, hypercapnia, acidosis, increased

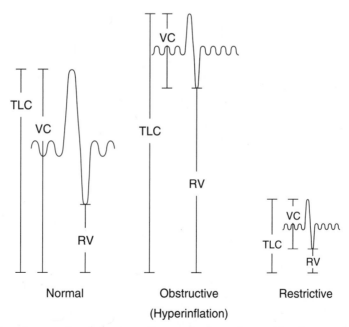

FIGURE 2–9. Examples of proportional changes of lung volumes and capacities characteristic of obstructive and restrictive lung diseases compared to normal. TLC = total lung capacity, VC = vital capacity, RV = residual volume. (From Clausen JL: Pulmonary function testing. *In* Kelly WN, et al., (eds.): *Textbook of Internal Medicine,* 2nd ed. Philadelphia, J.B. Lippincott Co., p. 1824, 1992. Used with permission.)

dead space volume, anxiety, and exercise and will be decreased in hypocapnia, alkalemia, respiratory center depression, and neuromuscular disorders with ventilatory muscle involvement.

— $\dot{V}E$ is the primary index of ventilation when used in conjunction with arterial blood gases.

- Respiratory, or physiologic, dead space (VD)
  — VD is that volume of the lungs that is ventilated but not perfused and is usually 125 to 175 ml.
  — VD can be divided into the conducting airways, or anatomic dead space, and the nonperfused alveoli, or alveolar dead space. Anatomic dead space is increased in larger individuals and in brochiectasis and emphysema and decreased in asthma, bronchial obstruction, and mucous plugging. VD is increased during exercise in individuals with normal pulmonary function and in individuals with pulmonary embolism and pulmonary hypertension.

- Ratio of dead space to tidal volume (VD/VT)
  — Normally, the derived value is 0.2 to 0.4.
  — VD/VT decreases in normal individuals during exercise because of increased cardiac output and enhanced perfusion of the alveoli at the lung bases (despite an absolute increase in VD) and increases in pulmonary embolism and pulmonary hypertension.

- Alveolar ventilation ($\dot{V}A$)
  — $\dot{V}A = f(VT - VD)$ and is usually about 4 to 5 L at rest, with large variations in healthy individuals. Decreased $\dot{V}A$ can result from absolute increases in dead space, as well as decreases in $\dot{V}E$.
  — $\dot{V}A$ is one of the major factors determining gas exchange, which is ultimately documented only by arterial blood gases.

Pulmonary Mechanics

Because studies of pulmonary mechanics (e.g., flow rates, compliance, and airway resistance) are dynamic in nature, their measurement validity is dependent on patient effort and cooperation. Tests of pulmonary mechanics are often performed before and after the administration of bronchodilators to determine the efficacy of their use.

- Spirometric and pulmonary mechanics measurements are described in Table 2–7.
- Typical flow curves obtained during forced expiration in obstructive and restrictive lung disease compared with normal function are depicted in Figure 2–10.
- Typical patterns for flow-volume loops for obstructive and restrictive dysfunction compared with normal function are shown in Figure 2–11.

Diffusion Studies

- The parameters that describe diffusing capacity include:
  - Carbon monoxide diffusing capacity (DLCO), which measures all factors that affect diffusion of gases across the alveolar-capillary membrane. Values decrease with anemia.
  - Transfer factor for carbon monoxide (TLCO), which has been proposed as more accurate terminology since the diffusion process includes the rate of reaction of carbon monoxide with hemoglobin as well as its diffusion across the alveolar-capillary membrane.
  - Diffusion constant (KCO), which indicates the rate of carbon monoxide uptake per minute, obtained from a semiplot of alveolar carbon monoxide concentration against time, assuming perfect mixing of the inspired and residual gas.
- Causes of abnormal diffusing capacity and the effect on the diffusion constant, KCO, are presented in Table 2–8.
- Patients with markedly abnormal diffusing capacity are more likely to have problems with oxygen desaturation during exertion.

OTHER MEASURABLE PARAMETERS

Maximum Respiratory Pressures

Measurements of the static pressures developed by inspiratory and expiratory muscle contraction are particularly valuable for determining the presence or absence of respiratory muscle weakness.

Chemical Control of Ventilation

The change in $\dot{V}E$ caused by breathing various concentrations of carbon dioxide (CO_2) under normoxic conditions (i.e., the CO_2 response) or various concentrations of oxygen (O_2) under isocapneic conditions (i.e., the O_2 response) is used to identify patients with chronic obstructive

TABLE 2–7. **Spirometric and Pulmonary Mechanics Measurements**

PARAMETER	COMMENTS
Forced vital capacity (FVC) (that volume that can be expired as forcefully and rapidly as possible after a maximal inspiration)	Normally FVC = vital capacity (VC) but may be less than VC, as in chronic obstructive pulmonary disease (COPD) where air trapping is exaggerated during forced expiration. Both FVC and VC are similarly ↓ in restrictive lung dysfunction (RLD).
Forced expiratory volume in 1 second (FEV$_1$) (the volume of gas expired over the first second of an FVC)	As a measure of flow, FEV$_1$ is valuable in assessing the severity of airway obstruction.
FEV$_1$/FVC (the forced expiratory volume in 1 sec expressed as a percentage of forced vital capacity)	Younger subjects can expire 50–60% of FVC in 0.5 sec, 75–85% in 1 sec, 94% in 2 sec, and 97% in 3 sec Older healthy subjects typically have FEV$_1$ of 70–75%.
Forced expiratory flow$_{200-1200}$ (FEF$_{200-1200}$) (the average rate of flow for the liter of gas expired after the first 200 ml during an FVC)	Also referred to as the maximal expiratory flow rate (MEFR$_{200-1200}$). A good index of airflow characteristics in the larger airways.
Forced expiratory flow$_{25-75}$ (FEF$_{25-75}$) (the average flow rate in L/sec during the middle half of an FVC, i.e., from 25%-75% of FVC)	Also referred to as the maximal midexpiratory flow rate (MMFR). Indicates the status of the medium-sized airways. ↓ Values seen in early stages of obstructive disease (OD).
Peak expiratory flow rate (PEFR) (the maximal flow rate attainable at any time during a FVC maneuver)	Even when measured with a pneumotachometer, PEFR is of limited value since even patients with COPD may develop high flow rates initially before obstruction develops.
Maximal voluntary ventilation (MVV) (the largest volume that a subject can breathe per minute by voluntary effort using rapid deep breaths)	Measures the status of the respiratory muscles, pulmonary compliance, and resistance offered by airways and tissues. Often extrapolated from values obtained in 10–15 sec ↓ Values seen in OD, neuromuscular disease. Values often normal in RLD.
Closing Volume (CV) (the volume at which closure of the small airways in the lower alveoli occurs during expiration)	Used to document pathologic changes in small airways (<2 mm in diameter) and to measure the uniformity of gas distribution within the lungs. ↑ Values seen in asthma, bronchitis, chronic smokers, the elderly. A change in slope of nitrogen curve by >2% indicates uneven alveolar ventilation.
Flow-volume loop (a graphic representation of the changes in flow and volume that occur during forced inspiration and expiration)	Although the initial third of the expiratory phase is effort dependent, the remainder of the curve is independent of patient effort and reproducible. Abnormal loops are seen in small airways disease (e.g., emphysema, asthma), large airways disease (e.g., tumors of trachea and bronchi), and moderately severe RLD. The highest point on the expiratory curve is the PEFR (see above)
Volume of isoflow (V$_{ISO}$V) (the volume at which the flow-volume loop obtained while breathing room air intersects with that obtained after breathing 80% helium/20% oxygen gas mixture when the two loops are superimposed)	↑ Values are due to ↑ resistance to laminar flow and indicate small airways disease. Low values are normal.

Continued on following page

Table 2-7. Spirometric and Pulmonary Mechanics Measurements *Continued*

PARAMETER	COMMENTS
Compliance (C) (the change in volume produced by a unit change in pressure for the lungs (C_L), the thorax (C_T), or the lungs-thorax system (C_{LT})	Measurements of C describe the elasticity of the lungs, thorax, and combination of two. C_L varies with the end-expiratory volume, or functional reserve capacity (FRC). Usually $\downarrow$ in pulmonary edema or congestion, atelectasis, pneumonia, loss of surfactant, other RLD, emphysema. C_L may be $\downarrow$ in COPD due to chronic hyperinflation; neurologic and neuromuscular disorders.
Airway Resistance (R_{aw}) (the pressure difference required for a unit of flow change)	Measurement of R_{aw} is helpful in distinguishing between RLD and OD; it is $\uparrow$ in acute asthmatic attack and other OD but not in RLD.

pulmonary disease (COPD) who increase ventilation to maintain a normal partial pressure of carbon dioxide (P_{CO_2}) versus those who do not, patients with chronic CO_2 retention who receive their primary stimulus for breathing from hypoxia, and those with little intrinsic lung disease who show markedly decreased response to hypoxemia or hypercapnia (e.g., myxedema, obesity-hypoventilation syndrome, idiopathic hypoventilation).

INDICATIONS FOR PFTS

- Identification of abnormal lung function
- Quantitation of severity and progression of disease
- Determination of the relationship of symptomatology to function
- Documentation of efficacy of therapy
- Evaluation of surgical risk and benefits

- Identification of likely site of pathological process (i.e., central versus peripheral airways in obstructive defects, or chest wall versus alveoli in restrictive defects)
- Establishment of the degree of impairment/ disability

INTERPRETATION OF PFT RESULTS

- For appropriate clinical interpretation of PFTs, pulmonary history and radiographic information are essential.
- PFT data are usually presented in both absolute terms with the predicted values (based on patient age, gender, height, weight, and race) included and as a percentage of the predicted compared with normal reference values. The level at which the result of an individual test should be considered abnormal is not universally accepted. Many facilities

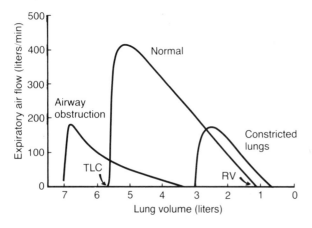

FIGURE 2-10. Effect of two different respiratory abnormalities, obstructive disease and restricted lung dysfunction, on the maximal expiratory flow-volume curve. (From Guyton AC: *Textbook of Medical Physiology,* 8th Ed. Philadelphia, W.B. Saunders Co., p. 455, 1991. Used with permission.)

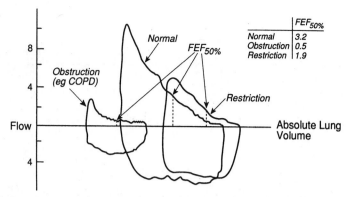

FIGURE 2-11. Examples of flow-volume loops in a patient with chronic obstructive disease and a patient with restrictive disease as compared with a normal individual. Volumes on the axis are absolute values to better demonstrate the relation of flows (e.g., FEF$_{50\%}$) to hyperinflation and restriction. (From Clausen JL: Pulmonary function testing. *In* Kelly WN, et al., (eds.): *Textbook of Internal Medicine*, 2nd Ed. Philadelphia, J.B. Lippincott Co., p. 1823, 1992. Used with permission.)

use a standard of 80% to 120% of normal reference values as normal and consider all other values abnormal; other facilities rely on some number of standard deviations (i.e., > ±1 to 2 s.d.) from the normal reference values.

- The diagnosis of obstructive pulmonary disease or restrictive pulmonary defects is based on the pattern of abnormal values exhibited, as seen in Figures 2-9, 2-10, and 2-11. Typical values for spirometric and airflow volume measurements for obstructive, restrictive, and combined defects are demonstrated in Table 2-9.
- The results of PFTs offer physical therapists valuable information, which has direct implications for rehabilitation:
  - The greater the degree of impairment, the greater the likelihood that the patient will exhibit abnormal physiologic responses to activity and will require treatment modifications.
  - The specific treatment modifications that are indicated vary according to the diagnosis and type of abnormality present (see Chapters 3 and 6).

ARTERIAL BLOOD GASES

Arterial and/or mixed venous blood is analyzed in order to obtain information related to a patient's oxygenation, ventilatory, and acid-base status. Values can be obtained by analysis of an arterial blood sample or by direct reading electrodes after arterial puncture or cannulation.

- Unless otherwise stated, a blood gas is usually assumed to be arterial in origin.
- The data obtained from arterial blood gases (ABGs) and normal values are listed in Table 2-10.
- Indications for ABGs measurements include:
  - Documentation of a patient's oxygenation, ventilatory, and/or acid-base status
  - Determination of a patient's oxygen-carrying capacity
  - Quantification of a patient's response to therapeutic interventions (e.g., supplemental oxygen, medications, etc.)
  - Documentation of severity and progression of disease processes
  - Quantification of a patient's responses to exercise
  - Documentation of intrapulmonary shunt
- The interpretation of ABGs is presented in detail in Chapter 5 (see pages 189 to 191); however, the following are abnormal conditions documented by ABGs:
  - *Hypoxemia* is defined as a Pa$_{O_2}$ < 80
  - *Alveolar hypoventilation* is indicated by a Pa$_{CO_2}$ > 45
  - *Alveolar hyperventilation* is indicated by a Pa$_{CO_2}$ < 35
  - *Ventilatory failure* is diagnosed if Pa$_{CO_2}$ > 50
  - *Acidemia* refers to a pH < 7.35, whereas *alkalemia* refers to a pH > 7.45, which can be

TABLE 2–8. **Causes of Decreased Diffusing Capacity and the Effect on the Diffusion Constant (KCO)***

CONDITION	EFFECT ON Kco	COMMENTS
Airway obstruction		
COPD	Usually ↓	Especially in emphysema.
Asthma†	Nl or ↑	
Pneumonectomy	↑	Caused by ↑ vascular volume of remaining lung.
Alveolar disease		
Fibrosing alveolitis	↓	Sometimes nl, but progressive ↓ Kco as fibrosis and vascular destruction ↑.
Asbestosis	↓	Same as above.
Sarcoidosis	Nl or slightly ↓	In early stages, diffusing capacity is more sensitive index of lung involvement than lung volumes.
Pulmonary vascular disorders		
Multiple emboli	↓	Kco may be preserved somewhat if there is alveolar collapse or consolidation.
R → L shunts	↓	
Cardiac conditions		
Mitral valve disease	↓	
Pulmonary edema	↓ or nl‡	
Extrapulmonary restriction		Probably caused by inability to achieve normal full inspiration. Diffusing capacity may be normal unless condition is severe.
Respiratory muscle weakness	↑	
Skeletal deformity	↑	
Pleural disease	↑	
Miscellaneous conditions		
Anemia: uncorrected	↓	Caused by ↓ reaction rate of CO with Hb.
Anemia: corrected	nl	Correction equation restores diffusing capacity and Kco to normal.§
Renal failure	↓	
Hepatic cirrhosis	↓	
Myxedema	↓	
Collagen vascular disease		
SLE	↓	Lung parenchymal involvement results in "shrinking lung" syndrome with ↓ in diffusing capacity and Kco.
Rheumatoid arthritis	↓	
Systemic sclerosis	↓	

*Diffusion capacity for carbon monoxide (CO) was obtained using the single breath technique with simultaneous measurement of alveolar volume and correction for current hemoglobin (Hb) level.
†Acute attack, mild to moderate in severity.
‡Few data available.
§To correct for abnormal hematocrit: multiply the diffusing capacity and Kco by 10.2 + [Hb], then divide by 1.7 × [Hb].
Nl = normal, SLE = systemic lupus erythematosis, ↑ = increased, ↓ = decreased.

either respiratory or metabolic in origin (see page 269).

- Sudden acute changes in the levels of $PaCO_2$ and pH are more dangerous than gradual chronic changes and tend to be associated with more signs and symptoms of abnormal function.
- Physical therapists should know the normal values for ABGs and have a basic understand-

ing of various blood gas abnormalities and their implications.

- Patients with oxygen saturations less than 86% to 90% require supplemental oxygen during exertion to avoid problems due to desaturation.
- Physical therapists should recognize the signs and symptoms of hypoxemia and hypercapnia (see page 89).

TABLE 2–9. **Patterns of Pulmonary Function Abnormalities**

FUNCTION	NORMAL	OBSTRUCTION	RESTRICTION	COMBINED
FVC	≥75–80% pred.	Nl–↓	↓	↓
FEV_1	≥75–80% pred.	↓	↓	↓
FEV_1/FVC	90% pred.	↓	Nl–↑	↓
FEF_{25-75}	≥75–80% pred.	↓	Nl–↓	↓
TLC	80–120% pred.	Nl–↑	↓	Nl–↓
RV	80–120% pred.	↑	Nl–↓	Nl, ↓, or ↑
RV/TLC	25–40%	↑	nl	↑

pred. = predicted normal value, nl = normal, ↓ = lower than normal, ↑ = higher than normal, FVC = forced vital capacity, FEV_1 = forced expiratory volume in 1 second, FEF_{25-75} = forced expiratory flow$_{25-75}$, RV = residual volume, TLC = total lung capacity.

OXIMETRY

Arterial oxygen saturation of hemoglobin (SaO_2) can be measured via a pulse oximeter (placed on the ear, finger, toe, or forehead), which uses a light-emitting diode (LED) to emit alternating red and infrared light hundreds of times per second, a photodiode signal detector to receive the signals, and a microprocessor to calculate the level of oxyhemoglobin saturation based on the intensity of the transmitted light.

- Patients with resting oxygen saturations less than 86% to 90% usually require supplemental oxygen during exertion to avoid further desaturation.
- Physical therapists should recognize the signs and symptoms of hypoxemia (see page 89).

PULMONARY EXERCISE TESTING

The same as cardiopulmonary exercise testing, described on page 12, pulmonary exercise testing may also include insertion of an arterial line for periodic blood gas analysis or the use of pulse oximetry for documentation of oxygen saturation.

- Pulmonary exercise testing often evaluates other available data, such as:
  - Breathing reserve (BR); calculated as maximal voluntary ventilation (MVV) − $\dot{V}_E$ at maximal exercise
  - Anaerobic threshold (AT)
  - Oxygen uptake–work rate (WR) relationship ($\Delta \dot{V}O_2/\Delta WR$) and oxygen difference
  - Respiratory dead space (V_D) and ratio to tidal volume (V_D/V_T)
  - Alveolar ventilation ($\dot{V}_A$)
  - Alveolar-arterial oxygen difference [$P(A-a)O_2$]
  - Arterial-end tidal carbon dioxide difference [$P(a-ET)CO_2$]
  - Ventilatory equivalents for oxygen ($\dot{V}_E/\dot{V}O_2$) and carbon dioxide ($\dot{V}_E/\dot{V}CO_2$)
  - Expiratory flow patterns
  - Plasma bicarbonate and acid-base responses
  - Lactate levels
- Conditions which are often associated with limited exercise performance and the measurements that deviate from normal are listed in Table 2–11.
- In some facilities physical therapists conduct and supervise pulmonary stress testing.

TABLE 2–10. **Parameters Measured During Arterial Blood Gas Analysis**

PARAMETER	NORMAL VALUE (RANGE)
Partial pressure of oxygen (PO_2, PaO_2)	97 mm Hg (>80)
Partial pressure of carbon dioxide (PCO_2, $PaCO_2$)	40 mm Hg (35–45)
Hydrogen ion concentration (pH)	7.40 (7.35–7.45)
Arterial oxygen saturation (SaO_2, % sat.)	>95%
Bicarbonate level (HCO_3^-)	24 (22–26)
Base excess/deficit (BE)	0 (−2 to +2)

TABLE 2–11. **Descriminating Measurements Seen During Pulmonary Exercise Testing in Common Disorders Associated with Limited Exercise Tolerance**

DISORDERS	DESCRIMINATING MEASUREMENTS DURING EXERCISE
Pulmonary	
Obstructive disease	↓ $\dot{V}O_2$ max, ↓ BR, abnormal expiratory flow pattern, ↑ VD/VT, ↑ $\dot{V}E/\dot{V}O_2$, ↑ P(a-ET)CO_2, ↑ P(A-a)O_2, ↑ HR reserve
Restrictive dysfunction	
↓ CL	↓ $\dot{V}O_2$ max, ↑ VT/IC ratio, $f > 50$, ↓ BR, ↑ VD/VT, ↑ P(a-ET)CO_2, ↓ PaO$_2$ and ↑ P(A-a)O_2 with ↑ work
↓ CT	↓ $\dot{V}O_2$ max, ↑ VT/IC ratio, $f > 50$, ↓ BR, normal Δ$\dot{V}O_2$/ΔWR, ↑ HR re-
Circulatory disorders	serve ↑ VD/VT, ↓ PaO$_2$, ↑ $\dot{V}E/\dot{V}O_2$, ↑ P(a-ET)CO_2, ↓ O_2 pulse, ↓ AT
Cardiac	
Coronary	abnl ECG, ↓ $\dot{V}O_2$ max, ↓ AT, ↓ O_2 pulse, ↓ Δ$\dot{V}O_2$/ΔWR, ↑ HR/$\dot{V}O_2$, ↑ BR
Valvular	↓ O_2 pulse, ↓ Δ$\dot{V}O_2$/ΔWR, ↓ $\dot{V}O_2$ max, ↑ BR
Myocardial	↓ O_2 pulse, ↓ Δ$\dot{V}O_2$/ΔWR, ↓ $\dot{V}O_2$ max, ↑ BR
Anemia	↓ O_2 pulse, ↓ AT, ↑ $\dot{V}E/\dot{V}O_2$; normal VD/VT, P(a-ET)CO_2, and P(A-a)O_2
Peripheral arterial disease	↓ $\dot{V}O_2$ max, ↓ AT, ↓ Δ$\dot{V}O_2$/ΔWR, ↓ HR$_{max}$, leg pain
Obesity	↑ O_2 cost of work, ↓ $\dot{V}O_2$ max and AT per body weight but not per height (unless extreme obesity), normal VD/VT and O_2 pulse according to height
Anxiety	Hyperventilation with regular respiratory rate, ↓ PaCO$_2$
Malingering	Hyperventilation and hypoventilation with irregular respiratory rate
Deconditioning	↓ O_2 pulse, ↓ AT

Data from Barnes, 1992,[2] and Wasserman et al., 1987.[25]
abnl = abnormal, AT = anaerobic threshold, CL = lung compliance, CT = thoracic compliance, IC = inspiratory capacity. For explanation of other abbreviations, see text.

INVASIVE DIAGNOSTIC TECHNIQUES

PULMONARY ANGIOGRAPHY

The injection of contrast material into the thoracic blood vessels allows morphologic findings to be recorded on x-ray film (similar to coronary angiography). Digital subtraction angiography uses a fluoroscope and image intensifier, along with a computer processing system, which subtracts out the background body parts and leaves only the intravascular contrast materials.

BRONCHOGRAPHY

Images of the airways can be obtained by instilling contrast medium directly into them and then obtaining radiographs or tomographs, as shown in Figure 2–12. The main indications for bronchography are suspected endobronchial disease which has not been identified using either bronchoscopy or CT (e.g., recurrent hemoptysis of unknown cause or presence of malignant cells in sputum without an identifiable source).

BRONCHOSCOPY

Using a flexible or rigid fiberoptic instrument, the larger airways down to the third or fourth divisions of the segmental bronchi can be directly visualized.

- Because fiberoptic bronchoscopy requires only topical anesthesia and the range of visible airways is greater, it is the most commonly used method.
- However, rigid bronchoscopy allows for greater airway patency, maintenance of ventilatory support, better removal of blood and secretions and tissue samples with less impairment of ventilation, greater ease and safety in removal of foreign bodies, and local tumor therapy (e.g., placement of radioactive seeds, laser therapy, and cryotherapy).
- If abnormalities are noted during bronchoscopy, additional diagnostic maneuvers, including brushings, biopsies, needle aspirations, and washings (see below) may be performed.

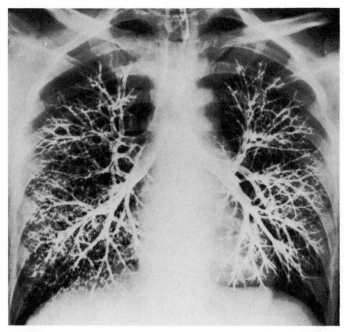

FIGURE 2-12. Normal bilateral bronchogram (posteroanterior view). The opaque medium coats the inner walls of the bronchial tree. (From Lillington GA: Roentgenographic diagnosis of pulmonary disease. *In* Burton GG, Hodgkin JE, Ward JJ (eds.): *Respiratory Care—A Clinical Guide to Clinical Practice,* 3rd Ed. Philadelphia, J.B. Lippincott Co., p. 240, 1991. Used with permission.)

- Brochoscopy can also be used as a therapeutic intervention, such as for the removal of retained secretions, removal of aspirated foreign bodies, difficult intubation, bronchodilation (using rigid bronchoscopy), and management of malignant obstruction (e.g., bronchodilation, placement of stents, laser therapy, brachytherapy).

BRONCHOALVEOLAR LAVAGE

During bronchoscopy a segment or subsegment of the lung can be lavaged, or washed out, in order to identify infectious microbes and examine types of cells and extracellular proteins present. The aspirated fluid from the lavage is then sent for microbiologic tests.

- Bronchoalveolar lavage (BAL) is commonly performed to confirm suspected bacterial, fungal, mycobacterial, *Pneumocystis, Legionella,* or viral infection.
- Examination of cellular composition and extracellular proteins is useful in the diagnosis of sarcoidosis, extrinsic allergic alveolitis, idiopathic pulmonary fibrosis, tuberculosis, and many other lung diseases.

BRONCHIAL BRUSHINGS

The acquisition of mucosal tissue samples from the tracheal or bronchial walls can be accomplished using a brush contained in a telescoping double catheter with a distal plug. The brush is swept over an area visually noted as abnormal on bronchoscopy, withdrawn into its inner sheath and then out of the lungs, and sent for microbiologic evaluation.

TRANSBRONCHIAL NEEDLE ASPIRATION/LUNG BIOPSY

Another diagnostic procedure designed to obtain tissue samples is transbronchial needle aspiration. Using a small-gauge needle or biopsy forceps passed through a rigid or, more commonly, a flexible fiberoptic bronchoscope, tissue samples can be acquired from within the walls of the trachea and major bronchi or through these structures to peribronchial lymph nodes. The samples are then sent for cytologic examination.

- The diagnostic yield is highest in diffuse lung diseases with specific recognizable histologic patterns (e.g., sarcoidosis, metastatic cancer, lymphoma, and lymphangitic carcinoma).
- Other diseases recognized by characteristic lesions, although with a lower level of sensitivity, include Wegener's granulomatosis, rheumatoid lung disease, lymphangiomyomatosis, eosinophilic granuloma, eosinophilic pneumonia, pulmonary alveolar proteinosis, and silicosis.

PERCUTANEOUS TRANSTHORACIC NEEDLE ASPIRATION/LUNG BIOPSY

In some cases, a needle is inserted through the skin to obtain tissue samples from peripheral lung and sometimes mediastinal masses. Material from fine needles is sent for cytologic and microbiologic examination only, whereas that from larger needles can also be studied histologically. This method produces a diagnostic yield in 80% to 90% of patients with lung cancer, but the yield is somewhat lower for benign disease.[4]

THORACENTESIS AND PLEURAL BIOPSY

The insertion of a needle into the pleural space allows for the removal of pleural fluid or acquisition of a pleural biopsy.

- The fluid is then analyzed for its total protein and lactic dehydrogenase concentrations, and possibly glucose and amylase levels, pH, complete blood cell count and differential, and reaction to Gram's stain.
- In addition, the fluid may be sent for cultures, cytologic study, immunoelectrophoresis, lipid studies, and immunologic studies (e.g., complement levels, antinuclear antibody, lupus erythematosus (LE) cells, and rheumatoid factor).

Rehabilitation activities should be postponed until a postprocedure chest radiograph has been taken and read because of the possibility of a procedure-related pneumothorax.

THORACOSCOPY/PLEUROSCOPY

The pleura can be directly visualized through a rigid endoscope, usually while the patient is under general anesthesia; multiple pleural biopsies are commonly obtained. This technique may be used as an alternative to open pleural biopsy when malignant disease is suspected and a diagnosis has not been made despite repeated thoracenteses and pleural biopsies.

MEDIASTINOSCOPY AND MEDIASTINOTOMY

Exploration of the mediastinum can be performed using an endoscopic instrument inserted through an anterior cervical or parasternal incision (i.e., mediastinoscopy) or by direct visualization via an anterior incision (i.e., mediastinotomy). These procedures are most commonly performed to assess whether there is mediastinal node involvement by lung cancer and to obtain a biopsy specimen of abnormal mediastinal lymph node tissue noted on radiography.

OPEN LUNG BIOPSY

In an open lung biopsy, pulmonary tissue samples are obtained through an exploratory thoracotomy.

- This technique is used in patients with hilar abnormalities where overlying vascular structures impede other approaches and when transbronchial biopsy has been unsuccessful in providing a diagnosis in chronic interstitial lung disease.
- Open lung biopsy is also useful in determining the nature of the underlying disease in pulmonary heart disease.
- Following surgery, two chest tubes are usually inserted: a lower one to drain fluids and an upper one, which requires a water seal and is often set to gentle suction, to evacuate air from the pleural space and create the negative pressure required for reexpansion of the lung.
  - At first there is marked bubbling from the water chamber if it is set to suction; however, the amount of bubbling diminishes as the air leak seals off.
  - If the water seal is set to suction, there should always be some bubbling. If the bubbling ceases, the tube has become kinked or blocked. If a change of position and release of the chest tube does not result in resumption of the bubbling, the nurse or physician should be notified. Likewise, a sudden increase in the amount of bubbling should be reported.
  - There is no contraindication to rolling onto the side where chest tubes are present; in fact, patients should be encouraged to inter-

mittently assume this position (with assistance) to preserve normal drainage and expansion of the unoperated lung.

- Ipsilateral shoulder range of motion is usually restricted as long as a chest tube is in place and must be encouraged once the tube is removed.

2.3 THERAPEUTIC INTERVENTIONS IN PULMONARY MEDICINE

Recent advances in pulmonary research continue to affect the therapeutic options that are available to patients with pulmonary diseases. Some of these are purely palliative, whereas others are actually curative. The more common interventions, as well as some of the newer ones, are described briefly in this section.

MEDICAL MANAGEMENT

The medical management of pulmonary disease includes pharmacologic agents, airway adjuncts, oxygen therapy, mechanical ventilation, bronchial hygiene and other physical therapy techniques, smoking cessation, pulmonary rehabilitation, and social services.

PHARMACOLOGIC THERAPY

The various medications used to treat pulmonary disease are described in Chapter 4. However, oxygen therapy is presented separately in this chapter.

AIRWAY ADJUNCTS

There are a variety of different types of accessory airways, which may be used to maintain or protect a patient's airway or to provide mechanical ventilation:

- An *oral pharyngeal airway* is a semirigid plastic tube or open-sided channel shaped to fit the natural curvature of the soft palate and tongue to hold the tongue away from the back of the throat and thus maintain the patency of the airway.
- A *nasal pharyngeal airway* is a soft latex or rubber tube commonly used to maintain airway patency and allow nasotracheal suctioning with less mucosal trauma to the nares and pharynx.
- The *endotracheal (ET) tube* is a semirigid plastic

tube inserted into the trachea through either the nose or mouth (i.e., an orotracheal tube or a nasotracheal tube) to provide an airway, protect the lungs from aspiration, and allow mechanical ventilation. Adult ET tubes usually have a low-pressure, large volume inflatable cuff near their distal end to prevent aspiration of secretions; neonatal and pediatric tubes usually do not have cuffs because of the small airway size

- An *esophageal obturator airway* is a unit consisting of a face mask, an attached plastic tube, and a distal cuff, which is used primarily by emergency medical technicians. The tube is inserted into the esophagus and the cuff is inflated; air enters the trachea through air ports in the midsection of the tube, which is positioned in the hypopharynx
- The *tracheostomy tube* is an artificial airway inserted into the trachea via an anterior cervical incision below the level of the vocal cords; most have inflatable cuffs, which are usually inflated to prevent aspiration, but may be deflated to assess a patient's ability to handle secretions, and so on. There are several types:
  - A *standard tracheostomy tube* has a neck flange, body, and usually a cuff (see page 63); some have a removable inner cannula. They are available in a variety of styles, sizes, and materials.
  - A *fenestrated tracheostomy tube* consists of a double cannula with an opening in the superior aspect of the outer cannula so air can pass through the vocal cords and upper airway when the inner cannula is removed, the tracheal opening is plugged, and the cuff is deflated.
  - The *speaking tracheostomy tube* has a separate pilot tube that directs compressed gas to an exit point just above the cuff so air passes through the vocal cords to allow speech.
  - A *tracheostomy button* is a short, straight, externally plugged tube extending from the anterior neck to the inner tracheal wall, which maintains the tracheal stoma for suctioning and emergency ventilation during weaning from prolonged mechanical ventilation.

OXYGEN THERAPY

Oxygen therapy is indicated for the treatment of hypoxemia and can be administered via a variety of devices, which achieve different concentrations of inspired oxygen, as shown in Table 2–12.

- As with any other drug, oxygen is prescribed so that the proper dose is administered; caution should be exercised to ensure adherence to the dose in order to provide maximal benefit with minimal toxicity.
- Since therapeutic oxygen is stored with all water vapor removed, it is necessary to add humidity to the oxygen in order to prevent irritation of the pulmonary mucosa.
- In addition, when the upper airway is bypassed (e.g., endotracheal intubation or tracheostomy) or when flow rates exceed 10 L/min, the oxygen must be heated to increase its water vapor carrying capacity.

The use of supplemental oxygen carries important implications for physical therapy:

- Patients should never exercise on less oxygen than they are receiving at rest.
- Therapists should be able to recognize the signs and symptoms of hypoxemia (see page 58) because the additional demands of rehabilitation activities may cause a patient's oxygenation status to deteriorate.
- If a patient's oxygenation status appears to deteriorate with activity, monitoring with a pulse oxymeter is indicated.
- A drop in oxygen saturation to < 86% to 90% (chronic versus acute disease, respectively) indicates that the patient needs more oxygen during activity; an order to institute oxygen therapy or increase the oxygen dose during exertion should be requested from the physician (be certain to return the flow back to resting level when treatment is completed).

INCENTIVE SPIROMETRY

Using a device that provides visual feedback about inspiratory effort (e.g., rising balls or cylinder, lights), the patient is encouraged to inhale as deeply as possible to achieve maximal inspiratory volume. This device is commonly used postoperatively to prevent or reverse atelectasis. Its major advantage is that once it is taught properly, the motivated patient can use it with little supervision. However, patients often use the device incorrectly; care must be exercised to take a

TABLE 2–12. Approximate F_{IO_2} Achieved with Different Oxygen Delivery Devices

DEVICE	OXYGEN FLOW RATE	F_{IO_2}
Nasal cannula*	1 L/min	0.24
	2 L/min	0.28
	3 L/min	0.32
	4 L/min	0.36
	5 L/min	0.40
	6 L/min	0.44
Simple face mask	5–6 L/min	0.35
	6–7 L/min	0.45
	7–10 L/min	0.55
Aerosol face mask	10–12 L/min	0.35–1.0†
Venturi mask‡	4 L/min	0.24–0.28§
	6 L/min	0.31
	8 L/min	0.35–0.40§
	10 L/min	0.50

Data from Baum and Wolinsky, 1989,[4] Brewis et al., 1990,[6] and Burton et al., 1992.[7]
*estimated F_{IO_2}, assuming normal minute ventilation (expired) ($\dot{V}E$).
†F_{IO_2} depends on setting
‡O_2 flow rates are minimums to be used with specific-sized orifice for desired F_{IO_2}
§F_{IO_2} depends on the size of the orifice or the entrainment ports, which vary among manufacturers.

slow deep breath using the diaphragm and lower chest rather than a quick inspiration using the upper chest.

INTERMITTENT POSITIVE PRESSURE BREATHING

Another device used to increase inspiratory volume, intermittent positive pressure breathing (IPPB), consists of a pressure-limited ventilator, which assists the patient's inspiration by delivering a rapid inflow of gas into the mouth until a preset pressure limit is reached.

- IPPB is contraindicated in patients with pneumothorax, bullous lung disease, asthma, recent esophageal or gastric surgery, cardiac dysfunction, or an uncooperative attitude.
- Once widely used, IPPB is now used mainly by the cooperative patient who is too weak to inspire effectively.

Physical therapists sometimes use IPPB during vibration and coughing to assist in secretion mobilization and clearance.

NEBULIZER TREATMENTS

In patients who are too ill to use their inhaler medications properly (see Chapter 4, page 141), nebulizers that produce suspended particulates can be used to carry medications into the airways. The medications are usually dissolved in 3 to 5 ml of saline and delivered into a mask or mouthpiece over approximately 10 minutes. The size of the particles determines their site of deposition (e.g., the oropharynx, trachea, or larger to smaller bronchi) so that only a small fraction of the medication is actually deposited in the lungs.

MECHANICAL VENTILATION

Mechanical ventilation involves the use of automatic cycling devices to generate air pressure and thus assist or take over the breathing function of a patient. The main indications for mechanical ventilation are ventilatory failure (e.g., central nervous system disease, neuromuscular disease, respiratory muscle fatigue) and hypoxemia (e.g., adult respiratory distress syndrome, cardiac failure, pulmonary embolism).

- There are many types of mechanical ventilators that can provide a variety of modes of ventilation, as described in Table 2–13.
  - Mechanical ventilation is associated with poor nutrition, psychologic depression, poor patient motivation, lack of restful sleep, and lack of mobility, which contributes to a vicious cycle of respiratory failure, as illustrated in Figure 2–13.
  - Complications associated with positive pressure ventilation include barotrauma, possible pneumothorax, diminished cardiac output, and hypotension.
- Physical therapy treatments involving a patient on a ventilator invariably trigger the ventilator alarms. Therapists should become familiar with the various ventilator settings and alarms so they will differentiate between real clinical problems and activity-induced false alarms (Table 2–14).

SUCTIONING

Suctioning involves the application of subatmospheric pressure through a flexible catheter or rigid tube for the removal of secretions from the airways. Indications for suctioning include loss of airway control, increased secretion production, inadequate cough, and thickened secretions.

- Suctioning can be performed in a number of ways:
  - Using a rigid oral suction tube to remove secretions from the oropharynx
  - Using a flexible catheter through the nares and nasopharynx into the trachea (nasotracheal suctioning)
  - Through artificial airways (e.g., nasopharyngeal airway, ET tube, tracheostomy tube [see page 57]) into the trachea
- Therapists who work with neurologic and ventilator-dependent patients should be familiar with, if not skilled in, suctioning techniques and other treatment procedures for secretion mobilization and clearance (see Chapter 6).

BRONCHIAL HYGIENE TECHNIQUES

A variety of bronchial hygiene techniques are performed by physical therapists and a number of other health care professionals involved in the care of patients with acute pulmonary dysfunction. These include bronchial drainage, chest percussion, vibration, shaking, assisted coughing techniques, and breathing exercises and are presented in Chapter 6.

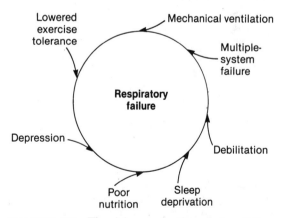

FIGURE 2-13. The vicious cycle of respiratory failure and mechanical ventilation. (From Holtackers TR: Physical rehabilitation of the ventilator-dependent patient. *In* Irwin S, Tecklin JS: *Cardiopulmonary Physical Therapy*, 2nd Ed. St. Louis, The C.V. Mosby Co., p. 374, 1990. Used with permission.)

TABLE 2–13. **Types and Modes of Mechanical Ventilation**

TYPE MODE	DESCRIPTION
Conventional Positive Pressure Ventilation: Volume or Time Cycled, Preset Tidal Volume (V_T)	
Controlled mechanical ventilation (CMV)	Delivers a preset V_T at a predetermined rate without regard to patient's spontaneous breathing pattern.
Augmented minute ventilation (AMV) or Assist control (A/C)	Delivers a preset V_T when the patient triggers the ventilator by spontaneous inspiratory effort; if less than required or no inspiratory effort is provided, the machine delivers a preset minute ventilation.
Intermittent mandatory ventilation (IMV)	Allows the patient to breathe spontaneously between the "mandatory" ventilator breaths, which are delivered at the preset rate regardless of the phase of the patient's spontaneous breathing. Mandatory minute ventilation (MMV) can be used with IMV to ensure a minimal minute ventilation with low IMV rates in case the spontaneous ventilation becomes inadequate.
Synchronous intermittent mandatory ventilation (SIMV)	As above except allows the mandatory breaths to be triggered by the patient's spontaneous inspiratory efforts.
Conventional Positive Pressure Ventilation: Flow or Time Cycled, Preset Peak Pressure	
Pressure support ventilation (PSV)	Augments the inspiratory phase of a patient's spontaneous ventilatory efforts with a preset amount of positive pressure.
Pressure control ventilation (PCV)	Delivers a preset number of breaths per minute with fixed inflation pressure and time but allows patient's pulmonary compliance to determine V_T.
Pressure control with inverse-ratio ventilation (PCIRV)	As above except with inspiratory time exceeding expiratory time to prevent collapse of the alveolar units; raises the mean airway pressure without increasing the peak inspiratory pressure.
Positive end-expiratory pressure (PEEP)	Applies a threshold-like resistance at end of exhalation to prevent early closure of the distal airways and alveoli.
Continuous positive airway pressure (CPAP)	Maintains pressure above ambient levels throughout the respiratory cycle in a spontaneously breathing patient.
Airway pressure-release ventilation (APRV)	Used in spontaneously breathing patients on high level of CPAP, it allows brief passive exhalation to occur by periodically releasing the CPAP so that functional reserve capacity (FRC) is reduced.
High Frequency Ventilation	
High-frequency positive-pressure ventilation (HFPPV)	Preset V_T (usually small) at cycling frequencies of 60–100 breaths/min.
High-frequency jet ventilation (HFJV)	Bursts of high-pressure (jet) gas flow directly into patient's trachea at rates of 60–150 bursts/min; delivered V_T is augmented by entrainment by a second humidified gas source; V_T and $\dot{V}_E$ are unknown.

Continued on following page

TABLE 2-13. **Types and Modes of Mechanical Ventilation** *Continued*

TYPE MODE	DESCRIPTION
High-frequency oscillation (HFO)	Active inspiration and expiration plus oscillation of gas in the respiratory tract at 600–1200 cycles/min (10–20 Hz).
Negative Pressure Ventilation	Intermittently applied subatmospheric pressure to the chest and abdomen.
Tank ventilator, "iron lung"	A rigid tank into which the patient's entire body except his head is placed.
Cuirass	A rigid shell which encloses the patient's chest.
Ventilation by Displacement of Abdominal contents	
Rocking bed	Patient is rocked back and forth head to toe through an arc of 45° so the force of gravity produces movement of the diaphragm.
Pneumobelt	Periodic inflation (and deflation) of a rubber bladder contained in a wide abdominal corset, forcing the diaphragm upward.

TABLE 2-14. **Ventilator Settings**

VENTILATOR SETTINGS	COMMENTS
Tidal volume	Typically set at 10–15 ml/kg of body weight.
Frequency (cycles/min)	Usually set at 8–16, depending on desired Pco_2 or pH.
Mode	Several are available: control, assist/control, IMV, SIMV, MMV, pressure support, sigh, inspiratory pause, CPAP.
Oxygen concentration (Fio_2)	Usually 100% initially unless it is apparent that a lower Fio_2 would provide adequate oxygenation ($Pao_2 \geq 60$ mm Hg); hopefully <40–50% within 20 min to ↓ toxicity.
Inspiratory flow rate (VI)	Typically set at 40–60 L/min unless patient has COPD when it is set at 80–100 L/min to allow more expiratory time.
Positive end-expiratory pressure (PEEP)	PEEP is generally initiated at 5 cm of H_2O and increased by increments of 2–5 cm to maintain the $Pao_2 \geq 60$ mm Hg.
Inspiratory time (TI)	The time interval between the start of inspiratory flow and the start of expiration.
Inspiratory triggering pressure (P_{tr})	The airway pressure that must be generated by the patient to initiate the ventilator inspiratory phase in assisted or intermittent ventilator modes.
Inspiratory triggering response time (T_{tr})	The time delay between triggering of the ventilator and the start of inspiratory flow.
Inspiratory triggering volume (V_{tr})	The volume change required to initiate the ventilator inspiratory phase.
Maximal safety pressure	The highest gauge pressure that is allowed during the inspiratory phase when the ventilator is malfunctioning so that the safety relief valve opens.

IMV = intermittent mandatory ventilation, MMV = mandatory minute ventilation, SIMV = synchronous intermittent mandatory ventilation. For explanation of other abbreviations, see text.

SMOKING CESSATION

Smoking is a major health problem in the United States; it is associated with increased risk of a number of medical problems, including lung cancer (the number one cause of death in smokers), atherosclerotic heart disease (the number one cause of death in the United States), stroke, COPD, adverse affects during pregnancy, peptic ulcers, cancer of the mouth, larynx, esophagus, stomach, breast, and bladder, respiratory tract infections, and increased prevalence of asthma, respiratory infections, and sudden infant death syndrome in infants and children living in a house where someone smokes.[4]

- Many techniques with a wide variability in success rates have been used to assist patients in smoking cessation, such as patient education programs, group counseling, hypnosis, acupuncture, aversive conditioning, behavior modification, and nicotine replacement therapy.
- The highest success rates (40% to 44% at 1 year) for the general public have been reported using a combination of nicotine replacement therapy and behavior modification.[23] Higher success rates are achieved in those who have suffered an acute myocardial infarction.[21]
- The advantages of smoking cessation include:
  - Decreased risk of stroke and heart attack, which begins to decrease immediately and returns to that of a nonsmoker in approximately 5 years
  - Decreased risk of developing lung cancer and emphysema almost to that of a nonsmoker in about 15 years
  - Decreased rate of deterioration of lung function
  - Increased survival in patients with COPD
  - Decreased respiratory infections
  - Financial savings
- Physical therapists can offer encouragement and support to their patients who are trying to quit smoking.

PULMONARY REHABILITATION

Pulmonary rehabilitation is an individually tailored, multidisciplinary treatment program that employs accurate diagnosis, therapy, emotional support, and education to stabilize or reverse both the physiologic and psychologic problems associated with pulmonary disease and attempts to return the patient to the highest possible functional capacity.[1]

- The essential components of a comprehensive program include:
  - Assessment by appropriate pulmonary rehabilitation team members
  - Patient training
  - Exercise
  - Psychosocial intervention
  - Follow-up
- The demonstrated benefits of pulmonary rehabilitation[19] are:
  - Decreased hospitalizations and use of medical resources
  - Increased quality of life
  - Decreased respiratory symptoms (e.g., dyspnea)
  - Improved psychosocial symptoms (e.g., decreased anxiety and depression, increased self-efficacy)
  - Increased exercise tolerance and performance
  - Increased ability to perform activities of daily living
  - Return to work for some patients
  - Increased knowledge about pulmonary disease and its management
  - Increased survival in some patients
- Because of our expertise in exercise prescription and modification, as well as our knowledge of pulmonary diseases and treatments, physical therapists are valued members of many multidisciplinary pulmonary rehabilitation teams.

SOCIAL SERVICES

Social services are often an important element in the care of pulmonary patients who have become debilitated. Some services that may be required include arrangements for home health services, home oxygen equipment, vocational rehabilitation, and patient and family support services.

SURGICAL INTERVENTIONS

As noted previously, surgery may play a role in the diagnosis of pulmonary disease. In addition, surgical interventions are used to treat some pulmonary diseases or their complications; for certain types of pulmonary disease, particularly localized primary lung cancer, surgery may be the best means of effecting a cure. The surgical procedures frequently used to treat pulmonary disease are listed below.

TRACHEOSTOMY

As illustrated in Figure 2–14, tracheostomy involves the insertion of a tube through the third tracheal ring or cricothyroid membrane (i.e., below the level of the vocal cords) into the trachea, usually for the purpose of allowing prolonged mechanical ventilation or providing airway protection or maintenance and sometimes relieving upper airway obstruction due to tumor, edema, trauma, or foreign body. Tracheostomy tubes eliminate the potential for vocal cord injury and offer a lower risk of tracheal damage than intubation with a nasotracheal or orotracheal tube.

CHEST TUBE/DRAIN PLACEMENT

When a pneumothorax develops, either spontaneously or as a result of a therapeutic intervention, chest tube placement may be required in order to evacuate air from the pleural space and restore the negative intrapleural pressure necessary for normal lung function. Chest drainage is also used to remove blood and serous fluids created by thoracic surgery and to evacuate an empyema.

- Intrapleural chest tubes require underwater seal and often gentle suction to remove air leaking from damaged lung tissue and create the desired negative intrapleural pressure.
  - Initially, there is marked bubbling from the water chamber if it is set to suction; however, the amount of bubbling diminishes as the air leak seals off.
  - If the water seal is set to suction, there should always be some bubbling. If bubbling ceases, the tube has become kinked or blocked; if a change in position and release of the chest tube does not result in bubbling, the nurse or physician should be notified. Likewise, a sudden increase in the amount of bubbling also should be reported.
  - There is no contraindication to rolling the patient onto the side where chest tubes are present; in fact, patients should be en-

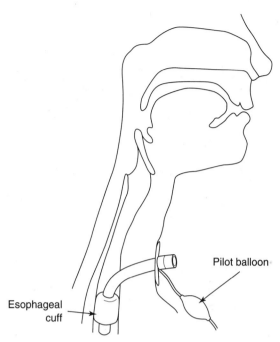

FIGURE 2-14. A tracheostomy tube in place. Note the endotracheal cuff to prevent aspiration of oral or gastric fluids and the pilot balloon, which is used to inflate the cuff.

couraged to intermittently assume this position (with assistance) to preserve normal drainage and expansion of the unoperated lung.
- An open tube inserted to drain an empyema is an intracavitary rather than an intrapleural drain, and thus it does not require water seal.

PULMONARY RESECTION/THORACOTOMY

Surgical resection of part or all of a lung may be indicated for the treatment of bronchogenic carcinoma, bronchiectasis, fungal infections, tuberculosis, and benign tumors.

- Resections are performed using an anterolateral or posterolateral thoracotomy incision (Fig. 2–15), involving:
  - An incision made through the intercostal space corresponding to the lesion,
  - Division of the muscle fibers of the serratus anterior and intercostal muscles, and sometimes the latissimus dorsi and rhomboid muscles, and

A

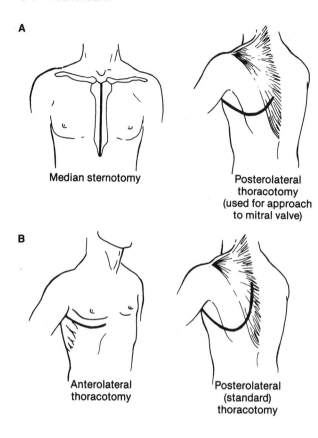

Median sternotomy

Posterolateral
thoracotomy
(used for approach
to mitral valve)

B

Anterolateral
thoracotomy

Posterolateral
(standard)
thoracotomy

FIGURE 2-15. Surgical incisions of the thorax. *(A)* The median sternotomy is commonly used for cardiac surgery, except for mitral valve surgery when the posterolateral thoracotomy is the usual approach. *(B)* Lung surgeries are usually performed via the anterolateral or posterolateral thoracotomy incision. (From Regan K, et al.: Physical therapy for patients with abdominal or thoracic surgery. *In* Irwin S, Tecklin JS: *Cardiopulmonary Physical Therapy,* 2nd Ed. St. Louis, The C.V. Mosby Co., p. 326, 1990. Used with permission.)

- Placement of chest tubes to evacuate accumulated fluid and air from the pleural space and to drain blood and serous fluid (see preceding topic).
- The surgical procedures are named for the portion of the lung removed:
  - *Wedge resection:* removal of a small localized lesion
  - *Segmentectomy:* excision of a bronchopulmonary segment
  - *Lobectomy:* resection of an entire lung lobe
  - *Bilobectomy:* removal of the middle lobe along with an upper or lower lobe
  - *Bronchoplastic/sleeve resection:* excision of a lobe and part of the main stem bronchus followed by the anastomosis of the lower lobe(s) to the proximal bronchus
  - *Pneumonectomy:* resection of an entire lung
- For the treatment of cancer, the amount of lung resected is not always related to the size of the tumor, but is determined by any extension of the tumor into adjacent pulmonary

lobes, lymph nodes, hilar structures, or blood vessels.
- Following pulmonary resection, two chest tubes are usually placed: one at the apex of the lung to remove air and one at the base and/or mediastinum to drain blood and serous fluid, as described previously.
- Because of significant postoperative pleural and musculoskeletal pain resulting from the operative position as well as the large number of muscles incised, deep breathing and coughing are very difficult for patients to perform. However, they are extremely important. Therefore, adequate pain medication is essential and any physical therapy treatments, which should always include deep breathing and coughing, will be more effective if coordinated with the pain medication schedule.
- Patients who have undergone thoracotomy for resection of lung tissue, or for any other reason, are prone to developing postural abnormalities and ipsilateral shoulder range of mo-

tion restrictions caused by splinting of the incision. Therefore it is important to encourage range of motion and postural exercises as healing occurs.

DECORTICATION

Decortication is the excision of the parietal pleura and residual clot and/or organizing scar tissue that forms after a hemothorax or empyema. The goal of the procedure is to allow expansion of the underlying lung tissue and to obliterate the pleural space to prevent further infection.

PLEURECTOMY

Pleurectomy consists of the stripping away and removal of the parietal pleura from the chest wall to obliterate the pleural space and thus prevent the reaccumulation of air or fluid. Obliteration of the pleural space, or *pleurodesis,* can also be achieved by instilling a sclerosing agent (i.e., quinicrine, tetracycline, nitrogen mustard, thiotepa, or bleomycin) into the pleural space, insufflating talc through a thorascope or at open pleural biopsy, or severely abrading the pleura at thoracotomy.

SURGERY FOR THE MANAGEMENT OF BULLAE

Surgery for the management of bullae consists of the excision or plication of dominant bullae in patients with significant emphysema. The goal is to allow the expansion and recruitment of better functioning lung tissue and to reduce intrathoracic volumes so the patient can breathe more comfortably at a lower functional residual capacity.

METASTASECTOMY

Metastasectomy is the excision of pulmonary metastases (which is performed in patients in which primary cancer has been completely controlled (usually by surgical excision)) and any other extrathoracic metastases, if present.

TRACHEAL RESECTION

The excision of a portion of the trachea with end-to-end anastomosis of the remaining trachea is most commonly performed for localized tumors and benign strictures. Resection is usually performed via a cervical incision. If resection of the carina or main stem bronchus is indicated, a right lateral thoracotomy is required.

REFERENCES

1. American Association of Cardiovascular and Pulmonary Rehabilitation (Connors G, Hilling L, Eds.): *Guidelines for Pulmonary Rehabilitation Programs.* Champaign, IL, Human Kinetics Publishers, 1993.
2. Barnes TA: *Respiratory Care Principles—A Programmed Guide to Entry-Level Practice,* 3rd Ed. Philadelphia, F.A. Davis Co., 1992.
3. Bates DV: *Respiratory Function in Disease,* 3rd Ed. Philadelphia, W.B. Saunders Co., 1989.
4. Baum GL, Wolinsky E (eds.): *Textbook of Pulmonary Diseases,* 4th Ed. Boston, Little, Brown & Co., 1989.
5. Behrman RE, Kliegman R: *Nelson Essentials of Pediatrics.* Philadelphia, W.B. Saunders Co., 1990.
6. Brewis RAL, Gibson GJ, Geddes DM (eds.): *Respiratory Medicine.* London, Baillière Tindall, 1990.
7. Burton GG, Hodgkin JE, Ward JJ (eds.): *Respiratory Care: A Guide to Clinical Practice,* 3rd Ed. Philadelphia, J.B. Lippincott Co., 1992.
8. Cherniack RM, Cherniack L: *Respiration in Health and Disease,* 3rd Ed. Philadelphia, W.B. Saunders Co., 1983.
9. Clough P: Restrictive lung dysfunction. *In* Hillegass EA, Sadowsky HS (eds.): *Essentials of Cardiopulmonary Physical Therapy.* Philadelphia, W.B. Saunders Co., 1994.
10. Farzan S: *A Concise Handbook of Respiratory Diseases,* 3rd Ed. Norwalk, CT, Appleton & Lange, 1992.
11. Flenley DC: *Respiratory Medicine,* 2nd Ed. London, Baillière Tindall, 1990.
12. Garritan SL: *Chronic obstructive pulmonary diseases. In* Hillegass EA, Sadowsky HS (eds.): *Essentials of Cardiopulmonary Physical Therapy.* Philadelphia, W.B. Saunders Co., 1994.
13. Guyton AC: *Textbook of Medical Physiology,* 8th Ed. Philadelphia, W.B. Saunders Co., 1991.
14. Hammon WE: Pathophysiology of chronic pulmonary disease. *In* Frownfelter DL: *Chest Physical Therapy and Pulmonary Rehabilitation,* 2nd Ed. Chicago, Year Book Medical Publishers, Inc., 1987.
15. Henson DJ, Morrissey WL: Acute respiratory failure: Mechanisms and medical management. *In* Irwin S, Tecklin JS: *Cardiopulmonary Physical Therapy,* 2nd Ed. St. Louis, The C.V. Mosby Co., 1990.
16. Hobson L, Dean E: Review of respiratory anatomy. *In* Frownfelter DL: *Chest Physical Therapy and Pulmonary Rehabilitation,* 2nd Ed. Chicago, Year Book Medical Publishers, Inc., 1987.

17. Hobson L, Dean E: Review of respiratory physiology. *In* Frownfelter DL: *Chest Physical Therapy and Pulmonary Rehabilitation,* 2nd Ed. Chicago, Year Book Medical Publishers, Inc., 1987.

18. Kelly WN (ed. in chief): *Textbook of Internal Medicine,* 2nd Ed. Philadelphia, J.B. Lippincott Co., 1992.

19. Ries AL: Position paper of the American Association of Cardiovascular and Pulmonary Rehabilitation: Scientific basis of pulmonary rehabilitation. *J. Cardiopulm. Rehabil.* 10:418-441, 1990.

20. Shaffer TH, Wolfson MR, Gault JH: Respiratory physiology. *In* Irwin S, Tecklin JS: *Cardiopulmonary Physical Therapy,* 2nd Ed. St. Louis, The C.V. Mosby Co., 1990.

21. Taylor CB, Miller NH: Smoking cessation in patients with cardiovascular disease. *Qual. Life. Cardiovasac. Care,* Spring: 229–236, 1989.

22. Tecklin JS: Common pulmonary diseases. *In* Irwin S, Tecklin JS: *Cardiopulmonary Physical Therapy,* 2nd Ed. St. Louis, The C.V. Mosby Co., 1990.

23. Tonneson P, Fryd V, Hansen M, et al.: Effect of nicotine chewing gum in combination with group counseling on the cessation of smoking. *N. Engl. J. Med.,* 318:15–18, 1988.

24. U.S. Department of Health and Human Services: Health consequences of smoking cessation report of the surgeon general. Washington D.C., U.S. Government Printing Office, 1990.

25. Wasserman K, Hansen JE, Sue DY, Whipp BJ: *Principles of Exercise Testing and Interpretation.* Philadelphia, Lea & Febiger, 1987.

26. Watchie J: Cardiopulmonary implications of specific diseases. *In* Hillegass EA, Sadowsky HS (eds.): *Essentials of Cardiopulmonary Physical Therapy.* Philadelphia, W.B. Saunders Co., 1993.

27. Wyngaarden JB, Smith LB Jr, Bennett JC: *Cecil Textbook of Medicine,* 19th Ed. Philadelphia, W.B. Saunders Co., 1992.

3

CARDIOPULMONARY PATHOLOGY

The purpose of this chapter is to describe the more common diseases and disorders that affect the cardiac and pulmonary systems and the clinical implications for physical therapy interventions. In addition, the cardiopulmonary complications associated with other medical diagnoses are presented, as well as recommendations for physical therapy treatment modifications. To provide optimal treatment, the reader is encouraged to study more detailed descriptions, such as those cited at the end of this chapter, for the patient diagnoses that are encountered.

3.1 CARDIOVASCULAR DISEASES AND DISORDERS

A brief description of the most common diseases and disorders affecting the cardiovascular system is presented in this section, including pathophysiology, clinical manifestations, and treatment. The clinical implications for physical therapy are offered for the more common diagnoses.

HYPERTENSION

Hypertension (HTN) is arterial blood pressure elevated above normal, as depicted in Table 3–1. When hypertension is not known to result from a specific identifiable cause, such as renal disease or endocrine disorders, it is called primary or essential HTN; on rarer occasions, a specific cause can be identified and it is called secondary HTN.

PATHOPHYSIOLOGY

- HTN causes an increased pressure load on the left ventricle (LV), which responds by developing left ventricular hypertrophy to decrease wall stress.

- Initially, normal LV systolic function is maintained by the hypertrophied LV, but *diastolic dysfunction* develops much earlier[27,83]:
  - LVH and the resultant prolonged relaxation time produce a stiffer LV (decreased compliance), causing higher LV end-diastolic pressure at any volume; this in turn increases the load on the left atrium (LA), which slows the ventricular filling rate and reduces the passive filling volume.
  - The stiffer LV becomes more dependent on active atrial contraction for adequate filling.
  - If there is inadequate filling volume (e.g., due to atrial arrhythmias or decreased filling time, such as tachycardia), stroke volume (SV) will decrease and symptoms of inadequate cardiac output and pulmonary congestion may develop.
  - Higher filling pressures increase the risk of subendocardial ischemia because coronary flow is inhibited.
- As HTN becomes more severe and/or prolonged, *systolic dysfunction* develops[27,49]:
  - If LVH is progressive, eventually the metabolic cost of maintaining the hypertrophied LV will exceed the heart's ability to meet it and SV will fall so that LV end-diastolic volume rises.
  - In the presence of LVH with its reduced compliance, this increase in end-diastolic volume will cause a rise in end-diastolic pressure, which will be reflected back to the LA and pulmonary vessels, thus creating the possibility of pulmonary edema if the pulmonary pressures rise high enough to cause transudation of intravascular fluid from the capillaries.
  - Initially systolic dysfunction is manifested as reduced LV functional reserve during exercise: later, symptoms may develop even at rest (i.e., congestive heart failure, CHF).

TABLE 3-1. **Classification of the Severity of Hypertension in Adults Aged ≥18 Years***

CLASSIFICATION†	HYPERTENSION (HTN) DBP (MM HG)	ISOLATED SYSTOLIC HTN SBP (MM HG)
High normal	85–89	140–159
Mild	90–104	—
Moderate	105–114	160–199
Severe	115–129	200–219

From 1988 Joint National Committee: The 1988 report of the Joint National Committee on Detection, Evaluation, and Treatment of High Blood Pressure. *Arch. Intern. Med.* 148:1023, 1989. Copyright 1989, American Heart Association.
*Classification based on the average of two or more readings on two or more occasions; DBP = diastolic blood pressure, SBP = systolic blood pressure.
†A classification of borderline or mild isolated systolic hypertension takes precedence over high-normal BP (DBP = 85–89 mm Hg), according to the level of SBP, when both are present in the same individual. Likewise, high-normal BP takes precedence over a classification of normal BP when only the DBP is elevated.

CLINICAL MANIFESTATIONS

- Generally asymptomatic, called "the silent killer"
- However, untreated or poorly managed HTN results in multiple complications:
  - Accelerated, malignant course
  - Cerebral vascular accidents
  - Hypertensive heart disease, CHF
  - Atherosclerotic heart disease
  - Renal failure, nephrosclerosis
  - Aortic aneurysm, simple or dissecting
  - Peripheral vascular disease
  - Retinopathy

TREATMENT

- Pharmacologic therapy (see Chapter 4)
  - β-Blockers
  - Diuretics
  - α-Adrenergic blockers
  - Centrally acting α-adrenergic agonists
  - Calcium channel blockers
  - Angiotensin converting enzyme (ACE) inhibitors
- Nonpharmacologic treatment
  - Weight reduction (systolic BP decreases 3 mm Hg for every kilogram of weight loss)
  - Alcohol moderation
  - Sodium restriction
  - Relaxation training
  - Exercise training

NOTE: Although these interventions may not eliminate the need for antihypertensive drugs, they often permit lower dosages and thus fewer side effects.

CLINICAL IMPLICATIONS FOR PHYSICAL THERAPY

- Clinical monitoring should be included as part of every physical therapy evaluation:
  - Almost half of the population with HTN do not know they have it.
  - Many patients stop taking their medications or do not take them correctly.
  - The exercise responses of patients with known HTN may be normal or abnormal[66]:
    — Although a patient may have normal BP at rest, his/her medications may not maintain their effectiveness in controlling BP during exercise.
    — In moderate HTN, there is often an exaggerated BP response to isometric and sometimes dynamic exercise because of blunted reduction in total peripheral resistance (TPR).
    — In more severe HTN, TPR may increase and cardiac output may decrease so that the systolic BP response may appear normal, hypertensive, blunted, flat, or hypotensive, depending on the balance between these two determinants.
    — Patients may develop angina and/or dyspnea on exertion.
- The side effects of medications and any exercise interactions should be known (see Chapter 4):
  - Many antihypertensive drugs are associated with hypotension, especially orthostatic and postexercise hypotension.
  - β-Blockers are associated with lower resting HR, blunted HR and BP responses to exer-

cise, muscle fatigue and cramps, and possible bronchospasm.
- Diuretic therapy may result in hypovolemia, hypokalemia, or hyperkalemia (and thus abnormal resting and exercise HR, BP, and ECG responses).
• Precautions and contraindications:
- If resting systolic BP >200 or diastolic BP >105, medical clearance should be obtained before initiating physical therapy. NOTE: the patient may exhibit an auscultatory gap (see page 187).
- If the patient has a history of retinopathy, renal failure, or LVH, BP must be controlled at rest and during exercise to avoid increased morbidity.
- If systolic BP increases to 250 or diastolic BP exceeds 110, exercise should be terminated.[1]
- Higher heart rates or arrhythmias may increase symptoms caused by diastolic dysfunction.
- Breath holding and the Valsalva maneuver should be avoided because of the BP elevations they induce.
• Physical therapy treatment modifications may be indicated:
- Use caution with quick changes of position, static standing, and whirlpool or Hubbard tank therapy because of potential for hypotension.
- Use caution with isokinetic, high-intensity isometric, and high-resistance exercises since they result in marked increases in BP, especially if associated with breath holding.
- Other treatment modifications, described in Chapter 6, may be indicated.
• Exercise training is very beneficial:
- Although controversy exists, the general consensus is that exercise training results in decreases in both systolic and diastolic BP of 10 to 20 mm Hg.
- Lower intensity exercise (50% to 65% of predicted maximum) may be more effective in achieving antihypertensive benefit than higher intensities.[33,36]
- Training HR ranges can be calculated using the standard formulas unless the patient is taking medications that affect HR; alternatively, a rating of perceived exertion (RPE) scale can be used.
• Physical therapists should encourage compliance with antihypertensive treatment(s).

ATHEROSCLEROTIC HEART DISEASE (CORONARY ARTERY DISEASE)

Atherosclerotic heart disease (ASHD), also known as coronary heart disease (CAD), is a progressive disease process characterized by irregularly distributed lipid deposits in the intimal layer of medium and large coronary arteries. Although the mechanisms of atherogenesis are not known, several risk factors, listed below, have been associated with an increased likelihood of developing CAD.

RISK FACTORS
• Male gender
• Family history of premature ASHD
• Hypertension
• Cigarette smoking (≥1/2 pack per day)
• Decreased high-density lipoprotein (HDL) cholesterol
• Increased low-density lipoprotein (LDL) or very low-density lipoprotein (VLDL) cholesterol)
• Diabetes mellitus
• Documented cerebrovascular or occlusive peripheral vascular disease
• Physical inactivity
• Obesity
• Stress
• "Type A" personality

CLINICAL MANIFESTATIONS OF ASHD
The clinical manifestations of ASHD evolve after many decades of progressive atherosclerosis and include myocardial ischemia, infarction, congestive heart failure (CHF), and sudden death.

Myocardial Ischemia
Myocardial ischemia is an abnormal state of cardiac function resulting from insufficient oxygen supply to meet the metabolic demands of the myocardium. The numerous factors that affect the balance between myocardial oxygen supply and demand are illustrated in Figure 3–1.

PATHOPHYSIOLOGY
Coronary atherosclerosis, coronary arterial spasm, or reduced coronary blood flow reduces myocardial oxygen supply so that it cannot meet myocardial oxygen demands, which results in:

• Myocardial irritability producing arrhythmias

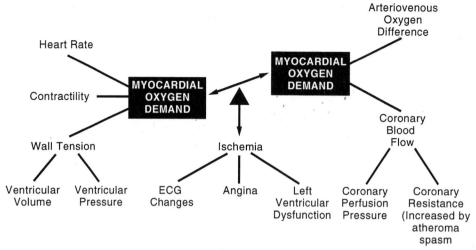

FIGURE 3–1. Factors that influence the balance between myocardial oxygen supply and demand. (From Wyngaarden JB, et al. (eds.): *Cecil Textbook of Medicine*, 19th Ed. Philadelphia, W.B. Saunders Co., 1990. Used with permission.)

- Impaired systolic ventricular function (i.e., diminished contractile function) resulting in reduced stroke volume
- Impaired diastolic function (i.e., impaired relaxation) causing prolongation of systole and reduced ventricular filling time, which decreases ventricular compliance and raises ventricular end-diastolic pressure so that coronary driving pressure is reduced even further (see HTN, preceding section)

CLINICAL MANIFESTATIONS

- *Angina pectoris*
  - Characteristic pain: pressure, heaviness, tightness
  - Location: substernal, shoulder, arm, throat, jaw, teeth
  - Precipitated by: exertion, stress, emotions, meals
  - Duration: minutes
  - Relieved by: rest, nitroglycerin
  - Pain free: between bouts
- Anginal equivalents (e.g., dyspnea, fatigue, lightheadedness, belching brought on by exertion or stress and relieved by rest or nitroglycerin)
- Arrhythmias caused by myocardial irritability
- Characteristic electrocardiographic (ECG) changes (e.g., ST depression, T wave inversion; see Fig. 1–10 and 1–22)

- Hypotension caused by impaired ventricular function

NOTE: Most patients have some episodes of "silent" ischemia (i.e., without any symptoms) and some patients have only "silent" ischemia (more commonly diabetic patients and elderly men).

Unstable angina is defined as an increase in frequency, duration, and/or severity of anginal discomfort superimposed on a preexisting pattern of exertional angina, with possible rest angina or pain on minimal exertion, or the new onset of angina, which is provoked by minimal exertion. It is usually a warning of impending infarction.

Prinzmetal's angina (also called atypical or variant angina) is chest pain, often severe, that occurs typically at rest rather than on exertion and results from myocardial ischemia caused by coronary artery spasm. The ECG usually shows ST elevation during the episodes of pain, and arrhythmias are common.

Myocardial Infarction

Myocardial infarction (MI) is the complete interruption of blood supply to an area of myocardium, resulting in necrosis.

PATHOPHYSIOLOGY

- Acute MI results in three concentric pathologic zones: the central area of myocardial necrosis and the surrounding areas of injury and ischemia (Fig. 3–2), which can give rise to:
  - Increased myocardial irritability, causing arrhythmias and possible sudden death
  - Systolic and diastolic dysfunction, leading to possible CHF or cardiogenic shock
  - Rupture of infarcted tissue producing a ventricular septal defect, cardiac rupture, or acute mitral regurgitation
  - Extension of infarction with expanded area of necrosis
  - Pericarditis, pulmonary or systemic emboli
- Over time, there is healing of the infarcted area, which initially undergoes coagulation necrosis, via formation of a fibrotic scar.
  - Myocardial wall motion may appear normal (e.g., subendocardial MI with scarring of only the innermost layer of the heart); or
  - Myocardial wall motion may be abnormal (e.g., transmural MI with full-thickness scar), as shown in Figure 3–3.

DIAGNOSIS

- Classic symptoms (see clinical manifestations)
- Acute injury pattern seen on a 12-lead ECG (see Fig. 1–9, page 11)
- Elevation of specific enzymes (CPK, AST, and LDH; see Table 8–10, page 275)
- ECG changes in MI evolve over time, as shown in Figure 3–4.

CLINICAL MANIFESTATIONS

- Severe crushing chest pain, with or without radiation to adjacent areas
- Diaphoresis
- Dyspnea
- Nausea
- Vomiting
- Lightheadedness, syncope
- Apprehension
- Weakness
- Denial
- Sudden death

NOTE: 20% to 25% of MIs occur without any symptoms ("silent" MIs).[1]

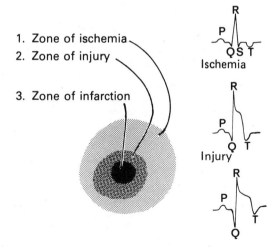

FIGURE 3–2. The zones of infarction and the electrocardiographic changes that correspond to them. (1) Ischemia causes acute inversion of the T wave. (2) Injury causes acute ST segment elevation. (3) Infarction causes permanent Q waves along with acute ST elevation. (From Underhill SL, et al.: *Cardiac Nursing.* Philadelphia, J.B. Lippincott, p. 206, 1983. Used with permission.)

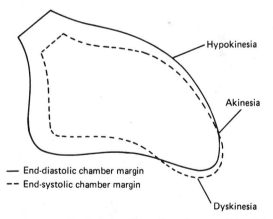

FIGURE 3–3. Regional wall motion abnormalities following MI: reduced motion of a myocardial wall segment is called hypokinesis, lack of motion of a segment of myocardium is termed akinesis, and paradoxic motion of a segment is known as dyskinesis. (From Alderman EL: Angiographic indicators of left ventricular function. *JAMA* 236:1055, 1976. Copyright 1976, American Medical Association. Used with permission.)

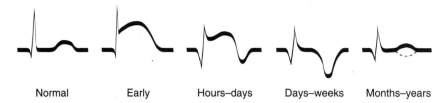

Normal   Early   Hours–days   Days–weeks   Months–years

FIGURE 3-4. Sequential ECG changes following acute MI. Initially, there is a Q wave with marked ST elevation. Over the next few days the Q wave gets deeper and wider, the ST segment moves toward the baseline, and the T wave becomes inverted. Within weeks of an acute MI, the ST segment is near the baseline and the T wave is deeply inverted. Finally, within months the T wave returns to a less inverted or somewhat upright position.

RISK FACTORS FOR INCREASED MORBIDITY AND MORTALITY FOLLOWING ACUTE MI[1]

- CHF
- Left ventricle ejection fraction <40%
- Large infarct size
- New bundle-branch block
- Mobitz II second- or third-degree heart block
- Anterior infarction
- Reinfarction or infarct extension
- Ventricular tachycardia or fibrillation
- Ventricular ectopy, especially if frequent or complex
- Supraventricular arrhythmias, excluding sinus bradycardia
- Postinfarction angina
- Inability to complete low-level exercise test
- Abnormal physiologic responses to low-level exercise test
- Diabetes mellitus
- Hypertension, or loss of preexisting hypertension
- Age >70 years
- Female gender

Congestive Heart Failure

Occasionally, ASHD is initially diagnosed when a patient demonstrates the signs and symptoms of CHF, which are discussed in detail in the following section.

Sudden Death

Not infrequently, a patient is discovered to have ASHD during autopsy for unexplained sudden death. In most of these cases, lethal arrhythmias associated with acute MI is the cause of death.

TREATMENT OF ASHD

- Pharmacologic therapy (see Chapter 4)
  - Antianginal medications
  - Antiplatelet therapy
  - Antiarrhythmic agents
  - Thrombolytic therapy
- Surgical interventions
  - Percutaneous transluminal coronary angioplasty (PTCA) (see page 25)
  - Coronary artery bypass graft (CABG) (see page 25)
  - Pacemaker insertion (see page 27)
  - Automatic implantable cardiac defibrillator (AICD) (see page 28)
  - Intracoronary stents (under investigation; see page 26)
  - Atherectomy (under investigation; see page 26)
- Other
  - Risk factor reduction (see page 24)
  - Cardiac rehabilitation (see page 24)

CLINICAL IMPLICATIONS FOR PHYSICAL THERAPY

- Patients should bring sublingual nitroglycerin (NTG) to physical therapy appointments.
  - Encourage patient to report chest discomfort and take NTG as directed.
  - Sublingual NTG can be used prophylactically if specific activity results in angina.
- The physiologic responses to activity should be monitored at least initially since they are quite variable in patients with CAD:
  - Patients may exhibit normal responses.
  - Patients may exhibit abnormal heart rate (HR) and/or blood pressure (BP) responses (see pages 174 and 188).
  - Patients may complain of angina or show other signs and symptoms of exercise intolerance (see page 194).
- Side effects of any medications and any exercise interactions should be known (see Chapter 4):

- β-blockers lower resting and exercise HR and BP, thus resulting in increased exercise tolerance in patients with angina; but they may cause muscle fatigue and cramps, as well as possible bronchospasm.
- Nitrates are associated with increased resting and possibly exercise HR, as well as hypotension, especially orthostatic and postexercise hypotension.
- The calcium channel blockers have different effects: verapamil and diltiazem lower HR and BP, whereas nifedipine lowers BP but causes reflex tachycardia; all are associated with the potential for hypotension.
- Physical therapy treatment modifications may be indicated, especially including brief rest breaks to reduce the cost of more strenuous rehabilitation activities (see Chapter 6).
- Exercise training is very beneficial (see page 223).

HEART FAILURE

Heart failure exists when the heart is unable to pump sufficient cardiac output to meet the body's metabolic demands at normal ventricular filling pressures, given adequate venous return.

LEFT VENTRICULAR FAILURE (CONGESTIVE HEART FAILURE)

Pathophysiology

Intrinsic myocardial disease (e.g., atherosclerotic heart disease, cardiomyopathy), excessive workload on the heart (e.g., hypertension, valvular disease, congenital defects), cardiac arrhythmias, or iatrogenic damage (e.g., alcohol, drug toxicity, irradiation) can result in the following:

- Systolic ventricular dysfunction results in reduced SV and increased end-diastolic volume (EDV) with a resultant drop in ejection fraction (EF, which equals SV/EDV).
- Increased LVEDV causes left atrial (LA) volume to expand with resulting LA dilatation.
- If the LV is less compliant (e.g., because of LVH), the expanded EDV will produce higher end-diastolic pressure (EDP), which will be reflected back to the LA, and pulmonary vessels and their pressures will be elevated; if pulmonary pressures rise high enough to cause transudation of intravascular fluid from the capillaries, dyspnea and possibly pulmonary

edema will develop (if the rate of transudation exceeds the rate of lymphatic drainage).
- In addition, the diastolic dysfunction (i.e., delayed ventricular relaxation) resulting from the LVH will cause an even greater rise in LVEDP.
- Elevated LVEDP inhibits diastolic coronary blood flow to the endocardium and thus increases the risk of subendocardial ischemia.
- Marked LV dilatation can result in functional mitral regurgitation.
- The patient's physiologic responses to physical activity will be altered:
  - Reduced stroke volume due to systolic dysfunction results in expanded LVEDV and possibly elevated EDP, which may result in increased pulmonary pressures, dyspnea, and possible pulmonary edema.
  - Redistribution of blood flow due to reduced cardiac output will cause a reduction of flow to the kidneys and skin initially and later to the brain, gut, and skeletal muscle.
  - Peripheral arteriovenous oxygen extraction will increase to compensate for reduced blood flow.

Clinical Manifestations

- Dyspnea, dry cough
- Orthopnea
- Paroxysmal nocturnal dyspnea (PND)
- Fatigue, weakness
- Pulmonary rales, "cardiac asthma"
- S_3 (third heart sound or ventricular gallop), and sometimes S_4 (fourth heart sound or atrial gallop) (see page 163)
- Enlarged heart, increased vasculature on chest x-ray examination
- Possible functional mitral and tricuspid regurgitation
- Signs and symptoms of acute pulmonary edema (marked dyspnea, pallor or cyanosis, diaphoresis, tachycardia, anxiety, agitation)

RIGHT VENTRICULAR FAILURE

Pathophysiology

Elevated pulmonary arterial pressures caused by LV failure, mitral valve disease, or chronic or acute pulmonary disease (i.e., cor pulmonale; see page 99) can result in:

- Increased pressure load on the right ventricle (RV), which causes RV dilatation with or without hypertrophy (i.e., RVH), depending on the acuteness and severity of the pressure load:

- If the pressure rises acutely (e.g., massive pulmonary embolism or acute mitral regurgitation), there will be RV dilatation and failure without RVH.
- If pulmonary HTN is a chronic problem (e.g., COPD), the RV will hypertrophy to decrease wall stress.
- Prolonged pulmonary HTN causes irreversible anatomic changes in the walls of the small pulmonary arteries so that the HTN becomes fixed, with resultant RV dilatation and RVH.
- Hypoxia, hypercapnia, and/or acidosis causes further pulmonary vasoconstriction with an even greater degree of pulmonary HTN, which again increases the workload on the RV.
- Eventually RVEDP increases, which will be reflected back to the right atrium (RA) and the venous system with resultant jugular venous distension (JVD), liver engorgement, ascites, and peripheral edema.
- Also, RVH reduces RV compliance, which may interfere with RV filling and reduce cardiac output.
- If there is a reduction in the pulmonary vascular bed, or an increase in cardiac output, HR (e.g., exercise), or blood volume, pulmonary HTN will worsen, producing increased signs and symptoms of RV failure.

Clinical Manifestations

- Dependent edema
- Liver engorgement (hepatomegaly)
- Ascites
- Fatigue
- Anorexia, bloating
- Right-sided S_3 (third heart sound)
- Accentuated P_2 (pulmonary component of the second heart sound)
- RV lift of sternum
- May be murmurs of pulmonary or tricuspid valve insufficiency
- Cyanosis
- JVD
- Weight gain

BIVENTRICULAR FAILURE

The elevated pulmonary pressures caused by LV failure can eventually cause RV failure as de-

scribed previously. The pathophysiologic effects and clinical manifestations are those associated with both LV and RV failure.

COMPENSATED HEART FAILURE

When a patient experiences heart failure but through activation of the various compensatory mechanisms (see below) or therapeutic interventions is able to return to a functional cardiac output, the heart failure is described as compensated. With increased workloads or progression of disease, the patient's status could again decompensate.

Compensatory Mechanisms Activated in Heart Failure

- Sympathetic nervous system stimulation results in increased HR, increased contractility, increased rate of ventricular relaxation, and arterial and venous constriction
- Activation of the renin-angiotensin-aldosterone system produces arterial vasoconstriction, increased sodium and water retention, and increased myocardial contractility
- Use of the Frank-Starling effect (i.e., cardiac dilatation) to increased SV
- Cardiac hypertrophy
- Increased peripheral oxygen extraction
- Anaerobic metabolism

TREATMENT OF HEART FAILURE

- Correct the underlying cause if possible (e.g., valve disease, arrhythmias)
- Pharmacologic therapies (see Chapter 4)
  - Inotropic agents (e.g., digitalis)
  - Preload reducers (e.g., diuretics)
  - Specific vasodilator therapy (e.g., enalapril, hydralazine, nitrates)
  - Diltiazem for microvascular circulatory abnormalities
  - β-Blockers to impede sympathetic nervous system (SNS) stimulation?
  - Relief of hypoxia (e.g., oxygen therapy, corticosteroids, bronchial hygiene, mechanical ventilation)
- Other
  - Rest
  - Low-sodium diet
  - Phlebotomy for HCT > 55% to 60% in cor pulmonale
  - Thoracentesis for pleural effusions (see page 56)

- Exercise training to increase peripheral efficiency (i.e., cardiac rehabilitation)
- Surgical interventions (refer to pages 30 and 31)
  - Intraaortic balloon counterpulsation if acute
  - Organ transplantation (i.e., heart transplantation for LV failure, heart-lung transplantation for cor pulmonale, lung transplantation for interstitial lung disease)
  - Pulmonary embolectomy for unresolved pulmonary embolus (PE)
  - LV assist device (LVAD) (under investigation)
  - Cardiomyoplasty (under investigation)

CLINICAL IMPLICATIONS FOR PHYSICAL THERAPY

- Physiologic responses to activity should be monitored:
  - Physiologic responses are often abnormal and can be correlated with the patient's symptoms; then symptoms can be used to monitor exercise intensity.
  - Physical therapists should know signs and symptoms of CHF, especially the early ones.
- Side effects of medications may cause problems (see Chapter 4):
  - Acute CHF may develop because of either inadequate or toxic drug levels.
  - Digitalis toxicity can cause arrhythmias, dizziness, confusion, and/or nausea.
  - Diuretics may result in hypovolemia, hypokalemia, or hyperkalemia.
  - Vasodilator therapy often causes hypotension, especially orthostatic and postexercise hypotension.
- Treatment modifications may be indicated:
  - Exercise and activity should be low level and progress slowly.
  - Frequent 1 to 2 minute rests interspersed with activity will make more demanding activities tolerable (e.g., upper extremity exercise, quadruped activities).
  - Rating of perceived exertion and signs and symptoms can be used to monitor exercise/activity intensity.
  - Instruction in energy conservation techniques is recommended (see page 204).
- Low-level, gradual exercise training is very beneficial in improving functional level, mainly via improved peripheral efficiency.

CARDIAC ARRHYTHMIAS

Any alteration in cardiac rhythm or conduction is termed an arrhythmia, or sometimes a dysrhythmia. Refer to pages 176 to 186 for descriptions of the various arrhythmias.

TYPES

Arrhythmias are classified according to:

- Site of origin (sinoatrial (SA) node, atria, atrioventricular (AV) node, ventricles)
- Type of cardiac activity (bradycardia, tachycardia, flutter, fibrillation)
- Presence of conduction block (SA node, AV node, bundle branches)

PATHOPHYSIOLOGY

Abnormal impulse generation (due to myocardial irritability or damage, drug toxicity, electrolyte disturbances, or idiopathic), abnormal impulse conduction (e.g., conduction blocks, accessory pathways), or a combination of both can result in a number of pathophysiologic outcomes, as illustrated in Figure 3–5.

CLINICAL MANIFESTATIONS

- Patient perception of arrhythmias varies widely; some patients feel every irregular heart beat, whereas others are not aware of them at all.
- The signs and symptoms that may be associated with arrhythmias include:
  - None
  - Palpitations, skipped beats, fluttering
  - Lightheadedness, dizziness
  - Syncope or near syncope
  - Chest discomfort
  - Weakness, fatigue
  - Dyspnea, possible pulmonary edema
  - Mental confusion, anxiety, agitation
  - Hypotension
  - Irregular and/or weak pulse
  - Sudden death

SIGNIFICANT VERSUS LESS SIGNIFICANT ARRHYTHMIAS

- The significance of an arrhythmia depends on its effects on:
  - HR
  - BP
  - Organ perfusion (e.g., cerebral, coronary, renal)
  - Ventricular function

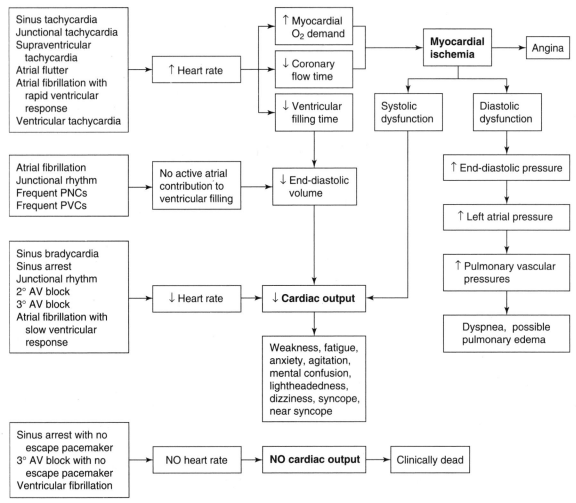

FIGURE 3–5. The possible pathophysiologic results of various arrhythmias. The major problems that can develop include myocardial ischemia, diminished cardiac output, or absolutely no cardiac output with clinical death. AV = atrioventricular, PNC = premature nodal complex, PVC = premature ventricular complex.

- The clinical significance of an arrhythmia is influenced by:
  - Duration of the arrhythmia
  - Cause of the arrhythmia and the presence or absence of underlying heart disease
    — More worrisome in patients with known cardiac disease, especially CAD
    — More worrisome in patients taking diuretics (may be increased or decreased potassium) or certain drugs (may indicate toxicity; e.g., digitalis, theophylline, aminophylline, dyphylline, oxitriphylline)

- The hemodynamic significance of an arrhythmia will be revealed by monitoring the HR and BP of the patient, as well as other signs and symptoms.

TREATMENT

- Treat identifiable causes of arrhythmias (e.g., electrolyte disturbances, drug toxicity)
- Antiarrhythmic drugs (see Chapter 4, pages 125 to 129)
- Cardioversion
- Pacemaker (see page 27)

- Automatic implantable cardioverter/defibrillator (AICD) (see page 28)
- Surgical excision (aneurysectomy, myectomy; see page 32)
- Chemical or surgical ablation (see page 32)

CLINICAL IMPLICATIONS FOR PHYSICAL THERAPY

- Physiologic responses to activity should be monitored:
  - Pulse should be monitored for rate and regularity versus irregularity.
    — Arrhythmias may increase, decrease, or remain the same during exercise.
    — Increasing arrhythmias during exercise are a cause for concern.
  - BP monitoring reveals hemodynamic significance of arrhythmias.
  - Patient may need holter/ambulatory monitoring.
- Side effects of medications may cause problems (see Chapter 4):
  - All antiarrhythmic agents have potential to increase arrhythmias.
  - Class I drugs may result in elevated resting and exercise heart rates, quinidine may mask ischemic ECG changes, and procainamide may cause a false positive exercise test.
  - Class II drugs (β-blockers) are associated with muscle fatigue and weakness and possible bronchospasm.
  - β-Blockers and calcium channel blockers often cause hypotension, especially orthostatic and postexercise hypotension.
- Treatment modifications may be indicated:
  - Be cautious if drugs cause hypotension, orthostatic intolerance; avoid sudden changes to upright positions.
  - Activity/exercise intensity may need to be restricted to avoid arrhythmias.
- Exercise training may be beneficial via improved ischemic threshold and/or decreased sympathetic tone.

VALVULAR HEART DISEASE

Malfunction of the heart valves, which is much more common on the left side of the heart than the right and often involves more than one valve, can lead to reduced effectiveness of cardiac function with decreased cardiac output and increased volume and pressure in the atria and vessels leading to them.

- Abnormal valve structure results in turbulent blood flow, which increases the hemodynamic stress on these structures and leads to progressive damage and dysfunction.
- Compensatory mechanisms, including ventricular hypertrophy, chamber dilatation, and peripheral processes, can help maintain the overall performance of the heart for many years, often decades, even when there is malfunction of more than one valve.
- Eventually, however, these compensatory mechanisms may become exhausted so that heart failure develops (see page 73).
- The pathophysiology and clinical manifestations of the various valvular abnormalities are described in Table 3–2.

TREATMENT

- Pharmacologic therapy
  - Digitalis to increase contractile state and/or control atrial fibrillation
  - Diuretics to ↓ preload and pulmonary venous congestion
  - Afterload reduction to ↑ cardiac output
  - Anticoagulation, if indicated
  - Treatment for pulmonary edema and shock if acute
- Other
  - Salt restriction
  - Endocarditis prophylaxis
  - Activity restriction if any of the following develop: severe aortic stenosis, moderate to severe aortic insufficiency with evidence of LVH, significant mitral or tricuspid stenosis, or acute mitral regurgitation
  - Cardioversion for new atrial fibrillation (if patient is anticoagulated)
- Surgical interventions (see page 29)
  - Urgent repair or valve replacement if acute
  - Balloon valvuloplasty or valvulotomy/commissurotomy for valvular stenosis
  - Valvuloplasty or annuloplasty for valvular incompetence
  - Valve replacement before irreversible deterioration in ventricular function develops

TABLE 3-2. **Valvular Heart Disease: Pathophysiology and Clinical Manifestations**

ABNORMALITY	PATHOPHYSIOLOGY	CLINICAL MANIFESTATIONS
Aortic Stenosis (AS)		
Etiology: congenital, senile calcification, inflammatory valvulitis, RF, severe atherosclerosis	Restricted opening of the AoV → ↑ Pressure load on LV →↑ LV systolic pressure, prolongation of ejection, + LVH → ↓ Compliance →↑ LV filling pressure after atrial systole. Dependence of adequate LV filling on atrial contraction. ↑ Risk of subendocardial ischemia. Initially, even with severe AS, there is normal cardiac output at rest but failure to ↑ on exertion. Prolonged severe AS → LV systolic dysfunction + LV dilatation →↑ pressures in lungs + right heart.	May be asymptomatic, even with significant AS, for many years. Once symptoms develop, prognosis is poor: Dyspnea, especially on exertion Angina pectoris Lightheadedness, syncope on exertion Sudden death Possible systemic emboli Harsh SEM at second ICS radiating to the neck, ↓ A₂ (aortic closure sound).
Aortic Insufficiency/Regurgitation (AI, AR)		
Etiology: congenital, RF, infective endocarditis, other (e.g., R. arthritis, SLE), aortic root disease	Incomplete closure of the AoV → regurgitation of blood from the Ao to the LV during diastole → ↑ Volume load on the LV during both systole and diastole. If chronic AI → LV dilatation + compensatory eccentric LVH →↑ total SV + possible ↑ forward SV if compensatory peripheral vasodilation. If severe acute AI →↑ total SV but ↓ forward SV →↑ LV end-diastolic volume +↑↑ LV end-diastolic pressure. If significant LVH →↓ LV compliance → dependence of adequate LV filling on atrial systole.	If chronic AI, gradual ↑ LV dilatation allows asymptomatic status for decades, then similar to AS (above), except for less angina and syncope. If acute AI, LV cannot adapt to sudden ↑ volume → S & S of LV failure Diastolic decrescendo murmur at LSB or sometimes RSB.
Mitral Stenosis (MS)		
Etiology: RF, congenital, other	Restricted opening of the MV → ↑ Pressure and volume load on the LA → LA dilatation + ↑ LA presssure →↑ pressure in the pulmonary vessels →↑ workload on RV → RVH. ↑ HR (e.g., uncontrolled a-fib, pregnancy, exercise, emotional stress, general anesthesia) →↓ diastolic flow time across tight MV →↑↑ LA pulmonary pressures → possible pulmonary edema. Adequate LV filling is dependent on atrial systole.	Often asymptomatic for 20–25 years, then gradually ↑ symptoms over 5 years: Dyspnea Fatigue Chest pain Chronic bronchitis Orthopnea Hemoptysis Palpitations Diastolic rumble, loud S₁ (first heart sound) unless there is severe calcification.

TABLE 3-2. **Valvular Heart Disease: Pathophysiology and Clinical Manifestations** *Continued*

ABNORMALITY	PATHOPHYSIOLOGY	CLINICAL MANIFESTATIONS
	Over time, ↑ pulmonary HTN → possible RV failure + TR (see below) + sometimes PR(see below).	
Mitral Regurgitation (MR) Etiology: LV dilatation, calcification, RF, infective endocarditis, papillary muscle dysfunction, chordal rupture, MVP	Regurgitation of blood from the LV into the LA during early systole →↑ volume load on LA + ↓ impedance to LV emptying. If acute, small LA cannot handle regurgitant flow →↑↑ LA pressure → pulmonary HTN + acute pulmonary edema. If chronic, ↑ LA absorbs regurgitant flow in most patients → normal or only slightly ↑ LA and pulmonary pressures at rest; if inadequate LA dilatation →↑ LA and pulmonary pressures.	If chronic, usually asymptomatic for decades (until LV fails) or for life if mild MR; then S & S of low cardiac output (e.g., chronic weakness, fatigue, lightheadedness, dizziness) and those of MS (see above) although less hemoptysis, systemic emboli, pulmonary HTN, and RV failure. If acute, S & S of LV failure. Loud, high-pitched pansystolic murmur transmitted to axilla, S_3 (third heart sound) is common.
Mitral Valve Prolapse (MVP) Etiology: hereditary, congenital, acquired	Ballooning of the MV leaflets into the LA during systole → Usually normal hemodynamics. Possible MR (see above).	Frequently asymptomatic. Otherwise, atypical chest pain, fatigue, palpitations, and/or dyspnea. Late systolic crescendo murmur, which is often preceded by one or more midsystolic clicks.
Pulmonary Stenosis (PS) Etiology: congenital, RF	Restricted opening of the PV → ↑ Pressure load on RV → RVH + dilatation: ↓ Compliance →↑ RV end-diastolic pressure →↑ RA and systemic venous pressures + dependence of adequate RV filling on atrial systole. Once RV systolic dysfunction develops →↓ cardiac output + eventual RV failure. If other coexisting lesions, there will be different problems: If ASD or PFO, may be L→R or R→L shunting. If VSD, usually is L→R shunting (see Chapter 7). If TR, ↓ forward output from RV.	May be asymptomatic if good RV function, sinus rhythm + no other lesions. Otherwise: Dyspnea, especially on exertion Fatigue, weakness Possible cyanosis S & S of RV failure Growth retardation in children Pulsations in throat Possible angina, syncope on exertion Harsh, diamond-shaped SEM at upper LSB, opening sound, S_4 (fourth heart sound) if severe PS.

Continued on following page.

TABLE 3-2. **Valvular Heart Disease: Pathophysiology and Clinical Manifestations** *Continued*

ABNORMALITY	PATHOPHYSIOLOGY	CLINICAL MANIFESTATIONS
Pulmonary Regurgitation (PR) Etiology: dilatation of PV (from pulmonary HTN) or PA, endocarditis, congenital, other	Regurgitation of blood from the PA into the RV during diastole → ↑ Volume load on RV. If coexistent pulmonary HTN →↑ RV failure. If infective endocarditis → septic pulmonary emboli, pulmonary HTN, + severe RV failure.	Tolerated well for decades unless pulmonary HTN is present. Otherwise, S & S of pulmonary HTN and/or RV failure. Diamond-shaped diastolic murmur along left parasternal border with ↑ on inspiration, possible ↑ P_2 (pulmonary closure sound).
Tricuspid Stenosis (TS) Etiology: RF, congenital, carcinoid	Restricted opening of the TV → a-fib → further ↑ RA and systemic venous pressures. ↓↓ Resting cardiac output with failure to ↑ during exercise. If TS + coexisting MS (not uncommon) →↓ RV flow →↓ severity of pulmonary HTN.	Dyspnea S & S of ↓ cardiac output c/o prominent pulsations in neck Systemic venous congestion (e.g., JVD, ascites, edema) Diamond-shaped diastolic murmur along lower left parasternal border at fourth ICS
Tricuspid Regurgitation (TR) Etiology: secondary to pulmonary HTN, congenital, RF, other	TR implies, as well as aggravates, severe RV failure. Systolic regurgitation into RA →↑ volume load on RA → RA dilatation + ↑ RA pressure with reflection to venous system → prominent venous *cv* wave. If a-fib →↑ RA volume and pressure + RV dilatation →↑ TR.	Well-tolerated if no pulmonary HTN; otherwise, similar to TS. Possible S & S of biventricular failure if due to left heart dysfunction. Holosystolic murmur at LSB with ↑ on inspiration. a-fib is common on ECG.

↑ = increased, ↑↑ = more markedly increased, ↓ = decreased, ↓↓ = more markedly decreased, → = results in, RF = rheumatic fever, AoV = aortic valve, L→R = left to right, LV = left ventricle/ventricular, LVH = left ventricular hypertrophy, ICS = intercostal space, R. = rheumatoid, SLE = systemic lupus erythematosis, Ao = aortic/aorta, S & S = signs and symptoms, LSB = left sternal border, R→L = right to left, RSB = right sternal border, MV = mitral valve, RV = right ventricle/ventricular, RVH = right ventricular hypertrophy, SEM = systolic ejection murmur, SV = stroke volume, HR = heart rate, a-fib = atrial fibrillation, LA = left atria/atrial, PV = pulmonary valve, PA = pulmonary artery, ASD = atrial septal defect, PFO = patent foramen ovale, VSD = ventricular septal defect, HTN = hypertension, TV = tricuspid valve, RA = right atrium, JVD = jugular venous distension, ECG = electrocardiography.

CARDIOMYOPATHIES

The cardiomyopathies consist of a diverse group of diseases involving a primary disorder of the myocardial cells with resultant myocardial dysfunction. Cardiomyopathies are classified according to the type of abnormal myocardial structure and function: dilated, hypertrophic, or restrictive. Table 3–3 presents a comparison of the features of the three types of cardiomyopathies.

DILATED CARDIOMYOPATHY

Dilated cardiomyopathy (DCM) is characterized by increased cardiac mass, dilatation of all four chambers with little or no wall thickening,

TABLE 3-3. **Comparison of the Three Types of Cardiomyopathies**

	DILATED	HYPERTROPHIC	RESTRICTIVE
Ventricular volume			
End-diastolic	↑	nl	↓–nl
End-systolic	↑↑	↓	nl
Ventricular mass	↑	↑↑↑	nl–↑
Mass/volume ratio	↓	↑↑	nl–↑
Systolic function			
Ejection fraction	↓–↓↓	nl–↑–↓	nl
Myocardial shortening	↓–↓↓	↑–↓	nl
Wall stress	↑	↓	↓
Diastolic function			
Chamber stiffness	↓	↑↑	↑↑
Filling pressure	↑↑	nl–↑	↑
Symptoms	CHF, fatigue, weakness	Dyspnea, angina, fatigue, syncope or presyncope	Dyspnea, fatigue, RV failure

↑ = mildly increased, ↑↑ = moderately increased, ↑↑↑ = markedly increased, ↓ = mildly decreased, ↓↓ = moderately decreased, CHF = congestive heart failure, nl = normal, RV = right ventricular.

impaired systolic function, and often symptoms of congestive heart failure (formerly called congestive CM).

Pathophysiology

Infectious and noninfectious inflammatory processes, toxins (e.g., alcohol, drugs), pregnancy/postpartum, metabolic disorders (e.g., endocrine, nutritional, altered metabolism), myocardial ischemia, or hereditary diseases (e.g., glycogen storage diseases, muscular dystrophies) may result in DCM with:

- Decreased SV and ventricular dilatation, which is compensated at rest by an increased HR, but impaired ability to increase cardiac output during exercise with resultant increased LV end-diastolic pressure (LVEDP)
- Dependence of cardiac reserve on preservation of RV function and systemic vasodilator reserve during exercise
- Eventual development of LV failure and later RV failure (see page 73)
- Decreased oxygen saturation, which results in increased arteriovenous oxygen difference
- Increased LV filling pressure, which increases the risk of subendocardial ischemia

Clinical Manifestations

- Dyspnea initially on exertion then at rest
- Nocturnal dry cough

- Signs and symptoms of LV failure
- Possible signs and symptoms of RV failure
- Chest pain on exertion
- Resting tachycardia
- LV impulse displaced lateral to the midclavicular line
- S_3-S_4 gallop rhythm (see page 163)
- Systolic murmurs of mitral and triscuspid regurgitation are common due to ventricular dilatation
- Atrial enlargement, decreased QRS, nonspecific ST-T changes on ECG
- Considerable cardiomegaly, possible LA and RA enlargement, and redistribution of blood flow on chest x-ray examination

Treatment

As described for heart failure (see page 74).

HYPERTROPHIC CARDIOMYOPATHY

Hypertrophic cardiomyopathy (HCM) is characterized by a considerable increase in cardiac mass (hypertrophy), which can be symmetrical or asymmetrical, without cavity dilatation and normal, or increased, systolic function. In addition, there may be LV outflow obstruction (hypertrophic obstructive cardiomyopathy, HOCM, formerly called idiopathic hypertrophic subaortic stenosis, IHSS).

Pathophysiology

- LVH results in diastolic dysfunction due to abnormal LV relaxation and distensibility, which leads to decreased LV compliance and increased LV filling pressures.
- Decreased LV compliance increases the dependence of LV filling on atrial systole.
- Hyperdynamic LV function produces rapid ejection and increased EF.
- Systolic anterior motion (SAM) of the mitral valve apparatus can result in contact with the intraventricular septum and outflow obstruction (see Fig. 1–14, page 15)
- Myocardial ischemia is common and may result from:
  - Impaired vasodilator reserve
  - Increased oxygen demands, especially if HOCM develops
  - Increased filling pressures with resultant subendocardial ischemia

Clinical Manifestations

- Varies widely, depending on extent and severity of morphologic abnormalities, rate of progression, and degree of obstruction
- May be asymptomatic or only mildly symptomatic
- Dyspnea
- Angina pectoris
- Fatigue
- Presyncope and syncope
- Palpitations
- Occasionally PND and symptoms of CHF
- LV lift; point of maximal impulse displaced laterally, abnormally forceful and enlarged; may be prominent presystolic apical impulse, systolic apical thrill
- Loud S_4 (fourth heart sound); harsh diamond-shaped systolic murmur if HOCM develops, which may radiate to lower sternal border, axillae, and base of heart; possible murmur of mitral regurgitation
- Briskly rising carotid pulse, which may decline in midsystole as outflow obstruction develops
- ST-T abnormalities and sometimes LV hypertrophy on ECG; may also be prominent abnormal Q waves in inferior and/or lateral leads; ventricular arrhythmias, supraventricular tachycardia, and occasionally atrial fibrillation

Treatment

- Pharmacologic (see Chapter 4)
  - β-Adrenergic blockers for angina, dyspnea, and presyncope
  - Calcium channel blockers to improve diastolic filling and to decrease myocardial contractility and outflow obstruction
  - Prophylactic antibiotics
- Surgical
  - Left ventricular septal myotomy-myectomy (LVMM) to relieve obstruction in HOCM (see page 32)
  - Mitral valve replacement to eliminate SAM in HOCM or to relieve severe mitral regurgitation (see page 29)
  - Laser myoplasty instead of LVMM (under investigation)
  - Pacemaker insertion to change pattern of depolarization so SAM does not coincide with contraction of the interventricular septum and outflow obstruction is prevented (under investigation)
- Other
  - Avoidance of strenuous exercise because of increased risk of sudden death

RESTRICTIVE CARDIOMYOPATHY

Restrictive cardiomyopathy is characterized by restriction of ventricular filling caused by endocardial or myocardial disease or both, which makes the ventricular walls excessively rigid.

Pathophysiology

- Decreased compliance due to endocardial or myocardial disease results in impaired ventricular filling, which leads to atrial enlargement and increased atrial pressures, which are reflected back to the filling vessels.
- Distortion of the ventricular cavity and involvement of the papillary muscles and chordae tendineae can cause mitral and/or tricuspid regurgitation.
- Partial obliteration of the ventricle by fibrous tissue and thrombus results in reduced SV and often compensatory tachycardia.
- Eventually systolic function becomes impaired.
- If there is LV involvement, pulmonary HTN is common.

Clinical Manifestations
- Exercise intolerance
- Weakness
- Dyspnea
- Increased central venous pressure leading to jugular venous distention, edema, enlarged liver, ascites
- S_3 and/or S_4 (see page 163)
- Possible inspiratory increase in venous pressure (Kussmaul's sign)
- Symptoms of CHF (see page 73)
- Diastolic dip and plateau (square root sign) in ventricular pressure pulse; prominent *a* wave, often of same amplitude as *v* wave
- Conduction disturbances, arrhythmias, ST-T abnormalities on ECG

Treatment
- Routine cardiac therapy (except as contraindicated in amyloidosis) (see Chapter 4)
  - Digitalis
  - Diuretics
  - Afterload reduction
  - Antiarrhythmics, AICD (under investigation)
  - Anticoagulation for atrial fibrillation
- Other specific treatments depend on cause
  - Corticosteroids (e.g., sarcoidosis, hypereosinophilia)
  - Cytotoxic drugs (e.g., hypereosinophilia, endomyocardial fibrosis)

OTHER CARDIAC DISORDERS

Cardiovascular disease sometimes results from infection or inflammation involving the cardiac structures, trauma, drug toxicity, or involvement of the heart by systemic diseases. Cardiomyopathy may result from these disorders and has already been discussed.

MYOCARDITIS

Inflammation of the myocardial wall most frequently results from streptococcal infection leading to rheumatic fever (see below) or viral infection, such as coxsackie B virus, but can also be caused by other bacterial, rickettsial, fungal, or parasitic infections, as well as allergic reactions, pharmacologic agents, and some systemic diseases. Myocarditis can be an acute or chronic process, may involve a limited area of my-

ocardium, or may be diffuse, and is often accompanied by pericarditis (see following page).

- The clinical manifestations of myocarditis are quite variable, ranging from asymptomatic to fulminent congestive heart failure (CHF); most patients have nonspecific cardiovascular complaints, including fatigue, dyspnea, palpitations, and precordial discomfort.
- Patient management includes treating the cause whenever possible, as well as the more prominent systemic manifestations, supportive care, and rest.
- Most patients recover completely, although some die and others develop a chronic dilated cardiomyopathy, as described on page 80.

RHEUMATIC FEVER

Acute rheumatic fever (ARF) most commonly affects children 5 to 15 years of age and therefore is discussed in Chapter 7 on page 238. Chronic rheumatic heart disease (RHD) may develop in some patients, particularly those with more severe carditis, and usually results in mitral and/or aortic valvular disease. There appears to be two different clinical groups: one that shows evidence of significant valvular disease with a higher percentage of death within the first 5 years after ARF and one that has relatively mild valve disease initially but develops slowly progressive dysfunction due to gradual wear and tear on the valve caused by turbulent flow through its defective structures. The pathophysiologic effect and clinical manifestations of RHD are presented under the specific valvular defect(s), as described on pages 77 to 80.

PERICARDITIS

Inflammation of the pericardium most commonly results from viral or bacterial infections, uremia, acute myocardial infarction, pericardiotomy associated with cardiac surgery, tuberculosis, malignancy, and trauma; but it may also be due to other infections, autoimmune disorders (e.g., connective tissue diseases), other inflammatory disorders (e.g., sarcoidosis, amyloidosis, inflammatory bowel disease), drug toxicity, chest irradiation, and hypothyroidism.

- Clinically, pericarditis is demonstrated by a range of signs and symptoms as it progresses from a simple inflammatory response with no cardiovascular compromise to cardiac tamponade (i.e., fluid filling the pericardial sac increases pericardial pressure causing cardiac compression and interference with diastolic ventricular filling, which results in very low cardiac output) and constrictive pericarditis (fibrotic, thickened, and adherent pericardium restricts diastolic filling). Typically, there is chest pain, dyspnea, a pericardial friction rub, and serial ECG abnormalities. There may be a pericardial effusion (fluid within the pericardial sac), which is often asymptomatic.

- Treatment of pericarditis consists of managing the underlying process, bedrest, and nonsteroidal antiinflammatory agents; pericardiocentesis or pericardial drainage may be indicated for pericardial effusion to evaluate fluid for presence of infectious agents and to prevent excessive accumulation of fluid; and surgical stripping of the pericardium (i.e., pericardiectomy) may be required for constrictive pericarditis.

INFECTIVE ENDOCARDITIS

Bacterial or fungal infection of the heart valves causes vegetations to form along the cusps, which interfere with proper opening and closing. Any abnormality of either a heart valve or the blood flow through a heart valve increases the risk of infective endocarditis (IE), although the degree of risk varies substantially according to the specific abnormality. The development of IE is associated with situations where infective organisms may be introduced directly into the blood stream (e.g., dental, urinary, or intestinal procedures, intravenous drug abuse, central venous catheter placement).

- The clinical manifestations of IE are highly variable and depend on the involvement of other organ systems due to embolization of valvular vegetation fragments, bacterial seeding of distant foci, or the development of immune complex-associated disease. Generally, there are symptoms suggestive of a "flu-like illness" and possibly the clinical manifestations of specific valvular lesions and/or CHF.
- Intracardiac infection can result in perforation of valve leaflets; rupture of the chordae tendinae, intraventricular septum, or papillary muscle; valve ring abscesses; occlusion of a valve orifice; coronary emboli; burrowing abscesses of the myocardium; and purulent pericardial effusions.
- Treatment is directed against the specific infective organism; surgical intervention (e.g., valve replacement or resection) is indicated if medical treatment is unsuccessful or for an unusual pathogen, myocardial abscess formation, refractory heart failure, serious embolic complications, or refractory prosthetic valve disease.
- Antibiotic prophylaxis is indicated for all patients with congenital or acquired valvular dysfunction, prosthetic heart valves, obstructive hypertrophic cardiomyopathy, a number of other congenital cardiac defects or shunt repairs, and for patients with previous endocarditis. It should be undertaken for all dental and respiratory procedures, gastrointestinal or genitourinary manipulation, and childbirth.

3.2 PULMONARY DISEASES AND DISORDERS

A brief description of the most common diseases and disorders affecting the respiratory system is presented in this section, including pathophysiology, clinical manifestations, and treatment. In addition, the clinical implications for physical therapy are listed for the major categories of obstructive and restrictive lung disease. To provide optimal treatment, the reader is encouraged to study more detailed descriptions of the disorders, which can be found in many references including those cited at the end of this chapter.

OBSTRUCTIVE LUNG DISEASES

Obstructive lung diseases are characterized by some degree of chronic airflow limitation, or increased airway resistance, which is particularly noticeable during prolonged forced expiration. Chest radiographs commonly show hyperinflated lungs and flattened diaphragms and possibly an enlarged right ventricle due to increased pulmonary artery pressure. Pulmonary function testing usually reveals increased total lung capacity, mainly caused by increased residual volume (see Fig. 2–9, page 47), normal or increased vital capacity, decreased flow rates at all lung volumes (see Figs. 2–10 and 2–11, page 51), and decreased diffusion capacity.

CHRONIC BRONCHITIS

Chronic bronchitis is an obstructive lung disease characterized by a chronic cough with excessive mucous production that is not due to known specific causes, such as bronchiectasis or tuberculosis, and that is present for most days of at least 3 months of the year for 2 or more consecutive years.

Pathophysiology

- Long-term irritation of the tracheobronchial tree (e.g., smoking, air pollution, occupational exposure, bronchial infection) causes hypersecretion of mucus and destruction of cilia, which results in a chronic productive cough and recurrent pulmonary infections. The end result consists of increased ventilation-perfusion ($\dot{V}/\dot{Q}$) mismatching and increased work of breathing.
- In addition, smoke irritation of the airways can result in bronchoconstriction.
- Over the years, hyperinflation of the lungs produces a barrel-shaped chest, which results in decreased efficiency of the respiratory muscles and increased work of breathing.
- During acute exacerbations (e.g., due to upper respiratory infection), sputum production is increased and more secretions are retained, resulting in further increased $\dot{V}/\dot{Q}$ mismatching and further increased work of breathing, which creates the potential for ventilatory muscle fatigue and even ventilatory or respiratory failure (see page 98).
- As the disease progresses, chronic hypoxemia causes hypoxic vasoconstriction in the lungs, which results in higher pulmonary artery (PA) pressure (especially during exertion) plus polycythemia (i.e., increased red blood cell count), both of which increase the work of the heart. The RV will hypertrophy, and late in the disease right heart failure (i.e., cor pulmonale; see page 99) may develop.

Clinical Manifestations

- Insidious onset of smokers' cough, which progresses to chronic productive cough
- Progressive exertional dyspnea, with possible respiratory distress late in the disease

- Increased respiratory symptoms with irritants, cold, damp or foggy weather, and acute pulmonary infections
- Possible wheezing
- Stiff, barrel-shaped chest with moderate or greater disease
- Hypoxemia and eventually increased P_{CO_2} and acidemia with moderate to severe disease
- Clinical manifestations of cor pulmonale and/or respiratory failure when end-stage disease develops
- Sometimes referred to as "blue bloaters" because of stocky body build and cyanosis

EMPHYSEMA

Emphysema consists of several diseases that ultimately result in permanent overdistension of the air spaces distal to the terminal nonrespiratory bronchioles accompanied by attenuation and destruction of the alveolar walls. Abnormal air spaces, called bullae and blebs, may be seen on chest radiograph. The most common causes of emphysema include cigarette smoking and occupational exposure (see page 88), which typically produce centrilobar destruction. A rarer cause is alpha-1 protease inhibitor (α_1-PI) deficiency (also called α_1-antitrypsin deficiency), which tends to cause panlobar emphysema.

Pathophysiology

Repeated inflammation of the airways along with the development of partial or complete bronchiolar obstruction results in:

- Air trapping and alveolar overdistension, which causes fragmentation of the intra-alveolar elastic tissue and rupture of the attenuated interalveolar septa (Fig. 3–6), leads to coalescence of several alveoli and bullae formation.
- Release of proteases by inflammatory neutrophils causes progressive lung destruction.
- As the disease progresses, hyperinflation of the lungs produces a barrel-shaped chest, which results in decreased efficiency of the respiratory muscles and increased work of breathing.
- Loss of functional alveoli results in gross $\dot{V}/\dot{Q}$ mismatching throughout the lungs, which increases the physiologic dead space and acts like a shunt; hyperventilation of the well-ventilated, well-perfused alveoli, which

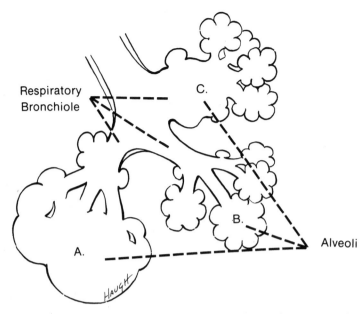

FIGURE 3–6. Emphysema. *(A)* Panlobar emphysema with it's characteristic destructive enlargement of the alveoli, *(B)* normal respiratory bronchiole and alveoli, and *(C)* centrilobar emphysema with its characteristic enlargement and destruction of the respiratory bronchiole. (From Hammon WE: Pathophysiology of chronic pulmonary disease. In Frownfelter DL: *Chest Physical Therapy and Pulmonary Rehabilitation,* 2nd Ed. Chicago, Year Book Medical Publishers, Inc., p. 93, 1987. Used with permission.)

must occur to maintain normal blood gases, increases the work of breathing and creates the potential for ventilatory muscle fatigue and ventilatory failure late in the disease (see page 98).

- Also, increased $\dot{V}/\dot{Q}$ mismatching produces increased hypoxemia and possibly carbon dioxide retention, resulting in an increased respiratory rate and use of the accessory muscles and even greater work of breathing. Thus, with moderate to severe disease, hypoxemia and hypercapnia worsen, resulting in more hypoxic vasoconstriction and further increased PA pressure, which may lead to cor pulmonale (see page 99).

- In addition, the loss of large portions of lung parenchyma decreases the number of pulmonary capillaries, which increases pulmonary vascular resistance leading to increased pulmonary HTN, and so on, as above.

- If a bulla ruptures, air will escape, which tracks along the tissue planes of the lungs and finally becomes localized in the subpleural areas as a bleb; if a bleb ruptures through the visceral pleura, the patient experiences a spontaneous pneumothorax.

Clinical Manifestations

- Progressive dyspnea, especially on exertion
- Cough, often severe, with variable degrees of productiveness
- Increased symptoms with acute respiratory infections
- With moderate to severe disease:
  - Diminished nutritional status, weight loss
  - Stiff, hyperinflated chest and increased use of accessory muscles
  - Possible spontaneous pursed-lip breathing
  - Distant breath sounds, especially at the bases with prolonged expiration; possibly end-expiratory high-pitched wheeze, especially on forced expiration
- Possible signs and symptoms of cor pulmonale and/or ventilatory failure when end-stage disease develops
- Sometimes called "pink puffers" because of increased work of breathing to maintain relatively normal arterial blood gases (ABGs).

ASTHMA

Asthma is a clinical syndrome characterized by airway hyperreactivity to various external and internal stimuli and manifested as recurrent episodes of intermittent reversible airway obstruction.

- When the provocative stimuli are immunologic in origin, in which mast cells, sensitized by immunoglobulin E (IgE) antibodies, degranulate and release bronchoactive mediators following exposure to specific antigens, asthma is called extrinsic, or atopic. Extrinsic asthma is most commonly seen in children.
- When the cause is not clearly related to allergy, as in adult-onset asthma, it is said to be intrinsic, or nonatopic.
- Factors that may precipitate an acute asthmatic attack are listed in Table 3–4.

Pathophysiology

- Hyperreactivity of the airways to various stimuli results in bronchial smooth muscle contraction and hypertrophy, inflammation of the mucosa, and overproduction of viscous, tenacious mucus.
- There may be an immediate (within minutes or seconds) versus a late (4 to 10 hours after exposure) hypersensitivity reaction.
- If respiratory distress continues without response to treatment, *status asthmaticus* is present and hospitalization is required.

Clinical Manifestations

- Recurrent paroxysmal attacks of cough, chest tightness, and difficult breathing, often accompanied by wheezing
- Thick, tenacious sputum, which may be difficult to expectorate
- Symptom-free between attacks versus chronic state of mild asthma, with symptoms particularly noticeable during periods of exertion or emotional excitement.
- Hyperinflated lungs with distant breath sounds, prolonged expiration; high-pitched wheezes throughout both lungs during acute attacks.
- Variable degree of respiratory distress (e.g., increased use of accessory muscles, intercostal retractions, nasal flaring) during acute attacks.
- Pulmonary function tests (PFTs) will show markedly reduced FEV_1, $FEF_{25\%-75\%}$, and V_{max} at all lung volumes and increased total lung capacity (TLC) during acute attacks; during remission, airway resistance is usually increased and maximal expiratory flow rates are lower than expected.
- Hypoxemia with hypocapnia is common during acute attacks; normal or increased P_{CO_2} is a serious sign indicating ventilatory insufficiency.

BRONCHIECTASIS

Bronchiectasis is an obstructive lung disease characterized by permanent abnormal dilation and distortion of one or more of the medium-sized bronchi and bronchioles. It is usually manifested clinically as a chronic cough, often with copious sputum production.

TABLE 3–4. **Factors That May Precipitate Acute Asthma**

TYPE OF ASTHMA	IRRITANT OR INDUCING STIMULI
Nonatopic (intrinsic)	Inhaled irritants (e.g., smoke, dusts, pollution, sprays) Weather (e.g., high humidity, cold air, fog) Respiratory infections (e.g., common cold, bronchitis) Drugs (e.g., aspirin, other analgesics) Emotions (e.g., stress) Exercise
Atopic (extrinsic)	Pollens (e.g., tree, grass, ragweed) Animal danders Feathers Mold spores Household dust Food (e.g., nuts, shellfish)

Pathophysiology

- Bronchial obstruction (caused by infection, aspiration, tumor, foreign body) produces atelectasis, which increases the intrathoracic pressure required to overcome greater elastic resistance and causes dilation of the bronchi.
- Also, prolonged bronchial obstruction increases the risk of secondary infection, which results in destruction of the bronchial walls and dilation of the bronchi leading to reparative laying down of fibrous tissue; this further increases the traction on the bronchi and creates even more distortion.
- With increased obstruction and additional secretion production, there is greater $\dot{V}/\dot{Q}$ mismatching and increased work of breathing, creating the potential for ventilatory muscle fatigue and ventilatory failure later in the disease (see page 98).
- In addition, as the disease progresses, increased $\dot{V}/\dot{Q}$ mismatching results in increased hypoxemia and possibly carbon dioxide retention, which increases the respiratory rate and use of the accessory muscles and thus the work of breathing, leading to further increased hypoxemia and P_{CO_2}, increased hypoxic vasoconstriction, and further increased PA pressure. Thus there is the potential for cor pulmonale (see page 99).

Clinical Manifestations

- Productive cough with variable amounts (often copious) of purulent sputum
- Possibly asymptomatic between episodes of acute infection
- Blood streaking of sputum or frank hemoptysis
- Possible intercurrent upper respiratory infection
- Dyspnea if both lungs are extensively involved
- Possible clubbing of digits
- Variable or no distinctive chest x-ray findings
- PFTs are extremely variable
  - No significant changes if bronchiectasis is minimal
  - Increased or decreased lung volumes if disease is more advanced
  - Mildly increased airflow resistance with decreased FEV_1, $FEF_{25\% -75\%,}$ and V_{max} at all lung volumes

- Possible hypoxemia even in mild disease
- If diffuse disease is present, there may be possible severe hypoxemia with hypercapnia and acidemia, as well as signs and symptoms of pulmonary HTN, RVH, and possibly cor pulmonale with more severe disease.

CYSTIC FIBROSIS

Cystic fibrosis (CF) is a genetic disorder characterized by dysfunction of the exocrine glands, with abnormal secretions in the respiratory tract, sweat glands, mucosal glands of the small intestine, the pancreas, and bile ducts of the liver. Abnormally thick, tenacious mucus along with impaired mucociliary clearance results in chronic obstructive pulmonary disease and frequent respiratory infections. Because CF is predominantly a disease affecting children, it is described in detail in Chapter 7 (see page 244). However, more effective medical management is allowing greater numbers of patients to survive into adulthood. In addition, some patients have received lung transplantations.

OCCUPATIONAL AIRWAYS DISEASE

Airway disease can result from occupational exposure to specific agents. There are three categories: occupational asthma, asthma-like syndromes, and chronic irreversible airflow obstruction (see bronchiolitis obliterans on page 97).

- Agents associated with occupational airways disease include:
  - Animal protein (e.g., hair, dander, and urine of animals, insects, birds, fish)
  - Enzymes (e.g., detergents, spices)
  - Plant proteins (e.g., organic dusts, flour, coffee, tea, castor bean)
  - Vegetable gums (e.g., used in printing)
  - Epoxy resin, ethylenediamine
  - Complex platinum salts, nickel, cadmium, vanadium, tungsten
  - Isocyanates
  - Formaldehyde, piperazine
  - Plicatic acid in Western red cedar

Pathophysiology

An acute inflammatory or allergic process produces hyperreactive airways and chronic inflammation of airways, which results in increased $\dot{V}/\dot{Q}$ mismatching and therefore increased work of breathing (similar to pathophysiology of asthma, see page 87).

TREATMENT OF COPD

- Medications (see Chapter 4)
  - β-Adrenergic agonists (bronchodilators)
  - Xanthine derivatives (bronchodilators)
  - Anticholinergic drugs (prevent bronchoconstriction)
  - Corticosteroids (antiinflammatory)
  - Cromolyn sodium (prevents bronchospasm)
  - Mucolytic agents (to thin mucous)
  - Antibiotics (for treatment of infections)
- Physical therapy (see Chapter 6)
  - Bronchial drainage
  - Bronchial hygiene techniques
  - Breathing exercises
  - Chest mobility, posture, shoulder range of motion (ROM) exercises
  - Relaxation training
  - Exercise training
- Pulmonary rehabilitation
- Supportive measures
  - Supplemental oxygen
  - Nutritional support
- Surgical interventions
  - Excision or plication of dominant bullae (see page 65)
  - Lung or heart-lung transplantation (see page 30)

CLINICAL IMPLICATIONS FOR PHYSICAL THERAPY

- Pretreatment with a bronchodilator may be beneficial for improving exercise tolerance.
- Patients should never exercise on less oxygen than they are using at rest.
- Physical therapy evaluation of patients with diagnosed or suspected pulmonary disease should include assessment of the following:
  - Airway clearance
  - Chest wall and shoulder mobility
  - Strength of skeletal muscles and diaphragm
  - Posture
  - Gait
  - Movement patterns
  - Physiologic responses to exercise (e.g., HR, BP, respiratory rate, oxygen saturation, and signs and symptoms of intolerance)
- Physical therapists must be able to recognize the clinical manifestations of hypoxemia (see Table 3–5), as well as those of respiratory muscle fatigue (see Table 3–6).
- Side effects of medications may affect exercise responses (see Chapter 4).
  - Increased resting and exercise HRs may be seen in patients on caffeine-derivative bronchodilators.
  - Increased arrhythmias, nervousness, confusion, and/or tremors may indicate bronchodilator toxicity.

TABLE 3–5. **Clinical Manifestations of Hypoxemia**

Decreased P_{O_2}
Central cyanosis with or without peripheral cyanosis
Tachycardia, arrhythmias
Mild hypertension or hypotension
Peripheral vasoconstriction
Poor judgement, motor incoordination, slower reaction times
Restlessness, confusion, agitation, paranoia
Fatigue, somnolence, apathy
Dizziness
Headache
Polycythemia if chronic
If severe, hypoventilation, or apnea, bradycardia, myocardial depression, shock, depression of medullary respiratory centers

---

TABLE 3–6. **Clinical Manifestations of Respiratory Muscle Fatigue**

Rapid, shallow breathing
Out-of-phase or incoordinated chest wall movements (paradoxical breathing, respiratory alternans; see page 158)
↑ Accessory muscle activity
Dyspnea
Signs and symptoms of hypoxia (see Table 3–5)
Signs and symptoms of carbon dioxide narcosis
  Flushed/red skin coloring
  Tachycardia
  Hypertension or hypotension
  Diaphoresis
  ↓ Mental status, confusion, drowsiness, coma
  Headache
  Muscular twitching, coarse myoclonic jerking, asterixis
  Papilledema if chronic

- Corticosteroids cause increased catabolism, so physical therapists must observe for skin breakdown and use caution regarding overstressing bones and musculoskeletal structures.
- Individualized treatment program should include (see also Chapter 6):
  - Identification of triggers for dyspnea
  - Incorporation of breath control with activities (e.g., inspiration with extension, expiration with flexion)
  - Activity and exercise modifications, as indicated:
    — Preexercise bronchial hygiene treatment for patients with increased secretions
    — Alternating exercise intervals and rest periods
    — Dyspnea positions
    — Use of pulse oximetry to monitor for oxygen desaturation, possible use of or increased dose of oxygen during exertion (requires physician order)
    — Pursed-lip breathing
    — Postexercise or ambulation cough encouragement
  - Identification of difficult/problem situations in a diary followed by brainstorming to come up with solutions and alternatives
  - Relaxation techniques
  - Exercise training
    — Respiratory muscle training
    — General endurance training
- Relaxation should be incorporated into the patient's lifestyle:
  - Pace activities throughout day
  - Maintain a positive attitude
  - Seek support and understanding
  - Take time daily for the "relaxation response"
- Preventative health measures should be encouraged:
  - Adequate hydration
  - Good nutrition: patients should
    — Eat small meals more frequently
    — Watch fats and protein when increasing activity
    — Avoid gas-producing foods
    — Use dietary supplement (e.g., Ensure) if patient experiences weight loss or poor appetite
    — Enjoy yogurt to replace "good" bacteria
  - Compliance with medications and other treatments

- Self-monitoring
- Early treatment if signs of problems occur
- Regular endurance exercise
- Flu and pneumonia prevention

RESTRICTIVE LUNG DYSFUNCTION

An abnormal reduction in pulmonary ventilation can result from any cause of reduced lung compliance (e.g., pulmonary fibrosis, edema, or inflammation; atelectasis, pneumothorax) or restricted thoracic compliance (e.g., respiratory muscle weakness, paralysis, or incoordination; impaired ventilatory drive, thoracic deformity). Chest x-ray findings are extremely variable in restrictive lung dysfunction (RLD) because of the diverse nature of the abnormalities that produce it. Pulmonary function testing usually reveals markedly decreased TLC caused by restriction in almost all volumes (see Fig. 2–9, page 47), normal or decreased flow rates (see Figs. 2–10 and 2–11, page 51), and decreased diffusing capacity. The general characteristics of RLD will be presented first, followed by more detailed information on some of the specific diseases and disorders that result in RLD.

PATHOPHYSIOLOGY

- Decreased chest wall or lung compliance, or both, results in decreased pulmonary compliance and RLD:
  - If a lung is less compliant, it will be stiffer and require increased transpulmonary pressure to expand it to any given volume.
  - If the chest wall is less compliant, thoracic expansion will be reduced, although lung compliance may be normal.
- Thus, decreased pulmonary compliance results in a faster respiratory rate, greater work of the inspiratory muscles, especially the diaphragm, and recruitment of accessory muscles so that the work of breathing will be markedly increased.
- The greater the severity of restriction, the more dependent the individual will be on respiratory rate as the only means to increase minute ventilation to meet increased metabolic demands for oxygen.
- In addition, reduced pulmonary compliance produces ventilation/perfusion $(\dot{V}/\dot{Q})$ mismatching and intrapulmonary right-to-left shunt, which further increases the work of

breathing, creating the potential for ventilatory muscle fatigue and ventilatory failure as the disease progresses in severity (see page 98).

- Furthermore, chronic hypoventilation seen in moderately severe disease results in hypoxemia, leading to hypoxic vasoconstriction and increased PA pressures (especially during exertion) plus polycythemia (i.e., elevated red blood cell count); this further increases the workload on the RV and produces RVH and possible eventual cor pulmonale (see page 99).

CLINICAL MANIFESTATIONS

- Dyspnea
- Cough, usually dry sounding and nonproductive
- Weight loss
- Tachypnea
- Hypoxemia with associated signs and symptoms (see page 89)
- Decreased lung volumes and diffusion capacity on PFTs
- Decreased breath sounds
- Abnormal chest x-ray findings (often with reticulonodular pattern)
- Possible signs and symptoms of ventilatory failure if severe dysfunction
- Possible signs and symptoms of pulmonary HTN, RVH, and cor pulmonale if severe dysfunction

TREATMENT

- Supportive measure
  - Supplemental oxygen
  - Antibiotic therapy
  - Nutritional support
  - Nocturnal ventilatory assistance (e.g., constant positive airway pressure [CPAP], pneumobelt, cuirass)
- Specific corrective measures (e.g., reversal of drug-induced central nervous system [CNS] depression, treatment of pulmonary edema)
- Physical therapy interventions (see Chapter 6) as indicated by patient status
  - Postural drainage
  - Bronchial hygiene techniques
  - Breathing exercises
  - Coughing techniques
  - Respiratory muscle training
  - Chest mobility, posture exercises
  - Exercise training

CLINICAL IMPLICATIONS FOR PHYSICAL THERAPY

- Physiologic monitoring during every physical therapy initial evaluation may identify patients with RLD (most of whom will not be diagnosed).
- The more severe the degree of restriction, the more dependent the patient will be on respiratory rate as the only means to increase ventilation.
- Physical therapists should be able to recognize the signs and symptoms of hypoxemia, as well as those of ventilatory muscle fatigue (see page 89).
- The physical therapy treatment program should include the following:
  - Low-level activity initially with gradual progression
  - Periodic rest periods to increase patient tolerance of more vigorous activities
  - Coordination of breathing with activity
  - Techniques to increase pulmonary compliance
    — Breathing exercises
    — Thoracic mobility and posture exercises
    — Soft tissue mobilization (under investigation)
  - Bronchial hygiene techniques if secretion management is a problem
  - Relaxation techniques
  - Creative problem solving in dealing with problem areas
  - Exercise training
    — Respiratory muscle strength and/or endurance training, if appropriate
    — General endurance training
- Relaxation techniques should be incorporated into the patient's lifestyle (see page 221).
- Preventative health measures should be encouraged per page 90.

SOME COMMON DISORDERS THAT RESULT IN RLD

Chest Trauma

Chest trauma commonly causes injuries to the chest wall and lungs. Lung contusion and flail chest are two types of common closed chest trauma. Open chest trauma results in pneumothorax, which is presented on page 95.

PATHOPHYSIOLOGY

- Lung contusion results in localized edema, hemorrhage into the parenchyma, and increased secretion production.

- Parenchymal congestion and additional fluid in the alveoli leads to $\dot{V}/\dot{Q}$ mismatching and hypoxemia, the degree of which is dependent on the extent and severity of injury.
- The inability to maintain adequate oxygenation often necessitates mechanical ventilation.
- Fracture of two or more adjacent ribs in at least two places or separation from the sternum allows for an area of chest wall that is no longer rigid.
  - The severity of the injury depends on the number of ribs that are fractured, as well as flail, and the presence of any lung injury, such as pneumothorax or hemothorax.
  - The negative pressure created by inspiration causes the flail segment to be sucked inward, so the mediastinum shifts to the other side to equalize the pleural pressures and allow both lungs to expand, although not properly. Then during expiration the higher pressure forces the flail area to push out.
  - The result is overall hypoventilation and hypoxemia.
  - Underlying lung contusion further compromises pulmonary function and contributes to the level of respiratory distress that is frequently observed.

CLINICAL MANIFESTATIONS
- Chest pain, especially on inspiration
- Tachypnea
- Respiratory distress
- Hypoxemia with hypercapnia
- Tachycardia

TREATMENT
- Maintain oxygenation (supplemental oxygen, mechanical ventilation)
- Analgesia
- Breathing exercises
- Possible surgery for internal fixation of flail segment
- Extracorporeal membrane oxygenation (ECMO) if all else fails (under investigation)

Adult Respiratory Distress Syndrome

Adult respiratory distress syndrome (ARDS) is a serious clinical syndrome caused by acute lung injury and characterized by severe hypoxemia, increased permeability of the alveolar capillary membrane, pulmonary edema, and atelectasis. Also called noncardiogenic pulmonary edema, shock lung, increased permeability pulmonary edema, and posttraumatic pulmonary insufficiency.

PATHOPHYSIOLOGY
Trauma, sepsis, aspiration, drug overdose, inhaled toxins, shock, massive blood transfusions, pneumonia, and other abnormalities result in:

- Increased permeability of the alveolar capillary membrane leads to increased exudation of fluid and plasma proteins into the interstitial tissue and then into the alveoli, causing marked reductions in lung compliance and all lung volumes and capacities and tremendously increasing the work of breathing, etc., as described on page 90.
- Also, reduced surfactant production along with edema in the interstitial spaces results in significant atelectasis, which exerts increased pressure on the adjacent bronchioles and alveoli and leads to further atelectasis.
- Refer to page 90 for general pathophysiologic features of RLD.
- In addition, edema produces narrowing of the airways, which increases airway resistance causing an obstructive disorder as well.
- ARDS is very difficult to resolve and results in death in 40% to 60% of patients.[5,10,11] However, it may resolve completely with normal pulmonary function in some patients, while others enter a subacute phase following ARDS with alveolar fibrosis and capillary obliteration leading to chronic RLD.

CLINICAL MANIFESTATIONS
- Respiratory distress, tachypnea
- Symmetrical, bilateral, diffuse, fluffy infiltrates on chest x-ray examination
- PO_2 <60 mm Hg, PCO_2 usually increased also
- Decreased breath sounds with wet rales, possible wheezing and rhonchi
- Tachycardia, possible arrhythmias
- Symptoms of hypoxemia (see page 89)
- Possible cyanosis

TREATMENT
- Treat primary cause
- Support adequate gas exchange and tissue

oxygenation (often requires positive end-expiratory pressure [PEEP]; see page 60)
- Support nutritional status and fluid balance
- Prevent and treat complications (nosocomial infections, barotrauma, etc.)

Atelectasis

Atelectasis is characterized by a collapse of alveoli so that they become airless. Atelectasis is most commonly caused by obstruction of an airway (e.g., by mucous or tumor), compression of alveoli (e.g., by pleural effusion, pneumothorax, or marked elevation of the diaphragm), or lack of surfactant.

- Atelectasis occurs only if there is blood flow to the affected alveoli.
- It can involve a localized area of the lung, an entire lobe, or an entire lung.

PATHOPHYSIOLOGY

- Complete obstruction of airway produces entrapment of air within alveoli; then the slow absorption of the gases into the pulmonary capillary blood results in collapse of the alveoli with hypoxic vasoconstriction of that area of the lung to maintain a near normal $\dot{V}/\dot{Q}$ ratio.
- Refer to page 90 for the general pathophysiologic features of restrictive lung dysfunction (RLD).

CLINICAL MANIFESTATIONS

- Few or no symptoms if atelectasis evolves slowly
- If acute collapse of a large section of lung:
  - Profound dyspnea
  - Severe hypoxemia (see page 89)
  - Tracheal and mediastinal shift toward the affected side, with elevated diaphragm, as demonstrated in Figure 3–7.

TREATMENT

- Removal of obstruction
  - Bronchoscopic or surgical removal of aspirated foreign object
  - Excision of tumor
  - Vigorous chest percussion and vibration to mobilize mucous obstructions
- Treatment of underlying disorder if not obstructive atelectasis
  - Chest tube insertion for pneumothorax

- Pleurocentesis for drainage of pleural effusion
- Deep breathing exercises (segmental expansion, diaphragmatic), increased mobility

Interstitial Pulmonary Fibrosis

Fibrosis results from the tissue repair process that follows any disease involving inflammation or necrosis of tissue. In addition, pulmonary fibrosis is often idiopathic, possibly due to viral, genetic, or immune-mediated disorders. The distribution of fibrous tissue in the lungs varies in different disease processes, and the resulting scar tissue may be confined to a small segment or lobe of a lung, or disseminated throughout one or both lungs.

PATHOPHYSIOLOGY

Pulmonary fibrosis results in:

- Reduced lung compliance, which increases the work of breathing and contributes to $\dot{V}/\dot{Q}$ mismatching, etc., as described on page 90.
- Impaired diffusion of oxygen across the alveolar-capillary membrane leads to hypoxemia with or without hypercapnia, which eventually creates the potential for cor pulmonale (see page 99)

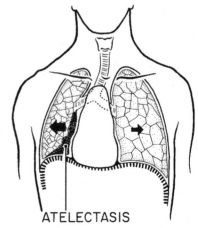

ATELECTASIS

FIGURE 3–7. A diagram showing atelectasis with elevated hemidiaphragm and mediastinal shift toward the affected side. (From Cherniack RM, Cherniack L: *Respiration in Health and Disease,* 3rd Ed. Philadelphia, W.B. Saunders Co., p. 175, 1983. Used with permission.)

- Possible eventual respiratory failure as described on page 98

CLINICAL MANIFESTATIONS

- Insidious or acute onset dyspnea on exertion (DOE), which may progress to resting dyspnea
- Possible repetitive, nonproductive cough
- Fatigue
- Loss of appetite, weight loss
- Tachypnea
- Diffuse reticulonodular pattern in involved areas on chest x-ray examination, or results may be normal
- Decreased P_{O_2}, during exercise initially, later at rest; usually normal P_{CO_2}
- Bibasilar end-inspiratory rales, possible decreased breath sounds on auscultation
- Possible cyanosis late in disease
- Digital clubbing
- Possible signs and symptoms of cor pulmonale and/or respiratory failure (see page 99)

Pneumonia

An inflammatory process of the lung parenchyma, as a result of infection (e.g., bacterial, viral, protozoal, mycoplasmas, psittacosis) in the lower respiratory tract can cause some or all of the alveoli to be filled with fluid and blood cells (i.e., pneumonia). Conditions associated with an increased risk of developing pneumonia include chronic airway obstruction, pulmonary edema, unconsciousness, and compromised immune status.

PATHOPHYSIOLOGY

- Bacterial infection results in inflammation and increased porosity of the pulmonary membranes so that there is an outpouring of edema fluid as well as capillary fluid and blood cells into the alveoli; this extends the infection to the adjacent alveoli, causing consolidation of an area of lung (Fig. 3–8); surface area for gas exchange is reduced, leading to $\dot{V}/\dot{Q}$ mismatching and decreasing diffusing capacity with resultant hypoxemia and hypercapnia. Resolution occurs via phagocytosis by polymorphonuclear leukocytes, and then deposition of fibrin in the inflamed area.
- Viral infection results in destruction of the cilia and mucosal surface of the respiratory epithelial cells and loss of mucociliary function, which increases the risk of bacterial in-

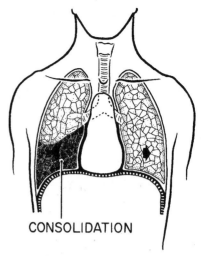

CONSOLIDATION

FIGURE 3–8. A diagram showing pneumonia with consolidation of the right lower lobe. Because the alveolar air is replaced by exudate, there is little, if any, change in the size of the affected lung. (From Cherniack RM, Cherniack L: *Respiration in Health and Disease,* 3rd Ed. Philadelphia, W.B. Saunders Co., p. 176, 1983. Used with permission.)

fection; viral infection reaching the alveoli results in possible edema, hemorrhage, hyaline membrane formation, and even ARDS.
- Refer to page 90 for the general pathophysiologic features of RLD.

CLINICAL MANIFESTATIONS

- Pleuritic chest pain or chest discomfort
- Cough, possibly productive
- Dyspnea
- Fever, possibly shaking chills
- Other constitutional symptoms (e.g., fatigue, weakness, malaise, coryza, headache, pharyngitis)
- Antecedent upper respiratory infection
- Signs or symptoms of hypoxemia (see page 89)
- Moist crackles versus signs of pulmonary consolidation
- Infiltrates or dense consolidation on chest radiograph
- Increased white blood cell count

TREATMENT

- Appropriate antimicrobial therapy
- Deep breathing and cough, bronchial drain-

age, percussion and vibration if patient's cough is productive
- Supportive measures (e.g., oxygen, replacement of fluids)

Pleural Effusion

The accumulation of fluid within the pleural space causes a pleural effusion.

- The fluid may be a transudate (e.g., CHF, hepatic cirrhosis, renal disease, hypoproteinemia, myxedema, and pulmonary embolus), which results from increased hydrostatic pressure within the pleural capillaries; or
- The fluid may be an exudate (e.g., infection, pleural malignancy, pulmonary embolism or infarction, acute pancreatitis, drug toxicity, and immune-mediated diseases, such as rheumatoid arthritis, systemic lupus erythematosis, sarcoidosis), which is caused by increased permeability of the pleural surfaces so that protein and excess fluid move into the pleural space.
- When the pleural fluid is grossly purulent or contains pyogenic organisms, it is called an *empyema.*

PATHOPHYSIOLOGY

The degree of functional impairment depends on the size of the pleural effusion.

- Increased pleural fluid results in compression of the underlying lung tissue, leading to atelectasis, which reduces lung compliance and increases the work of breathing, and so on, as described on page 98.
- The increased pressure caused by the accumulating fluid results in mediastinal shift away from the affected side (see Fig. 3–9).
- If perfusion is normal, there will be a shunt-like venous admixture and $\dot{V}/\dot{Q}$ mismatching, which causes hypoxemia, but P_{CO_2} will remain normal because of hyperventilation of the remaining alveoli.
- Refer to page 90 for the general pathophysiologic features of RLD.

CLINICAL MANIFESTATIONS

The severity of symptoms depends on the rate of fluid accumulation more than the size of the pleural effusion.

- Possibly asymptomatic versus

- Dyspnea
- Chest discomfort (varying from a dull ache to excruciatingly severe, sharp, stabbing pain) aggravated by deep inspiration or coughing
- Possible fever, shaking chills, night sweats
- Decreased or absent breath sounds, decreased or absent vocal fremitus; possible bronchial breath sounds and whispered pectoriloquy at upper level of effusion, especially if there is compression of lung tissue overlying a patent bronchus
- Decreased resonance to percussion

TREATMENT

- Observe for natural reabsorption
- Segmental expansion and diaphragmatic breathing exercises to prevent underlying atelectasis; increased mobility
- Thoracentesis

Pneumothorax

The presence of air or gas in the pleural space creates a pneumothorax, which occurs via disruption of either the visceral or parietal pleura (e.g., chest wall trauma, bronchopleural fistula, rupture of subpleural bleb, spontaneous rupture of alveoli or an infected abscess, gas-producing anaerobic organisms in the pleural space, or iatrogenic trauma).

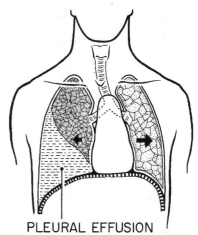

PLEURAL EFFUSION

FIGURE 3–9. A diagram showing a large right pleural effusion with marked compressive atelectasis and mediastinal shift away from the affected side. (From Cherniack RM, Cherniack L: *Respiration in Health and Disease,* 3rd Ed. Philadelphia, W.B. Saunders Co., p. 176, 1983. Used with permission.)

PATHOPHYSIOLOGY

The degree of functional impairment depends on the size of the pneumothorax.

- Air in the pleural space abolishes negative intrapleural pressure and results in the collapse of the underlying lung, causing decreased TLC, vital capacity, and residual volume and creating a shunt-like venous admixture with $\dot{V}/\dot{Q}$ mismatching and resultant early hypoxemia; later, blood is diverted away from the involved lung, and $\dot{V}/\dot{Q}$ matching is improved so there is less hypoxemia.
- In addition, accumulation of air in a hemithorax increases the pressure/tension on the mediastinum, causing it to shift away from the side of pneumothorax.
- If paradoxical chest movement develops, there is shunting of air back and forth between the normal and collapsed lung, which produces increased physiologic dead space.
- In severe cases there will be alveolar hypoventilation with hypoxemia and hypercapnia.
- In a tension pneumothorax, air leaks into the pleural space during inspiration but cannot exit during expiration, resulting in progressive increased positive pleural pressure. Eventually there is complete collapse of the lung with mediastinal shift to the contralateral side, which interferes with venous return to the heart and causes reduced cardiac output, tachycardia, and shock.
- Refer to page 90 for the general pathophysiologic features of RLD.

CLINICAL MANIFESTATIONS

The severity of symptoms depends on the size of the pneumothorax and the degree of collapse of the underlying lung. When there are symptoms, they are abrupt in onset.

- Asymptomatic with no abnormal physical findings if pneumothorax is small; otherwise
- Marked unilateral chest pain
- Respiratory distress, marked if large pneumothorax
- Irritated cough
- Cyanosis
- Cold, clammy skin
- Rapid thready pulse
- Low blood pressure
- Decreased or no movement of hemithorax

- Deviation of mediastinum toward contralateral side
- Hyperresonance on percussion
- Decreased or inaudible breath sounds with decreased or absent vocal fremitus
- Chest x-ray film showing denser-appearing underlying lung tissue; thin, fine line at periphery; and uniform translucency with complete absence of lung markings in area of pneumothorax; possible overexpansion of the affected rib cage with flattening of the hemidiaphragm if pneumothorax is large

TREATMENT

- Observation (i.e., allow natural reabsorption) if small
- Air aspiration
- Chest tube insertion (see page 63)
- Segmental expansion breathing exercises

Pulmonary Emboli and Infarction

An embolus causing occlusion of blood flow through a pulmonary artery can arise from the right side of the heart, a venous thrombosis (e.g., from a lower extremity, upper extremity, or pelvic region), or nonthrombotic materials (e.g., amniotic fluid, fat, air, bone spicules, and fragments of organs).

FACTORS ASSOCIATED WITH INCREASED RISK OF VENOUS THROMBOSIS

- Prolonged bedrest, especially if there is cardiac disease, CHF, lower extremity fracture, limb paralysis, or multiple trauma
- Postoperative state
- Pregnancy
- Oral contraceptive use
- Varicose veins
- Carcinoma
- Obesity
- Cardiac valve dysfunction or prosthetic replacement
- Polycythemia vera or other blood diseases
- Sickle cell disease

PATHOPHYSIOLOGY

The severity of the hemodynamic and respiratory alterations depends on the size of the embolus and the previous cardiopulmonary status. Occlusion of a small pulmonary artery may go unnoticed, but larger emboli can result in:

- Severe pulmonary hypertension, increased systemic pressure, distension of the RA and RV and engorgement of the peripheral veins, and decreased cardiac output
- Death versus gradual resolution of pulmonary hypertension with increasing LV output
- Pulmonary infarction, especially if there is CHF, compromised bronchial circulation, alveolar hypoventilation, or pulmonary infection
- Refer to page 90 for the general pathophysiologic features of RLD.

CLINICAL MANIFESTATIONS

- Acute dyspnea
- Chest pain
- Unexplained vascular collapse or syncope
- Rapid feeble pulse
- Hypotension
- Signs of cerebral ischemia
- Accentuated P_2 (pulmonary component of second heart sound) with decreased physiologic splitting
- Prominent a wave in the jugular pulse
- Positive $\dot{V}/\dot{Q}$ scan (see Fig. 2–8, page 46)

TREATMENT

- Supportive therapy (e.g., supplemental oxygen, analgesics, vasoactive drugs)
- Prevention of further embolization
- Surgical embolectomy if massive PE
- Once stable, deep breathing exercises with prolonged expiration

Pulmonary Edema (Cardiogenic)

Flooding of the pulmonary interstitial space and alveoli by transudative fluid from the pulmonary capillaries commonly results from elevated left heart pressures reflected back to the lungs.

PATHOPHYSIOLOGY

- As the LV fails, SV and cardiac output decrease leading to increased LA pressure and increased impedance to blood flow through the pulmonary vessels, which causes pulmonary capillary pressure to rise; if the pulmonary pressure becomes high enough, fluid will transudate into the interstitial space, causing flooding of the alveoli and pleural space (i.e., pleural effusions) and resulting in dramatically reduced lung compliance, increased $\dot{V}/\dot{Q}$ mismatching, increased airway resistance, impaired gas exchange, and increased work of breathing, and so on, as described on page 90.

- Reduced peripheral tissue perfusion due to poor cardiac output results in significant tissue hypoxia and lactic acidosis.

CLINICAL MANIFESTATIONS

See LV failure on page 73.

TREATMENT

The treatment of pulmonary edema/CHF is listed on page 74.

OTHER CAUSES OF RLD

- Neurologic and neuromuscular disorders (e.g., spinal cord injury, amyotrophic lateral sclerosis, Guillain-Barré syndrome, polio, myasthenia gravis, muscular dystrophy, cerebrovascular accident, diaphragmatic paralysis) (see page 106)
- Collagen vascular and connective tissue disorders (e.g., ankylosing spondylitis, rheumatoid arthritis, systemic lupus erythematosus, polymyositis, progressive systemic sclerosis/scleroderma) (see page 106)
- Occupational lung disease (see page 88)
- Infant respiratory distress syndrome, bronchopulmonary dysplasia (see Chapter 7)
- Others (e.g., sarcoidosis, obesity, ascites, diabetes mellitus, trauma, surgery, CNS depression by drugs, thoracic deformities, drug or radiation toxicity)

COMBINED RESTRICTIVE AND OBSTRUCTIVE DEFECTS

Patients sometimes have more than one cardiopulmonary disorder, which may result in a clinical picture consistent with both restrictive and obstructive abnormalities; for example, a patient with emphysema and CHF or an obese patient with asthma. In addition, some pulmonary disorders may produce combined defects, as in bronchiolitis obliterans, presented below.

BRONCHIOLITIS OBLITERANS

Bronchiolitis obliterans is a fibrotic disease affecting the smaller airways, which is characterized by necrosis of the respiratory epithelium in the affected bronchioles.

Pathophysiology

Severe respiratory infections, particularly in childhood, recurrent aspiration, exposure to toxic fumes or inorganic dusts, extrinsic allergic alveolitis, viral infection, connective tissue disorders, or following bone marrow, heart, or heart-lung transplantation can result in:

- Epithelial necrosis leads to the entry of fluid and debris into bronchioles and alveoli, which causes pulmonary edema as well as partial or complete obstruction of the small airways.
- If there is complete obstruction, the gradual absorption of trapped air will produce atelectasis.
- If the disease is severe or widespread, a significant inflammatory response may develop with resultant bronchiolar and alveolar fibrosis, which leads to $\dot{V}/\dot{Q}$ mismatching, decreased lung compliance (restrictive lung dysfunction), impaired gas exchange, and chronic obstructive ventilatory defects in many patients.

Clinical Manifestations
- Cough, possibly productive
- Dyspnea
- Wheezing
- Tachypnea
- Intercostal retractions
- Possible fever
- Possible restrictive and obstructive defects shown on PFTs, or one of these defects may dominate

Treatment
- Prevention
- Possible response to steroids if treated early

PULMONARY HYPERTENSION

When pulmonary arterial pressure exceeds 30/15 mm Hg, pulmonary hypertension (HTN) exists. Pulmonary HTN can result from chronic pulmonary disease, impedance to pulmonary blood flow (e.g., mitral stenosis), obstruction or obliteration of the pulmonary vasculature (e.g., acute PE, pulmonary fibrosis, emphysema, kyphoscoliosis), active pulmonary vasoconstriction (e.g, primary pulmonary HTN), LV failure (e.g., systemic HTN, ischemic heart disease, cardiomyopathy), or increased pulmonary blood flow (e.g., ventricular septal defect, patent ductus arteriosus).

PATHOPHYSIOLOGY

Increased pulmonary arterial pressure creates a pressure load on the RV, which responds with RV hypertrophy (RVH) with or without dilatation; eventually, RV failure can develop, which is referred to as cor pulmonale if it develops as a result of chronic or acute pulmonary disease.

CLINICAL MANIFESTATIONS
- Dyspnea on exertion
- Weakness, fatigue
- Possible palpitations
- Exertional chest pain
- Possible syncopal episodes
- Hemoptysis
- Possible signs and symptoms of right heart failure (see page 74)
- Loud P_2 (pulmonary component of second heart sound) with increased physiologic splitting, possible murmur of tricuspid regurgitation
- Chest x-ray findings of RVH, bulging PA, and prominent hilar vessels with normal or increased intrapulmonary vascular markings

TREATMENT
- Supplemental oxygen (see page 57)
- Vasoactive drugs (see Chapter 4)
- Specific treatment for underlying disease
- Heart-lung transplantation (see page 30)

CARDIORESPIRATORY FAILURE

Severe acute pulmonary dysfunction and chronic obstructive and restrictive lung diseases can result in respiratory failure, cor pulmonale, or both.

RESPIRATORY FAILURE

A defect in pulmonary gas exchange leading to severe hypoxemia with or without hypercapnia is called respiratory failure.

- Hypoxemia without hypercapnia occurs when there is failure of oxygenation but hyperventilation of functional alveoli is able to eliminate excess carbon dioxide (due to its greater ease of diffusion), as in the early stages of COPD and some forms of RLD or an acute asthmatic attack
- Hypercapnic respiratory failure, or sometimes referred to as ventilatory failure, develops when there is true alveolar hypoventilation, causing poor gas exchange.

- Respiratory failure can be acute or chronic in nature.

Pathophysiology

- Hypoxemia results in the activation of numerous compensatory mechanisms in an attempt to improve tissue oxygenation (e.g., hypoxic vasoconstriction, use of accessory muscles of respiration, elevated HR, increased arteriovenous oxygen extraction); when these fail, respiratory failure is present.[41]
- Hypercapnia leads to hyperventilation in an attempt to eliminate excess carbon dioxide; when either respiratory chemoreceptor insensitivity to hypercapnia or respiratory muscle fatigue develop, P_{CO_2} will progressively rise, producing severe dyspnea, then lethargy, followed by semicoma, anesthesia, and death.

Clinical Manifestations

- Signs and symptoms of hypoxemia (see Table 3–5, page 89)
- Signs and symptoms of ventilatory muscle fatigue (see Table 3–6, page 89)
- Signs and symptoms of underlying disease or disorder

Treatment

- Ventilatory support (e.g., oxygen supplementation, mechanical ventilation)
- Treatment of cause if acute

COR PULMONALE

Right heart failure due to chronic or acute pulmonary disease is called cor pulmonale. Cor pulmonale most commonly results from COPD, but other causes include any RLD, primary pulmonary arterial disease, thrombotic disorders (e.g., sickle cell disease), embolic disorders, pulmonary resection, high-altitude disease, and congenital developmental defects.

Pathophysiology

RV failure is presented on page 73.

Clinical Manifestations

The signs and symptoms of RV failure/cor pulmonale are listed on page 74. Also the reader should refer to the causative diagnosis.

Treatment

- Treat underlying cause (e.g., PE, acute infection in COPD)

- Supportive therapy (e.g., oxygen, vasoactive drugs, mechanical ventilation)
- Heart-lung transplantation if chronic

LUNG CANCER

Lung cancer results from a malignant neoplasm that starts in the lung tissue. Most primary lung cancers originate from the bronchial mucosa and are referred to as bronchogenic carcinoma. Malignant tumors in the lungs can also be metastatic.

PATHOPHYSIOLOGY

- Obstruction or compression of bronchi results in atelectasis, pneumonia, and/or lung abscess.
- Obstruction or compression of blood vessels causes $\dot{V}/\dot{Q}$ abnormalities and sometimes a superior vena cava syndrome.
- Compression of nerves causes pain.
- Involvement of the pleura produces pleural effusion.
- Metastasis often leads to chest wall pain, with resultant hypoventilation.

CLINICAL MANIFESTATIONS

Most patients with lung cancer experience a prolonged period without symptoms. When symptoms do develop, they are frequently nonspecific and vary depending on location, size, rapidity of growth, cell type, and presence of underlying pulmonary disease. They may include:

- Cough
- Dyspnea
- Hemoptysis
- Chest pain
- Wheezing
- Dysphagia
- Weight loss
- Anorexia
- Weakness, fatigue
- Bone and joint pain
- Edema of face and upper extremities
- Hoarseness
- Neurologic symptoms

TREATMENT

- Surgical resection
- Chemotherapy
- Radiation therapy
  - Curative
  - Palliative

3.3 CARDIOPULMONARY COMPLICATIONS OF OTHER DISEASES AND DISORDERS

Cardiac and/or pulmonary dysfunction may also develop in association with other systemic diseases and various other disorders, as summarized in Tables 3–7 and 3–8. These include disorders of the pericardium (e.g., pericarditis and pericardial effusion), myocardium (e.g., cardiomyopathy, myocarditis), endocardium/valves (e.g., valvular inflammation or dysfunction), coronary arteries (e.g., atherosclerosis, coronary ischemia, vasculitis), and electrocardiographic abnormalities (e.g., arrhythmias, conduction disturbances, ST-T changes). Common pulmonary manifestations include pleural effusion, infection, pneumonitis, vasculitis, and respiratory muscle dysfunction. A more complete presentation of these diseases and their cardiopulmonary effects is beyond the scope of this book but can be found elsewhere.[82]

DIABETES MELLITUS

Diabetes mellitus (DM) is a chronic metabolic disease characterized by hyperglycemia, which results from inadequate or absent insulin production (type I DM, or insulin dependent, IDMM) or insulin resistance at the cellular level

TABLE 3–7. **Cardiac Abnormalities Associated with Other Diseases**

DISEASE/DISORDER	PL	M	E/V	CA	ECG	COMMENTS
Diabetes mellitus	−	+	−	+ +	+	HTN is common, "silent" myocardial ischemia and infarction, ↑ CHF, autonomic dysfunction.
Chronic renal failure	+	+	−	+ +	+	HTN is common, ↑ CHF.
Obesity	−	+	−	+	+	HTN is common, ↑ CHF.
Peripheral vascular disease	−	+	−	+ +	+	Since ↑ atherosclerosis, CAD and cerebrovascular disease are likely.
Collagen vascular diseases						
Rheumatoid arthritis	+ +	+	+	+	+	Usually not clinically significant.
Systemic lupus erythematosus	+ +	+/−	+ +	+	+/−	HTN is common, ↑ CHF.
Polyarteritis nodosa	+	+ +	−	+ +	+	HTN is common, ↑ CHF.
Ankylosing spondylitis	−	+/−	+ +	−	+	Sclerosing inflammatory lesions of AoV
Progressive systemic sclerosis	+	+ +	−	+ +	+	HTN is common, ↑ CHF.
Marfan's syndrome	−	−	+ +	+	−	Aortic dissection is common.
Neurologic and neuromuscular disorders						
Cerebrovascular accident	−	−	−	+ +	+	If due to atherosclerosis.
Myasthenia gravis	−	+	−	−	+	Rare CHF.
Muscular dystrophy	−	+ +	−	−	+ +	Especially Duschenne's.
Friedreich's ataxia	−	−	−	+	+	↑ CHF.
Sickle cell disease	−	+	−	+ +	+/−	Cardiomegaly, arteritis, ischemia.
Cancer (sequelae to treatment)						
Radiotherapy to the chest	+ +	+	+/−	+	+	Varies with treatment techniques.
Chemotherapy	+ +	+	−	+	+	Varies with specific agents.
Bone marrow transplantation	−	+/−	−	−	+ +	Varies with chemotherapeutic agents employed.

PL = pericardial, M = myocardial, E/V = endocardial/valvular, CA = coronary arteries, ECG = electrocardiographic changes, arrhythmias, conduction disturbances, HTN = hypertension, CHF = congestive heart failure, CAD = coronary artery disease, AoV = aortic valve, + = convincing association, + + = common occurrence, +/− = possible association, − = no documented association.

(type II DM, or noninsulin dependent, NIDDM). The major actions of insulin are the inhibition of glucose production by the liver and the promotion of glucose metabolism within the cells. Insulin is also important for the synthesis of glycogen, fat, and protein; a deficiency of insulin results in an inability to use glucose as fuel and increases lipolysis of stored fat (triglycerides) with the mobilization of free fatty acids for use as fuel.

TABLE 3–8. **Pulmonary Abnormalities Associated with Other Diseases**

DISEASE/DISORDER	PL	P	I	V	MM	COMMENTS
Diabetes mellitus	−	+	−	+	−	Sleep related breathing problems
Chronic renal failure	+	+	−	−	+/−	Fluid overload, immunosuppression
Obesity	−	−	−	−	+/−	Sleep apnea, obesity hypoventilation syndrome
Peripheral vascular disease	−	+	−	−	−	↑ Incidence of COPD
Collagen vascular diseases						
Rheumatoid arthritis	++	+	+	+/−	−	RLD, rare intrapulmonary nodules
Systemic lupus erythematosus	++	+	+	+/−	+	RLD, possible hypoxemia
Polyarteritis nodosa	−	−	−	+/−	−	Pulmonary problems only if allergic angiitis or granulomatosis
Ankylosing spondylitis	−	+/−	+	−	−	Ankylosing of thoracic cage, RLD
Progressive systemic sclerosis	++	+	+	++	−	RLD, pulmonary hypertension
Neurologic and neuromuscular disorders						
Hemiplegia cerebrovascular accident	−	−	+/−	−	++	Weakness or spastic paralysis, RLD
Spinal cord injury	−	−	+	−	++	Weakness or paralysis corresponding to level of lesion, RLD
Parkinson's disease	−	−	+/−	−	++	Dyskinetic breathing, possible OD
Amyotrophic lateral sclerosis	−	−	++	−	++	Bulbar paralysis, possible OD
Guillain-Barré syndrome	−	−	+	−	++	Temporary paralysis, RLD
Myasthenia gravis	−	−	+	−	++	RLD, possible respiratory failure
Muscular dystrophy	−	−	+	−	++	Chronic alveolar hypoventilation, RLD, eventual respiratory failure
Friedreich's ataxia	−	+	+/−	−	+	Scoliosis, chest deformity, possible cor pulmonale
Sickle cell disease	−	−	++	++	−	Pulmonary thrombosis
Cancer (sequelae to treatment)						
Radiotherapy to the chest	−	+	+	+/−	−	Radiation pneumonitis, fibrosis, RLD
Chemotherapy	−	+	+	−	−	IP with many agents, RLD
Bone marrow transplantation	−	++	++	−	−	Possible IP, GVHD, RLD, OD

COPD = chronic obstructive pulmonary disease, PL = pleural, P = parenchymal, I = interstitial, V = vascular, MM = respiratory muscles, RLD = restrictive lung dysfunction, OD = obstructive disease, IP = interstitial pneumonitis, GVHD = graft-versus-host disease, + = convincing association, ++ = common occurrence, +/− = possible association, − = no documented association.

- The treatment of DM is aimed at controlling hyperglycemia and thus minimizing the secondary problems associated with the disease. Individualized according to patient disease and metabolic status, treatment may include education, diet modification, insulin, oral hypoglycemic agents, and exercise. Refer to Chapter 4 for information on insulin and the hypoglycemic agents (see page 142).
- Exercise is important, particularly in the treatment of type II DM, because it elicits an increased sensitivity and responsiveness of the peripheral tissues to insulin. These alterations compensate for the exercise-induced reduction in insulin secretion and increment in counterregulatory hormone secretion. Secretion of the counterregulatory hormones, particularly glucagon, results in enhanced hepatic glucose production and mobilization of muscle glycogen and free fatty acids.
- The primary problem associated with insulin therapy, and to a lesser degree the hypoglycemic agents, is hypoglycemia, which becomes a greater risk during or following exercise. In type I DM, the metabolic responses to activity are influenced by the level of insulin at the onset of exertion.
  - Commonly, an excess of insulin exists at the onset of exercise (see Fig. 4–3), which inhibits hepatic glucose production and thus promotes the development of hypoglycemia. Factors associated with exercise-induced hypoglycemia include inadequate food intake preceding exercise, rapid absorption of depot insulin from an injection site near exercising muscle, and exercising at the time of peak insulin effect.
  - However, when there is an insulin deficiency with marked hyperglycemia at the onset of exercise, glucose uptake by the exercising muscle is impaired, and the additional glucose being produced by the liver (which exceeds peripheral utilization) results in even greater hyperglycemia. In addition, the excessive mobilization of free fatty acids may lead to accelerated ketogenesis and ketoacidosis, which can lead to coma and death.

CARDIOPULMONARY COMPLICATIONS OF DM

Morbidity and mortality are directly related to the level of blood glucose control and usually entail blood vessel abnormalities (angiopathies), as well as peripheral and autonomic neuropathies. Abnormalities of the small blood vessels (microangiopathies caused by thickening and/or damage to the basement capillary membrane) result in retinopathy (leading to blindness) and nephropathy (causing renal failure), whereas those involving the large vessels (macroangiopathies due to atherosclerosis) produce coronary artery, cerebrovascular, and peripheral vascular disease.[55,60] The combination of peripheral neuropathy and atherosclerotic occlusive disease leads to the prevalence of lower extremity tissue necrosis and infection, and sometimes amputation.

- Cardiovascular disease is the major cause of death in patients with DM.[47,54]
  - Hypertension (HTN) is approximately twice as prevalent in diabetic persons and accelerates both the microvascular and macrovascular complications associated with DM.
  - CAD is more prevalent in diabetic patients, although it often presents atypically. Myocardial ischemia and infarction may occur "silently," that is, with little or no discomfort; or ischemia may be manifested as shortness of breath or fatigue that comes on with exertion and resolves immediately with rest (i.e., angina equivalents).
  - Mortality resulting from acute MI is two to three times higher in diabetic persons than nondiabetic persons and results from arrhythmias or pump failure.
  - CHF is common later in the disease and may result from CAD, HTN, or a diabetic cardiomyopathy.
- Pulmonary disorders associated with DM include a higher incidence of pulmonary infections and sleep-related breathing problems. In addition, diabetic ketoacidosis is related to hyperventilation, pneumomediastinum, and mucous plugging of the major airways.

IMPLICATIONS FOR PHYSICAL THERAPY INTERVENTION

Because of the prevalence of cardiovascular complications in DM and the abnormal metabolic responses to exercise, caution is required in providing physical therapy treatment to patients with DM. The following recommendations are offered:

- Physiologic monitoring of heart rate (HR), blood pressure (BP), and signs and symptoms should be included in all physical therapy evaluations and may be indicated during treatment sessions if abnormalities are noted. In addition, blood glucose monitoring before, during, and after exercise may be helpful, especially initially.
  - Resting HRs are often elevated in diabetic patients with autonomic dysfunction, although their responses to standing, deep breathing, and the Valsalva maneuver are minimal and those to exercise are blunted.[70,80]
  - A drop in BP of >20 mm Hg diastolic or >30 mm Hg systolic when a patient quickly moves from supine to standing is indicative of autonomic dysfunction.
  - Patients without autonomic dysfunction often have hypertensive BP responses to exercise but are hypotensive following exercise.
- Therapists should take precautions to avoid exercise-induced hypoglycemia:
  - Avoid scheduling appointments at the time of peak insulin effect or have the patient eat a carbohydrate snack 30 minutes before exercising.
  - Start with moderate workloads and increase intensity gradually.
  - Use a consistent pattern of exercise (time of day, duration, and intensity)
  - Make sure the patient uses an injection site away from exercising muscle.
  - Know the signs and symptoms of hypoglycemia (Table 3–9).
  - Have 5 to 10-g carbohydrate snacks, such as orange juice or a candy bar, available for each 30 to 45 minutes of exercise.
- When blood glucose levels are high prior to therapy, adjustments in treatment are indicated:[26,58]
  - If blood glucose is 250 to 300 mg/dL, the patient should not perform any vigorous or prolonged exercise.
  - If values are >300 mg/dL, the patient should not perform any exercise.
- Because diabetics, especially those with type I DM, tend to have blunted HR responses to exercise and engage anaerobic metabolism at lower HRs. Exercise HRs should not exceed 50% to 60% of the predicted maximum unless the patient has a good level of physical fitness.[28]
- Exercise for control of blood sugar and weight in type II DM should be of longer duration (45 minutes) and only moderate intensity (50% to 60% of maximal HR).
- Special attention should be directed toward maintaining adequate fluid replacement and taking proper care of feet, including good footwear, careful hygiene, and daily inspection.
- Patients should be counseled to *never* exercise alone, because of the potential for hypoglycemia.

RENAL FAILURE

Renal failure results in the accumulation of water, crystalloid solutes, and waste products, which leads to altered electrolyte and acid-base balances, gastrointestinal distress, severe anemia, and multiple other abnormalities involving the skin and the respiratory, cardiovascular, neurologic, musculoskeletal, endocrine, genitourinary, and immune systems.

- The treatment options for patients with chronic renal failure (CRF) include conservative management of symptoms, dialysis, and transplantation.

TABLE 3-9. **Signs and Symptoms of Hypoglycemia**

ADRENERGIC*	NEUROGLUCOPENIC†
Weakness	Headache
Sweating	Hypothermia
Tachycardia	Visual disturbances
Palpitations	Mental dullness
Tremor	Confusion
Nervousness	Amnesia
Irritability	Seizures
Tingling of mouth and fingers	Coma
Hunger	
Nausea‡	
Vomiting‡	

*Caused by increased activity of the autonomic nervous system.
†Caused by decreased activity of the central nervous system.
‡Unusual.

- Because the clearance of metabolic waste products and other substances by the kidneys remains superior to that achieved by dialysis until renal function deteriorates to 10% to 20% of normal, conservative management (e.g., control of diet, fluid balance, BP, mineral metabolism, and symptoms of uremia) is employed as long as possible.
- When the symptoms or complications of CRF become unacceptable, dialysis is indicated and most commonly accomplished using hemodialysis or continuous ambulatory peritoneal dialysis (CAPD). However, dialysis fails to adequately provide the regulatory and endocrine functions normally afforded by the kidneys and is associated with renal osteodystrophy, anemia, vascular access infections and thromboses, pericarditis, and ascites.
- Therefore, the treatment of choice, particularly in younger patients, is kidney transplantation. It offers the best opportunity for normalization of renal function and lifestyle.

CARDIOPULMONARY COMPLICATIONS OF CRF

Several cardiopulmonary complications are seen in CRF.

- The cardiovascular complications associated with CRF include hypertension, pericarditis with pericardial effusion, accelerated atherosclerosis, and CHF.[63,77]
  - Hypertension is both a cause and a consequence of renal disease and greatly aggravates renal dysfunction in CRF.
  - Pericarditis and pericardial effusion occasionally produces cardiac tamponade (diminished cardiac output resulting from impaired filling resulting from excessive fluid in the pericardial sack).
  - Accelerated atherosclerosis is related to both HTN and the hyperlipidemia seen in CRF.
  - Heart failure can develop as a result of fluid overload, HTN and/or ASHD.
- Pulmonary abnormalities are also observed in patients with renal failure.
  - Fluid overload, hypoalbuminemia, and capillary damage can result in pulmonary edema, whereas impaired immune status is responsible for pulmonary infections and secondary hyperparathyroidism may lead to pulmonary calcification.
- In addition, the treatment of renal failure is frequently associated with pulmonary complications: hypoxemia is seen with hemodialysis; pleural effusions and an elevated diaphragm are common with peritoneal dialysis; and opportunistic pulmonary infections may develop in transplant patients because of immunosuppression.

CLINICAL IMPLICATIONS FOR PHYSICAL THERAPY

Patients with CRF are usually very debilitated and tolerate exercise poorly. However, carefully monitored exercise training can increase physical work capacity and offers numerous other benefits as well: improved lipid profiles, enhanced BP control, normalization of insulin sensitivity and glucose metabolism, increased red blood cell mass, increased muscle strength, and improvements in mood, level of depression, and psychosocial functioning. Important considerations include:

- Compliance with exercise programs is increased if the sessions are scheduled on dialysis days; exercise has been safely performed (in limited patients) before, during, and after dialysis.[32,38,64,69,73]
- Physiologic monitoring is critical, especially in dialysis patients, whose fluid volume status and electrolyte balance varies tremendously from day to day, and in transplant patients, who frequently develop HTN as a side effect of their immunosuppressive drugs.[71]
- Exercise intensity should be low initially, and the workout should be performed in short intervals with frequent brief (1 to 2 minute) rests as needed.
- The exercise intervals should increase gradually with decreasing number of rest periods; the eventual goal is 30 to 45 minutes of continuous exercise.
- Aerobic activities, particularly those that are non-weight-bearing, are recommended.
- A rating of perceived exertion (RPE) scale (see page 172) may be more consistent than HR levels for monitoring exercise intensity.

OBESITY

Obesity is defined as an accumulation of adipose tissue so that body mass index (BMI) is greater than 30 kg/m² or body fat exceeds 25% for males or 30% for females. An increasing problem in the United States, obesity is associated with a number of complications, including cardiovascular disease, osteoarthritis, gastrointestinal problems, endometrial and breast cancers, glucose intolerance, type II DM, and pulmonary dysfunction.

CARDIOPULMONARY COMPLICATIONS

The major complications associated with obesity are cardiovascular, though there may also be pulmonary dysfunction.

- The cardiovascular complications associated with obesity include HTN, atherosclerotic heart disease (ASHD) (probably due to the increased incidence of HTN, hyperlipidemia, and glucose intolerance), CHF (caused by LVH, which results from the increment in blood volume, SV, cardiac output, and filling pressures required to meet the metabolic needs of the excessive adipose tissue), and a cardiomyopathy of obesity.[52]
- Obesity, especially if massive, causes a restriction to thoracic expansion because of the additional weight loading the chest wall and resisting diaphragmatic descent during inspiration. In addition, sleep apnea may be exhibited, particularly in moderately to severely obese males, aged 40 to 60 years, causing hypersomnolence during the day and sleep apnea at night. Finally, about 5% of massively obese individuals develop the obesity hypoventilation syndrome with characteristic hypoxemia, hypercapnia, cyanosis, polycythemia, and somnolence. The resulting biventricular hypertrophy eventually progresses to pulmonary and systemic congestion.

CLINICAL IMPLICATIONS FOR PHYSICAL THERAPY

When prescribing exercise for obese individuals, the physical therapist needs to consider some specific factors to maximize safety and effectiveness:

- Because of the increased prevalance of HTN and ASHD, physiologic monitoring of exercise response is indicated, at least initially.
- An endurance exercise program should be prescribed for all patients to increase energy expenditure, reduce cardiovascular risk factors, and improve functional efficiency.
  - Intensity should be lower than anaerobic threshold, or around 50% to 60% of maximum, to promote the use of free fatty acids as fuel.
  - Duration and frequency should be prescribed so that a total of 1750 to 2000 calories are expended per week in a fairly even distribution.
  - The goal is to perform 45 to 60 minutes of moderate-intensity aerobic activity at least 3 to 5 days per week.
- Non-weight-bearing exercise programs (e.g., swimming, cycling, water aerobics) are recommended to minimize the stress placed on joints affected by osteoarthritis.
- Patients should be encouraged to increase their general level of activity during their daily routines whenever possible.

PERIPHERAL VASCULAR DISEASE

Atherosclerosis is a disease process that affects not only the coronary arteries but also the peripheral and cerebral vessels. The blood supply to the lower extremities becomes impaired by peripheral vascular disease, or more specifically atherosclerotic occlusive disease, and when it is not adequate to meet the demands of the limb(s), ischemia develops. The resulting pain, or intermittent claudication, occurs on exertion initially but as the disease progresses may develop at rest and be associated with skin changes.

CLINICAL IMPLICATIONS FOR PHYSICAL THERAPY

Because the same disease process is involved, patients with peripheral vascular disease usually have ASHD, although it may not be diagnosed. Therefore, the recommendations printed on page 72 apply to these patients as well; however, there are also some concerns specific to these individuals:

- Patients with intermittent claudication have moderate to severe impairment in walking ability but benefit significantly from exercise training.[21,43,59]
- Patients with atherosclerotic occlusive disease may exhibit precipitious rises in BP during exercise because of the atherosclerosis and diminished vascular bed.
- A subjective gradation of pain for expressing the discomfort of claudication can be very useful and is described in Table 3–10. It is generally recommended that patients avoid exercising with pain above grades 1 to 2 because more stressful exercise elicits anaerobic metabolism, which may exacerbate the claudication pain.
- Workouts should be performed in short intervals with brief rests as needed and should progress according to the description in Chapter 6 (see page 198).
- Lower exercise intensities are suggested because they maximize the potential length of the training sessions.

OTHER SPECIFIC DISEASES AND DISORDERS

A wide variety of other medical diagnoses may be associated with cardiopulmonary complications that may affect patient tolerance of rehabilitation activities.

COLLAGEN VASCULAR DISEASES

The collagen vascular diseases are a diverse group of systemic diseases that are characterized by diffuse and variable abnormalities of the vasculature and inflammatory lesions involving the joints, muscles, and connective tissue. Included in these diseases are systemic lupus erythematosus (SLE), rheumatoid arthritis (RA), polyarteritis nodosa, ankylosing spondylitis, and progressive systemic sclerosis (PSS), also called scleroderma.

- Inflammation of the vasculature is common in all of these diseases and can result in renal disease and HTN, CAD with possible myocardial infarction, Raynaud's phenomenon, and obliterative disease of the pulmonary arteries. HTN evokes compensatory left ventricular hypertrophy, which can eventually give rise to congestive heart failure.
- Inflammation of the serous membranes fre-

TABLE 3–10. Claudication Pain Scale for Subjective Rating of Intensity

GRADE	DESCRIPTION
1	Definite discomfort or pain, but minimal
2	Moderate discomfort or pain, but attention can be diverted with ease
3	Intense pain, attention can only be diverted by catastrophic events
4	Excruciating and unbearable pain

quently leads to pericarditis and pleural effusions (SLE, RA, and polyarteritis nodosa), whereas inflammation of other structures sometimes causes pancarditis (SLE), diffuse myocarditis (severe RA), endocarditis with valvular disease (SLE, RA), sclerosis of the aortic valve area and/or conduction system (ankylosing spondylitis), and interstitial pneumonitis with resultant RLD (SLE, RA, PSS).
- In addition, pulmonary nodules occasionally develop in RA, and chronic infiltrative and fibrotic changes can be seen in the upper lung lobes in ankylosing spondylitis. Diaphragmatic weakness is relatively common in SLE and is manifested as dyspnea, especially when the patient is recumbent.[23]
- Involvement of the kidneys, brain, and heart cause the most serious morbidity.

CONNECTIVE TISSUE DISEASES

Abnormalities of connective tissue can affect the great arteries, cardiac valves, skeletal system, and skin and are characteristic of a number of diseases, including Marfan's syndrome, Ehlers-Danlos syndrome, osteogenesis imperfecta, and homocystinuria. The effects of these diseases can range from minimal cardiovascular dysfunction, as with mitral valve prolapse and mild aortic root dilatation, or severe problems, such as severe aortic or mitral insufficiency or aortic dissection and aneurysm. Pulmonary dysfunction can occur as a result of skeletal abnormalities, such as scoliosis or pectus excavatum, frequent respiratory infections, and hemoptysis.

NEUROMUSCULAR DISEASES AND NEUROLOGIC DISORDERS

A number of disorders affecting the neurologic or neuromuscular systems are associated with cardiac and pulmonary dysfunction. These include spinal cord injury, cerebrovascular accident (CVA), Parkinson's disease, amyotrophic lateral sclerosis (ALS), Guillain-Barré syndrome, myasthenia gravis, the muscular dystrophies, and Friedreich's ataxia. The incidence and severity of dysfunction in all of these disorders varies widely.

- Cardiac dysfunction may occur as a result of cardiomyopathy (the muscular dystrophies, myasthenia gravis, Friedreich's ataxia), disorders of impulse formation and conduction (the muscular dystrophies), or the usual cardiovascular problems affecting same-aged peers, such as HTN and ASHD (Parkinson's disease, myasthenia gravis). Not surprisingly, most patients with CVA have ASHD, though many have not been diagnosed.[17,42] Arrhythmias are common in almost all diagnoses. Autonomic dysfunction is most obviously manifested as orthostatic hypotension.
- Pulmonary abnormalities are usually related to respiratory muscle paralysis, weakness, or incoordination, causing hypoventilation and reduced cough force, bulbar muscle weakness resulting in aspiration pneumonia, and cardiomyopathy leading to pulmonary edema. Respiratory muscle fatigue is usually the final event responsible for respiratory failure in the neuromuscular disorders, but may be delayed by nocturnal ventilatory assistance (e.g., cuirass, rocking bed; see page 61).

HEMATOLOGIC DISORDERS

Many hematologic disorders can lead to cardiopulmonary dysfunction because of impaired oxygen-carrying ability, reduced immune function, or coagulopathy (see Table 8–4, page 271).

Anemia

Anemia is defined as a reduced circulating red cell mass relative to an individual's gender and age and can result from excessive destruction of red cells, loss by hemorrhage, impaired red cell production, or a combination of these.

- The clinical manifestations of anemia depend on the cause of anemia, extent, rapidity of onset, and presence of other medical problems that compromise an individual's health. The most common complaints are fatigue,

headache, and exertional dyspnea, although patients with ASHD may experience myocardial ischemia even with mild anemia.
- Compensatory mechanisms that are available to preserve tissue oxygenation consist of reduced oxygen-hemoglobin affinity, increased cardiac output, decreased peripheral vascular resistance, reduced blood viscosity, slower circulatory time, enhanced oxygen extraction, and redistribution of blood flow. Higher cardiac output is probably due to diminished LV afterload and increased SV rather than elevated HR, at least until anemia is severe.
- Notably, CHF can develop in severe anemia even in the absence of cardiac disease, but is usually due to the increased workload being imposed on an unhealthy heart.

Sickle Cell Disease

Sickle cell disease (SCD) is a genetic disease found most commonly in blacks, which is characterized by structurally abnormal hemoglobin, resulting in red cells that are "sickle" shaped, less pliable, and "sticky." Hemolytic anemia develops when the abnormal red cells become trapped and destroyed in the spleen, and tissue ischemia and infarction occur when small capillaries and venules are occluded. These painful crises frequently involve the spleen, CNS, bones, liver, kidneys, and lungs.

- Cardiopulmonary dysfunction is common in SCD:
  - As with anemia, cardiac output and tissue oxygen extraction increase, but in SCD the reduction in oxygen content of the red cells causes even further sickling and compounds the cardiopulmonary complications.
  - Biventricular hypertrophy and dilatation lead to cardiomegaly with dyspnea on exertion and systolic cardiac murmurs.[40]
  - Arteritis can involve the cardiac and pulmonary vessels leading to thrombosis; pulmonary infarction and myocardial degeneration, necrosis, and fibrosis can occur.
  - CHF may develop late in the disease.
  - In addition, there is an increased incidence of pneumococcal pneumonia, which is a major cause of morbidity and mortality in children.

AIDS

Acquired immune deficiency syndrome (AIDS) is a syndrome characterized by severe immunodeficiency caused by infection of CD4 (T4) lymphocytes with human immunodeficiency virus (HIV). Pulmonary involvement is the major cause of morbidity and mortality in individuals with AIDS and consists of opportunistic infections (often with *Pneumocystis carinii* (PCP) or *Mycobacterium avium-intracellulare* (MAI)), as well as interstitial pneumonitis, AIDS-related malignancies, and ARDS. Multiple pulmonary complications coexist simultaneously in about 20% of patients.

SEQUELAE TO CANCER TREATMENTS

The development of more aggressive treatments for a number of malignancies has yielded higher survival rates and survival periods but has also increased the frequency of cardiac and pulmonary toxicity.

Radiation Therapy

Radiation therapy to the chest, as for the treatment of Hodgkin's disease, lymphoma, and lung and breast cancer, necessarily exposes the heart and lungs to varying degrees and dosages of radiation, depending on the extent of disease.

- The most common sign of cardiotoxicity is pericarditis with pericardial effusion, which is occasionally severe, requiring pericardiocentesis for relief of cardiac tamponade or pericardiectomy for constrictive pericarditis. Other more rare cardiac manifestations of radiation toxicity include acute MI caused by radiation-induced or accelerated coronary artery disease, restrictive cardiomyopathy and electrocardiographic changes resulting from endocardial fibrosis, mitral regurgitation resulting from papillary muscle dysfunction, and aortic regurgitation as a consequence of endocardial valvular thickening.[62]
- Radiation-induced pulmonary toxicity can occur within a few months of completing treatment or much later. Acute radiation pneumonitis occurs in 3% to 5% of patients who receive chest irradiation but about 20% of patients with Hodgkin's disease and massive mediastinal involvement (mass occupying > one third of the chest diameter).[62] Most patients require no treatment, but about 5% develop severe pneumonitis and require hospi-

talization and aggressive supportive care. Many individuals then develop late radiation fibrosis with RLD, which is usually mild but can occasionally lead to cor pulmonale and respiratory failure if a large volume of lung is involved.

Chemotherapy

A number of chemotherapeutic agents have been associated with cardiac and pulmonary toxicity.

- The most well-known agents linked with cardiac toxicity are the anthracycline antibiotics, doxorubicin (Adriamycin) and daunorubicin (Cerubidine).
  - Acute toxicity can be manifested by arrhythmias and conduction disturbances, LV dysfunction and possibly CHF caused by cardiomyopathy, a pericarditis-myocarditis syndrome, sudden death, and myocardial ischemia and infarction.
  - Late cardiotoxicity occurs in the form of a chronic cardiomyopathy, which can develop up to 20 years after treatment.[75]
- Other chemotherapeutic agents have been associated with cardiotoxicity: amsacrine (AMSA), azathioprine, methotrexate, paclitaxel, and mechlorethamine may cause arrhythmias; cyclophosphamide (Cytoxan) in high doses can result in acute lethal pericarditis-myocarditis on rare occasions and cardiomyopathy in some individuals; mitoxantrone can cause a dilated cardiomyopathy in 5% of patients at cumulated doses >160 mg/m^2; and 5-fluorouracil (5-FU), the vinca alkaloids (vinblastine and vincristine), paclitaxel, and high-dose interleukin-2 (IL-2) therapy have been reported to cause myocardial ischemia and/or infarction in a few individuals.[31,34,79,81]
- The most frequent manifestation of pulmonary toxicity associated with chemotherapy is interstitial pneumonitis (IP). Although bleomycin is the drug usually related to IP, a number of other agents have also been implicated, including busulfan, cyclophosphamide (Cytoxan), chlorambucil, carmustine (BCNU), mitomycin, methotrexate, and procarbazine.[76] In addition, an unexplained pulmonary edema occurs in up to 38% of patients treated with cytosine arabinoside.[39]

Bone Marrow Transplantation

Bone marrow transplantation (BMT) is being used in the treatment of leukemia, aplastic anemia, lymphoma, Hodgkin's disease, breast cancer, certain immunodeficiency states, and some genetic disorders, such as SCD and thalassemia major. BMT is achieved by infusing bone marrow from an identical twin (syngeneic BMT) or an individual with similar, although not identical, genetic markers (allogeneic BMT), or by reinfusing an individual's own bone marrow that was obtained during a period of remission or was treated in vitro to remove any contaminating cells (autologous BMT).

- Pulmonary and cardiac toxicity, which are common, significantly limit the success of BMT. They can result from the radiation and chemotherapy used to treat the primary disease, the chemotherapy and total body irradiation used to prepare the patient for transplantation, or the drugs used to prevent graft versus host disease (GVHD).[6]
  - Pulmonary toxicity is the major cause of morbidity and mortality following BMT and can occur early or late.[20] The most frequent and dangerous pulmonary complication is interstitial pneumonitis (IP), which is manifested clinically by cough, dyspnea, and hypoxemia. IP is more prevalent following allogeneic BMT, but also occurs in autologous and syngeneic transplant recipients.[45,48,65,85] Other indicators of pulmonary toxicity, which occur in some allogeneic BMT patients, include obstructive small airways disease and RLD (usually in patients who had previous IP).[14,18,29,67] In addition, patients who receive autologous BMTs sometimes develop diffuse alveolar hemorrhage (DAH) or ARDS.[8,68]
  - Cardiotoxicity is often manifested by ECG abnormalities, such as arrhythmias and conduction disturbances and pericardial effusion, which are usually asymptomatic but occasionally cause major problems.[13,56] Also, some patients develop chemotherapy-induced cardiomyopathies.[3] Recently, exercise testing was used to evaluate the cardiac function of children undergoing BMT, which documented significantly reduced cardiac reserve both before and after transplantation.[57] This dysfunction appears to persist, and may even worsen, over time.

CLINICAL IMPLICATIONS FOR PHYSICAL THERAPY

Based on the information presented in this last section, it should be obvious that many patients with a wide variety of primary medical problems can have cardiopulmonary dysfunction, even though most will not be formally diagnosed. Yet, the symptoms of dysfunction are often nonspecific, such as shortness of breath, lightheadedness, and fatigue; or there may be no symptoms at all, as in hypertension. Furthermore, many patients will not complain of any symptoms of exercise intolerance because they have gradually limited their physical activity in order to avoid discomfort.

The general implications of all these diseases are similar to those already presented in this chapter. More specific recommendations can be found under other diagnoses applicable to a particular patient, such as HTN or RLD.

- To determine if a patient has any cardiopulmonary dysfunction, the physical therapist must evaluate the patient's physiologic responses to activity.
- The therapist should be aware of any medications an individual is taking and how they might affect the exercise responses.
- Endurance exercise training (see Chapter 6, page 197) should be included in the physical therapy plan for every patient who is not already performing regular aerobic exercise, except for those who are acutely ill or have debilitating neuromuscular diseases that are adversely affected by exercise. Endurance exercise facilitates the other components of almost every physical therapy program and offers a number of additional health benefits as well.

REFERENCES

1. American College of Sports Medicine: *Guidelines for Exercise Testing and Prescription,* 4th Ed. Philadelphia, Lea & Febiger, 1990.
2. Andreoli TE, Carpenter CC, Plum F, Smith LH, Jr: *Cecil Essentials of Medicine,* 2nd Ed. Philadelphia, W.B. Saunders Co., 1990.
3. Baello EB, Ensberg ME, Ferguson DW, et al.: Effect of high-dose cyclophosphamide and total body irradiation on left ventricular function in adult patients with leukemia undergoing allogeneic bone marrow transplantation. *Cancer Treat. Rep.* 70: 1187–93, 1986.

4. Bates DW: *Respiratory Function in Disease,* 3rd Ed. Philadelphia, W.B. Saunders Co., 1989.

5. Baum GL, Wolinsky E (eds.): *Textbook of Pulmonary Diseases,* 4th Ed. Boston, Little, Brown & Co., 1989.

6. Bearman SI, Applebaum FR, Buckner CD, et al.: Regimen-related toxicity in patients undergoing bone marrow transplantation. *J. Clin. Oncol.* 6:1562–68, 1988.

7. Bradley WG, Daroff RB, Fenichel GM, Marsden CD (eds.): *Neurology in Clinical Practice.* Boston, Butterworth-Heinemann, 1991.

8. Braude S, Apperley J, Krausz T, et al.: Adult respiratory distress syndrome after allogeneic bone marrow transplantation: Evidence for a neutrophil independent mechanism. *Lancet* 1:1239–1242, 1985.

9. Braunwald E (ed.): *Heart Disease—A Textbook of Cardiovascular Medicine.* Philadelphia, W.B. Saunders Co., 1992.

10. Brewis RAL, Gibson GJ, Geddes DM (eds.): *Respiratory Medicine.* London, Bailliére Tindall, 1990.

11. Burton GG, Hodgkin JE, Ward JJ (eds.): *Respiratory Care. A Guide to Clinical Practice.* 3rd Ed. Philadelphia, J.B. Lippincott Co., 1992.

12. Cahalin L: The effects of aerobic exercise upon hypertension. *Cardiopulm. Rec.* 3(2):1–3, 1989.

13. Cazin B, Gorin NC, Laporte JP, et al.: Cardiac complications after bone marrow transplantation. A report on a series of 63 consecutive transplantations. *Cancer* 57:2061–2069, 1986.

14. Chan CK, Hyland RH, Hutcheon MA: Pulmonary function following bone marrow transplantation. *Clin. Chest Med.* 11:323–332, 1990.

15. Cheng TO (ed.): *The International Textbook of Cardiology.* New York, Pergamon Press, 1986.

16. Cherniack RM, Cherniack L: *Respiration in Health and Disease,* 3rd Ed. Philadelphia, W.B. Saunders Co., 1983.

17. Chimowitz MI, Mancini GBJ: Asymptomatic coronary artery disease in patients with stroke—prevalence, prognosis, diagnosis, and treatment. *Curr. Concepts Cerebrovasc. Dis. Stroke* (American Heart Assoc). 26:23–27, 1991.

18. Clark JG, Crawford SW, Madtes DK, et al.: Obstructive lung disease after allogeneic marrow transplantation: Clinical presentation and course. *Ann. Intern. Med.* 111:368–376, 1989.

19. Clough P: Restrictive lung dysfunction. *In* Hillegass EA, Sadowsky HS (eds.): *Essentials of Cardiopulmonary Physical Therapy.* Philadelphia, W.B. Saunders Co., 1993.

20. Cordonnier C, Bernaudin J-F, Bierling P, Huet Y, Vernant J-P: Pulmonary complications occurring after allogeneic bone marrow transplantation. A study of 130 consecutive transplanted patients. *Cancer* 58:1047–1054, 1986.

21. Creasy TS, McMillan PJ, Fletcher EWL, Collin J, Morris PJ: Is Percutaneous Transluminal angioplasty better than exercise for claudication?—Preliminary results from a prospective randomised trial. *Eur. J. Vasc. Surg.* 4:135–140, 1990.

22. Davidson MB: *Diabetes Mellitus Diagnosis and Treatment,* 3rd Ed. New York, Churchill Livingstone, 1991.

23. Dickey BF, Myers AR: Pulmonary manifestations of collagen vascular diseases. *In* Fishman AP (ed.): *Pulmonary Diseases and Disorders.* New York, McGraw-Hill, 1988.

24. Farzan S: *A Concise Handbook of Respiratory Diseases,* 3rd Ed. Norwalk, CT, Appleton & Lange, 1992.

25. Flenley DC: *Respiratory Medicine,* 2nd Ed. London, Bailliére Tindall, 1990.

26. Foster C, Jacobson MM, Pollock ML: Exercise for the diabetic patient. *In* Pollack ML et al. (eds.): *Heart Disease and Rehabilitation,* 2nd Ed. New York, John Wiley & Sons, 1986.

27. Frohlich ED: The heart in hypertension. *In* Genest J, et al. (eds.), *Hypertension—Physiopathology and Treatment.* New York, McGraw-Hill Book Co., 1983.

28. Fujita Y, Kawaji K, Knamori A, et al.: Relationship between age-adjusted heart rate and anaerobic threshold in estimating exercise intensity in diabetics. *Diabetes Res. Clin, Pract.* 8:69–74, 1990.

29. Fyles G, Chan CK, Hyland RH, Virdee M, Hutcheon MA, Messner HA: Restrictive ventilatory defect after allogeneic bone marrow transplantation. *Am. Rev. Respir. Dis.* 137(Suppl):313, 1988.

30. Garritan SL: Chronic obstructive pulmonary disease. *In* Hillegass EA, Sadowsky HS (eds.): *Essentials of Cardiopulmonary Physical Therapy.* Philadelphia, W.B. Saunders Co., 1993.

31. Ginsberg SJ, Comis RL: The pulmonary toxicity of antineoplastic agents. *Semin. Oncol.* 9:34–51, 1982.

32. Goldberg AP, Geltman EM, Gavin JR III, Carney RM, Hagberg JM, Delmez JA, Naumovich A, Oldfield MH, Harter HR: Exercise training reduces coronary risk and effectively rehabilitates hemodialysis patients. *Nephron* 42:311–316, 1986.

33. Gordon NF, Scott CB, Wilkinson WJ, et al.: Exercise and mild hypertension—Recommendations for adults. *Sports Med.* 10:390–404, 1990.

34. Gottdiener JS, Applebaum FR, et al.: Cardiotoxicity associated with high-dose cyclophosphamide therapy. *Arch. Intern. Med.* 141:758–763, 1981.
35. Guyton AC: *Textbook of Medical Physiology,* 8th Ed. Philadelphia, W.B. Saunders Co., 1991.
36. Hagberg JM, Mountain SJ, Martin WH, et al.: Effects of exercise training on 60–69 year old essential hypertensives. *Am. J. Cardiol.* 64:348–353, 1989.
37. Hammon WE: Pathophysiology of chronic pulmonary disease. *In* Frownfelter DL: *Chest Physical Therapy and Pulmonary Rehabilitation,* 2nd Ed. Chicago, Year Book Medical Publishers, Inc., 1987.
38. Harter HR, Goldberg AP: Endurance exercise training—An effective therapeutic modality for hemodialysis patients. *Med. Clin. North. Am.* 69:159–175, 1985.
39. Haust HM, Hutchins GM, Moore GW: Ara-C lung: Noncardiogenis pulmonary edema complicating cytosine arabinoside therapy of leukemia. *Am. J. Med.* 70:256–261, 1981.
40. Hellenbrand W, Brown J, Covitz W, Gallagher D, Geer M, Leff S, Talner N: Cardiovascular performance in sickle cell disease. *Circulation* 68(Suppl 3):163, 1983.
41. Henson DJ, Morrissey WL: Acute respiratory failure—Mechanisms and medical management. *In* Irwin S, Tecklin JS: *Cardiopulmonary Physical Therapy,* 2nd Ed. St. Louis, The C.V. Mosby Co., 1990.
42. Hertser NR, Young JR, Beven EG, Graor RA, O'Hara PJ, Ruschhaupt WF III, deWolfe VG, Maljovec LC: Coronary angiography in 506 patients with extracranial cerebrovascular disease. *Arch. Intern. Med.* 145:849–852, 1985.
43. Hiatt WR, Regensteinier JG, Hargarten ME, Wolfen EE, Brass EP: Benefit of exercise conditioning for patients with peripheral arterial disease. *Circulation* 81:602–609, 1990.
44. Hurst JW, Schlant RC, Rackley CE, Sonnenblick EH, Wenger NK (eds.): *The Heart, Arteries and Veins,* 7th Ed. New York, McGraw-Hill Information Services Co., 1990.
45. Jochelson M, Tarbell NJ, Freedman AS, et al.: Acute and chronic pulmonary complications following autologous bone marrow transplantation in non-Hodgkin's lymphoma. *Bone Marrow Transplant.* 6:329–331, 1990.
46. Julian DG, Camm AJ, Fox KM, Hall RJC, Poole-Wilson PA (eds.): *Diseases of the Heart.* Toronto, Bailliére Tindall, 1989.
47. Kannel WB, McGee DL: Diabetes and cardiovascular disease. *JAMA* 241:2035–2038, 1979.
48. Kaplan EB, Pietra GG, August CS: Interstitial pneumonitis, pulmonary fibrosis, and chronic graft-versus-host disease. *Bone Marrow Transplant.* 9:71–75, 1992.
49. Kaplan NM: *Clinical Hypertension,* 4th Ed. Baltimore, Williams & Wilkins, 1986.
50. Katz WA (ed): *Diagnosis and Management of Rheumatic Diseases,* 2nd Ed. Philadelphia, J.B. Lippincott Co., 1988.
51. Kelly WN, et al. (eds.): *Textbook of Rheumatology,* 2nd Ed. Philadelphia, W.B. Saunders Co., 1985.
52. Keys A: Overweight, obesity, coronary heart disease and mortality. *Nutr. Rev.* 38:297–307, 1980.
53. Kloner RA (ed.): *The Guide to Cardiology,* 2nd Ed. New York, Le Jacq Communications, 1990.
54. Kozak GP: *Clinical Diabetes Mellitus.* Philadelphia, W.B. Saunders Co., 1982.
55. Krall LP (ed.): *World Book of Diabetes in Practice,* Vol. 3. New York, Elsevier Science Publishers BV, 1988.
56. Kupari M, Volin L, Soukas A, et al.: Cardiac involvement in bone marrow transplantation: electrocardiographic changes, arrhythmias, heart failure and autopsy findings. *Bone Marrow Transplant.* 5:91–98, 1990.
57. Larsen RL, Barber G, Heise CT, et al.: Exercise assessment of cardiac function in children and young adults before and after bone marrow transplantation. *Pediatrics* 89:722–729, 1992.
58. Leon AS: Patients with diabetes mellitis. *In* Franklin BA, et al. (eds.) *Exercise in Modern Medicine.* Baltimore, Williams & Wilkins, 1989.
59. Mannarino E, Pasqualini L, Menna M, Maragoni G, Orlandi U: Effects of physical training on peripheral vascular disease: A controlled study. *Angiology,* 40:5–10, 1989.
60. Marble A, Krall LP, Bradley RF, Christlieb AR, Soeldner JS (eds.): *Joslin's Diabetes Mellitus,* 12th Ed. Philadelphia, Lea & Febiger, 1985.
61. Mehta AD, Wright WB, Kirby B: Ventilatory function in Parkinson's disease. *Br. Med. J.* 1:1456–1457, 1978.
62. Myers CE, Kinsella TJ: Cardiac and pulmonary toxicity. *In* DeVita VT, Hellman S, Rosenberg SA (eds.): *Cancer—Principles and Practice of Oncology,* 2nd Ed. Philadelphia, J.B. Lippincott Co., 1985, pp. 2022–2032.
63. O'Rourke RA, Brenner BM, Stein JH (eds.): *The Heart and Renal Disease.* New York, Churchill Livingstone, 1984.

64. Painter PL, Nelson-Worel JN, Hill MM, Thornberry DR, Shelp WR, Harrigton AR, Weinstein AB: Effects of exercise training during hemodialysis. *Nephron* 43:87–92, 1986.
65. Pecego R, Hill R, Applebaum FR, Amos D, Buckner CD, Fefer A, Thomas ED: Interstitial pneumonitis following autologous bone marrow transplantation. *Transplantation* 42:515–517, 1986.
66. Pickering TG: Exercise and hypertension. *Cardiol. Clin.* 5(2):311–318, 1987.
67. Prince DS, Wingard JR, Saral R, et al.: Longitudinal changes in pulmonary function following bone marrow transplantation. *Chest* 96:301–306, 1989.
68. Robbins RA, Linder J, Stahl MG, et al.: Diffuse alveolar hemorrhage in autologous bone marrow transplant recipients. *Am. J. Med.* 87:511–518, 1989.
69. Ross DL, Grabeau GM, Smith S, Seymour M, Knierim N, Pitelli KH: Efficacy of exercise for end-stage renal disease patients immediately following high-efficiency hemodialysis: a pilot study. *Am. J. Nephrol.* 9:376–383, 1989.
70. Rybka J: *Diabetes Mellitus and Exercise.* ACTA Universitatis Carolinae Medica, Monograph CXVIII, 1987.
71. Scott JP, Hay IFC, Higenbottam TW, Evans D, Calne RY: Hypertensive exercise responses in ciclosporin-treated normotensive renal transplant recipients. *Nephron* 56:143–147, 1990.
72. Seiden MV, Elias A, Ayash L, Hunt M, Eder JP, Schnipper LE, Frei E III, Antman KH: Pulmonary toxicity associated with high dose chemotherapy in the treatment of solid tumors with autologous marrow transplant: an analysis of four chemotherapeutic regimens. *Bone Marrow Transplant.* 10:57–63, 1992.
73. Shalom R, Blumenthal JA, Williams RS, McMurray RG, Dennis VW: Feasibility and benefits of exercise training in patients on maintenance dialysis. *Kidney Int.* 25:958–963, 1984.
74. Sokolow M, McIlroy MB: *Clinical Cardiology,* 4th Ed. Los Altos, CA, Lange Medical Publications, 1986.
75. Steinherz LJ, Steinherz PG, Tan CTC, et al.: Cardiac toxicity 4 to 20 years after completing anthracycline therapy. *JAMA* 266:1672–1677, 1991.
76. Stover DE: Pulmonary toxicity. *In* DeVita VT, Hellman S, Rosenberg SA (eds.): *Cancer—Principles and Practice of Oncology,* 3rd Ed. Philadelphia, J.B. Lippincott Co., 1989, pp. 2162–2169.
77. Sweny P, Farrington K, Moorhead JF: *The Kidney and Its Disorders.* Oxford, Blackwell Scientific Publications, 1989.
78. Tecklin JS: Common pulmonary diseases. *In* Irwin S, Tecklin JS: *Cardiopulmonary Physical Therapy,* 2nd Ed. St. Louis, The C.V. Mosby Co., 1990.
79. Torti FM, Lum BL: Cardiac toxicity. *In* DeVita VT, Hellman S, Rosenberg SA (eds.): *Cancer —Principles and Practice of Oncology,* 3rd Ed. Philadelphia, J.B. Lippincott Co., 1989, pp. 2153–2162.
80. Vranic M, Wasserman D, Bukowiecki L: Metabolic implications of exercise and physical fitness in physiology and diabetes. *In* Rikfin H, Porte D, Jr. (eds.): *Ellenberg and Rifkin's Diabetes Mellitus —Theory and Practice,* 4th Ed. New York, Elsevier Science Publishing Co., Inc., 1990.
81. Wasserheit C, Speyer J: Recognizing cardiac effects of chemotherapy. *Contemp. Oncol.* April: 44–55, 1994.
82. Watchie J: Cardiopulmonary implications of specific diseases. *In* Hillegass EA, Sadowsky HS (eds.): *Essentials of Cardiopulmonary Physical Therapy.* Philadelphia, W.B. Saunders Co., 1993.
83. Wikstrand J: Diastolic function of the hypertrophied left ventricle. *In* Messerli FH (ed.): *The Heart and Hypertension.* New York, Yorke Medical Books, 1987.
84. Wilson JD, Braunwald E, Isselbacher KJ, Petersdorf RG, Martin JB, Fauci AS, Root RK (eds.): *Harrison's Principles of Internal Medicine,* 12th Ed. New York, McGraw-Hill, Inc., 1991.
85. Wingard JR, Sostrin MB, Vriesendorp HM, et al.: Interstitial pneumonitis following autologous bone marrow transplantation. *Transplantation* 46:61–65, 1988.
86. Wyngaarden JB, Smith LH Jr, Bennett JC (eds.): *Cecil Textbook of Medicine,* 19th Ed. Philadelphia, W.B. Saunders Co., 1992.

4

PHARMACOLOGY

COREEN WOODFORD, PHARM.D.

This chapter introduces the drugs used in the treatment of various cardiac and pulmonary conditions and examines in varying degrees the indications, mechanisms of action, and side effects of these agents. Included are drugs used in the treatment of hypertension, congestive heart failure, arrhythmias, angina, shock, and hyperlipidemia, as well as several respiratory diseases. A brief introduction and discussion of the medications used in organ transplantation and diabetes mellitus are also included.

The indications and other drug information presented in this chapter conform to those found in the medical literature or in the manufacturer's product literature. However, this chapter provides only the more important elements of pharmacology and is not intended to be a comprehensive drug information source. The manufacturer's current product information or other standard references should always be consulted for more detailed information. Regarding the discussions of adverse reactions, it should be noted that it is not possible to identify all the reactions reported in the literature; therefore, the approach here is limited to (1) very serious reactions, (2) very common reactions, and/or (3) reactions that potentially have a direct impact on the practice of physical therapy in the clinical setting.

Coreen Woodford, Pharm.D., is a former assistant professor of clinical pharmacy at the University of Southern California School of Pharmacy. She is currently a preceptor for Level IV USC pharmacy students in the community pharmacy clerkship at the San Marino Pharmacy, San Marino, California.

4.1 ANTIHYPERTENSIVE AGENTS

The objective of antihypertensive therapy is to achieve a normal blood pressure (BP) and thus reduce cardiovascular mortality and morbidity. Antihypertensive therapy protects against stroke, left ventricular hypertrophy, congestive heart failure, and progression to more severe hypertension (HTN). In addition to drug therapy, lifestyle modifications are also recommended and include weight reduction, sodium and alcohol restriction, smoking cessation, regular exercise, and a diet low in saturated fat.

- The stepped care approach begins with lifestyle modifications. If BP remains more than or equal to 140/90 mm Hg for 3 to 6 months, antihypertensive therapy is initiated. Therapy is started with one agent, the dosage is gradually increased, then agents are added or substituted with gradual increases in doses until the therapeutic goal is achieved, side effects become intolerable, or maximal dosages are reached.

DIURETICS

Diuretics can be divided into three general categories composed of thiazides and related drugs, loop diuretics, and potassium-sparing agents (Tables 4–1 and 4–2). All are used to treat HTN, congestive heart failure, and edema associated with various other disease states.

- Generally, therapy is initiated with a thiazide or other diuretic as first-line therapy. This therapy alone may control many cases of mild HTN.

113

TABLE 4–1. **Thiazides and Derivatives and Loop Diuretics**

GENERIC NAME	TRADE NAME
Thiazides and Derivatives	
Bendroflumethiazide	Naturefin
Benzthiazide	Exna
Chlorthalidone*	Hygroton
	Thalitone
Chlorothiazide	Diuril
Hydrochlorothiazide	Hydrodiuril
	Oretic
	Esidrix
Hydroflumethiazide	Diucardin
Indapamide*	Lozol
Methyclothiazide	Enduron
	Aquatensin
Metolazone*	Zaroxolyn
	Mykrox
Polythiazide	Renese
Quinethazone*	Hydromox
Trichloromethiazide	Metahydrin
	Naqua
	Diurese
Loop Diuretics	
Bumetanide	Bumex
Ethacrynic acid	Edecrin
Furosemide	Lasix
Torsemide	Demadex

*Chlorthalidone (phthalimide derivative), indapamide (indoline), metolazone, and quinethazone (quinazolin derivatives) are included here because of structural and pharmacologic similarities to the thiazides.

- Hydrochlorothiazide, either alone or in combination with potassium-sparing diuretics, remains the most commonly prescribed thiazide.
- All thiazides are equally effective in lowering BP.
- With the exception of metolazone, thiazides lose their hypertensive activity as renal function declines below a creatinine clearance of 30 mL/min.
- The mechanism by which thiazides lower BP is probably independent of their diuretic effect. Although diuresis initially occurs, plasma and extracellular fluid volume return to pretreatment levels and are accompanied by reduced peripheral vascular resistance.

- In general, loop diuretics are less effective than thiazides in treating HTN. Their use is limited primarily to those individuals who have a creatinine clearance less than 30 mL/min or who have concomitant edema.
- The potassium-sparing diuretics include triamterene, amiloride, and spironolactone; only spironolactone lowers BP. The use of potassium-sparing drugs is mainly to minimize the hypokalemia from thiazides.
- In addition to their use as first-line antihypertensive agents, thiazides continue to be important second-line agents. Their combination with a β-blocker, angiotensin converting enzyme inhibitor, or an α_1-receptor agonist results in additive BP control. There are several commercially available combination products that are not indicated in the tables addressing these products.

β-ADRENERGIC BLOCKING AGENTS

β-Adrenergic blocking agents may also be used as first-line drug therapy for HTN. The available β-blockers approved for administration in HTN are shown in Table 4-3.

- All β-blockers share one property, the blockade of β_1-receptors, which are responsible for increasing heart rate and contractility. However, cardioselective β-blockers exhibit a higher binding affinity for the cardiac β_1-receptors, with less effects on β_2-receptors located primarily in the bronchioles and in the peripheral vascular system. Cardioselectivity is a relative property and is predictable only at lower doses. As the dosage of any cardioselective drug is increased, β_2-receptors will be inhibited as well.
- Another property of β-blockers is intrinsic sympathetic activity (ISA). At low levels of sympathetic nervous system activity, β-blockers with ISA, such as pindolol, produce slight β-receptor stimulation. Clinically, this may result in less resting bradycardia compared with that with β-blockers that lack ISA.
- An additional potential action of β-blockers is concomitant α-blocking activity. Since stimulation of α_1-receptors can cause vasoconstriction or can decrease lipoprotein lipase activity, a β-blocker with α_1-blocking activity might be

TABLE 4-2. **Diuretics**

DRUG	MODE OF ACTION	PHARMACOLOGIC EFFECTS					ADVERSE REACTIONS
		PLASMA VOLUME	PERIPHERAL RESISTANCE	PLASMA RENIN ACTIVITY	CARDIAC OUTPUT		
Thiazides and derivatives* (see Table 4–1)	↑ excretion of Na and Cl and inhibits reabsorption in ascending loop of Henle and distal tubules.	↓	↓	↑	↓		Fluid/electrolyte imbalance, hyperglycemia, ↑ uric acid levels, and ↑ cholesterol, triglycerides, and LDL.
Loop diuretics† (see Table 4–1)	Inhibit reabsorption of Na and Cl in proximal and distal tubules and in loop of Henle	↓	↓	↑	↓		Fluid and electrolyte imbalance, hypotension, anorexia, vertigo, hearing loss, and weakness.
Potassium-sparing diuretics							
Sprionolactone (Aldactone)	Antagonizes aldosterone and prevents Na reabsorption in distal tubule.	↓	↓	↑	↔		Hyperkalemia, gastrointestinal upset, diarrhea, and possible cardiac irregularities.
Triamterene‡ (Dyrenium)	Exerts direct membrane effect in distal tubule and inhibits reabsorption of Na.	—	—	—	—		Hyperglycemia, ataxia, dizziness, and weakness.
Amiloride (Midamor)	Inhibits Na-K-ATPase in proximal and distal tubules.	↓	↓	↑	↓		

↑ = increase, ↓ = decrease, ↔ = no change.
*Indapamide exerts little or no effect on cardiac output.
†Torsemide may lead to ↓ loss of potassium compared with other loop diuretics.
‡Pharmacologic effects of triamterene are not reported directly but are probably similar to those of other diuretics.

more beneficial in individuals who have concomitant peripheral vascular disease or dyslipidemia. Labetalol is the only β-blocker that possesses this property.

• The exact mechanisms by which the β-blockers reduce BP remain unknown. By blocking stimulation of cardiac β_1-receptors, cardiac output may decrease and as a result BP decreases since it is a product of cardiac output and peripheral vascular resistance. Blockade of the β-receptors in the kidney might also decrease the release of renin, which might decrease BP.

ANTIADRENERGIC AGENTS

Antiadrenergic agents (central and peripheral adrenergic inhibitors) are considered supplemental antihypertensive agents and are used when the initial drug therapy fails to lower BP adequately. Diuretics are usually continued to provide synergistic effects and to prevent secondary fluid accumulation that may occur with the use of antiadrenergic agents alone. Combination therapy may also minimize untoward reactions, which are more common at the higher doses necessary when a single drug is used alone.

TABLE 4–3. β-Adrenergic Blocking Agents

DRUG	MODE OF ACTION			INDICATIONS				ADVERSE REACTION (CAN OCCUR WITH ANY OF THESE DRUGS)
	ADRENERGIC RECEPTOR BLOCKING	MEMBRANE STABILIZING	SYMPATHO-MIMETIC ACTIVITY	HTN	ARRHYTHMIA	ANGINA	MYOCARDIAL INFARCTIONS	
Acebutolol (Sectral)	β_1*	+	+	✓	✓			*General:* Most are mild and transient and rarely require withdrawal of therapy.
Atenolol (Tenormin)	β_1*	0	0	✓	✓	✓	✓	*Cardiovascular:* Bradycardia, CHF, ↑AV block, hypotension, paresthesia of hands.
Betaxolol (Kerlone)	β_1*	+	0	✓				
Bisoprolol (Zebeta)	β_1*	0	0	✓	✓	✓		*CNS:* Lightheadedness, depression, insomnia, fatigue, weakness, visual disturbances, hallucinations.
Esmolol (Brevibloc)	β_1*	0	0	✓	✓	✓		*Gastrointestinal:* Nausea, vomitng, abdominal cramping, diarrhea, constipation.
Metoprolol (Lopressor, Toprol)	β_1*	0†	0	✓	✓	✓	✓	*Endocrine:* Hyperglycemia, unstable diabetes, hypogycemia.
Carteolol (Cartrol)	β_1, β_2	0	+ +	✓		✓		*Genitourinary:* sexual dysfunction, impotence.
Nadolol (Corgard)	β_1, β_2	0	0	✓	✓	✓		*Musculoskeletal:* Joint pain, arthralgia, muscle cramps, tremor, twitching.
Penbutolol (Levatol)	β_1, β_2	0	+	✓				*Allergic:* Rash, pharyngitis, and agranulocytosis, respiratory distress.
Pindolol (Visken)	β_1, β_2	+	+ + +	✓	✓			
Propranolol (Inderal, Inderal LA)	β_1, β_2	+ +	0	✓	✓	✓	✓	
Timolol (Blocadren)	β_1, β_2	0	0	✓	✓		✓	
Sotalol (Betapace)	β_1, β_2	0	0		✓			
Labetalol (Normodyne, Trandate)	$\beta_1, \beta_2, \alpha_1$	0	0	✓				

0 = none, + = low, + + = moderate; + + + = high, ✓ = indicated, ↑ = increased.
*Inhibits β_2-receptors (bronchial and vascular) at higher doses.
†Detectable only at doses much greater than required for β-blockade.

- Decreased adrenergic tone results in reduced cardiac output and decreased peripheral vascular resistance.
- Methyldopa, guanabenz, guanfacine, and clonidine act mainly in the central nervous system (CNS), as shown in Table 4–4. Although reserpine has been used for years, other agents are now preferred. Guanadrel is a peripheral antiadrenergic agent similar to guanethidine.

α_1-RECEPTOR ANTAGONISTS

α_1-Receptor antagonists are now considered first-line antihypertensive drugs (Table 4–5). These agents include prazosin, terazosin, and doxazosin.

- The drugs in this class exert their antihypertensive effects by selectively inhibiting the postsynaptic α_1-receptors, which results in decreased peripheral resistance and vasodilation (see Table 4–5).
- Prazosin and related drugs have no direct effects on the α_2-receptors and usually are not associated with reflex tachycardia.
- In higher doses, sodium and water retention may occur resulting in the need for concurrent diuretic therapy.
- While generally well tolerated, the α_1-receptor antagonists are recognized to produce a "first-dose syndrome," characterized by severe hypotension, dizziness, or even syncopal episodes, that occurs within several hours of the

first dose or after subsequent increases in the dose. Patients must be warned about the potential for this side effect and should be instructed to take the first dose at bedtime and to be careful when standing from a supine or sitting position.

VASODILATORS

Vasodilators are also considered supplemental agents and are not suited for initial monotherapy (Table 4–6). Rather, they are usually part of a three-drug regimen, which includes agents acting by different mechanisms to maximize therapeutic effects.

- Hydralazine and minoxidil have direct vasodilating actions (Table 4–6); to prevent reflex tachycardia caused by decreased peripheral resistance, these agents are most effective when used with a diuretic and β-blocker.
- Minoxidil's undesirable side effects limit its use to severely hypertensive patients who do not respond to maximal doses of a diuretic and two other agents.

ANGIOTENSIN CONVERTING ENZYME INHIBITORS

Despite some initial concerns, angiotensin converting enzyme (ACE) inhibitors are very safe and effective in lowering BP and have gained broad acceptance as initial antihypertensive therapy.

- The drugs listed in Table 4–7 inhibit the activity of plasma ACE thereby blocking the conversion of angiotensin I to angiotensin II, which is a potent vasoconstrictor and stimulus for the release of aldosterone.
- ACE inhibitors also prevent the breakdown of bradykinin and may stimulate the synthesis of local vasodilators including prostaglandins.
- Although all these actions may contribute to the hypotensive effects of ACE inhibitors, local tissue angiotensin systems may also modulate much of the vascular response to these drugs.
- ACE inhibitors have been associated with significant hypotension in sodium- or volume-depleted individuals, but dermatologic reactions and cough are the more common adverse reactions associated with ACE inhibitors.

CALCIUM CHANNEL BLOCKERS

The calcium channel blockers, also classified as first-line antihypertensive agents, represent at least three distinct pharmacologic groups including nifedipine and other dihydropyridines, diltiazem, and verapamil, as shown in Table 4–8. Vasodilation, negative inotropic effects, and cardiac conduction effects are three major properties of the calcium channel blockers. Vasodilation is greatest with nifedipine, while negative inotropic properties predominate with verapamil. Heart rate is decreased and cardiac conduction is lowered by verapamil and, to a lesser extent, with diltiazem.

- The calcium channel blockers exert their antihypertensive activity by causing vascular smooth muscle relaxation. They specifically block voltage-sensitive calcium channels and decrease the movement of extracellular calcium into vascular smooth muscle cells.
- Adverse effects are usually a simple extension of their basic pharmacologic properties, with hypotension and dizziness common. Other possible side effects include headache, gastrointestinal upset, peripheral edema, flushing, angina, fatigue, weakness, congestive heart failure, dry mouth, thirst, and skin rash.

4.2 DRUGS USED IN TREATING CONGESTIVE HEART FAILURE

In treating congestive heart failure (CHF), the goals of therapy are to decrease cardiac work, increase cardiac output, and prevent known complications of CHF and its treatment. The cause of CHF and the degree of dysfunction are different for each patient, and these factors underscore the need for an individualized approach to treatment. Although ACE inhibitors, digitalis, and diuretics have complementary effects and are generally used in combination, a standard stepped care approach to treatment does not exist because of the various causes of CHF.

- It is generally recommended that diuretics be used for patients with edema.

Text continued on page 124

TABLE 4–4. Antiadrenergic Blocking Agents Used in the Treatment of Hypertension

DRUG	MODE OF ACTION	PHARMACOLOGIC EFFECTS					ADVERSE REACTIONS
		BLOOD PRESSURE	PLASMA RENIN ACTIVITY	HEART RATE	PERIPHERAL VASCULAR RESISTANCE	CARDIAC OUTPUT	
Centrally Acting Drugs							
Methyldopa (Aldomet)	Metabolized to norepinephrine and stimulates central inhibitory α-adrenergic receptors, false neurotransmission.	↓	↓	↓↔	↓↓	↓↔	Sedation, dizziness, angina, bradycardia, abnormal liver function and positive Coombs test, nasal stuffiness.
Clonidine (Catapres)	Inhibits sympathetic cardioaccelerator and vasoconstrictor centers. Also ↓ renal vascular resistance and ↓ excretion of aldosterone and catecholamines.	↓	↓	↓↓	↓↓	↓↔	Dry mouth, dizziness, sedation, constipation, weight gain, and CHF; rebound HTN on discontinuation if dosage is not tapered.
Guanabenz (Wytensin)	Stimulates α-adrenergic receptors and ↓ sympathetic outflow from brain. Also ↓ catecholamine levels.	↓	↓↓	↓↓	↓↓	↔	Sedation, dry mouth, dizziness, weakness, headache, angina, nausea, and nasal congestion.
Guanfacine (Tenex)	Stimulates central α-adrenergic receptors and ↓ sympathetic nerve impulses from vasomotor center to heart and blood vessels.	↓	↓↓	↓	↓↓	↔	Reactions are common but mild and tend to disappear with continued therapy; dry mouth, sedation, weakness, dizziness, constipation, and impotence.

Peripherally Acting Drugs

Drug	Mechanism						Adverse Reactions
Reserpine (Serpasil)	Depletes tissue stores of catecholamines (epinephrine and norepinephrine) from peripheral sites causing depression of sympathetic nerve function; inhibits carotid sinus reflex.	↓	↓↔	↓↓	↓↓	↓↓↔	Hypersecretion and ↑ intestinal motility, nausea, vomiting, dry mouth, angina, bradycardia, drowsiness, dizziness, muscle aches, and nasal congestion.
Guanethidine (Ismelin)	Inhibits release of norepinephrine at sympathetic neuroeffector junction; also directly depresses myocardium depleted of catecholamines.	↓	↓↔	↓↓	↓↓	↓↓↔	Frequent reactions resulting from sympathetic blockade; dizziness, weakness, and syncope resulting from postural or exertional hypotension. Frequent reactions from unopposed parasympathetic activity; bradycardia and diarrhea.
Guanadrel (Hylorel)	Inhibits norepinephrine from neuronal storage sites in response to nerve stimulation; does not inhibit parasympathetic nerve function nor does it enter the CNS.	↓	—	↓↓	↓↓	↔	Shortness of breath, palpitations, angina, cough, fatigue, headache, drowsiness, gastrointestinal upset, nocturia, peripheral edema, aching limbs, leg cramps, and visual disturbances.

↑↑ = increase, ↑ = slight increase, ↔ = no change, ↓ = slight decrease, ↓↓ = decrease, ↓↔ = slight decrease or no change, — = not reported, CHF = congestive heart failure, CNS = central nervous system.

TABLE 4-5. α-Receptor Antagonists

DRUG	MODE OF ACTION	PHARMACOLOGIC EFFECTS					ADVERSE REACTIONS (CAN OCCUR WITH ANY OF THESE DRUGS)
		BLOOD PRESSURE	PLASMA RENIN ACTIVITY	HEART RATE	PERIPHERAL VASCULAR RESISTANCE	CARDIAC OUTPUT	
Peripherally Acting Drugs							General: "First-dose" effect can cause marked hypotension and syncope with first doses. Also, nausea, dyspnea, palpitations, dizziness, asthenia, drowsiness, and headache.
Prazosin (Minipress)	General: Selectively block postsynaptic α-adrenergic receptors and dilate both resistance (arterioles) and capacitance (venous) vessels.	↓	↓↔	↑↔	↓↓	↑↔	
Terazosin (Hytrin)		↓	↔	↑	↓↓	↑	
Doxazosin (Cardura)		↓		↑	↓	↔	

↑↑ = increase, ↑ = slight increase, ↔ = no change, ↓ = slight decrease, ↓↓ = decrease, ↓↔ = slight decrease or no change, ↑↔ = slight increase or no change.

TABLE 4-6. Vasodilators

DRUG	MODE OF ACTION	PHARMACOLOGIC EFFECTS					ADVERSE REACTIONS
		BLOOD PRESSURE	PLASMA RENIN ACTIVITY	HEART RATE	PERIPHERAL VASCULAR RESISTANCE	CARDIAC OUTPUT	
Hydralazine (Apresoline)	Direct relaxation of vascular smooth muscle by interfering with calcium movement.	↓	↑↑	↑↑	↓↓	↑↑	Headache, palpitations, tachycardia, angina, gastrointestinal upset, syncope, arthralgia. May cause lupus erythematosus.
Minoxidil (Loniten)		↓	↑↑	↑↑	↓↓	↑↑	Pericardial effusion, angina, edema, CHF, and enhanced growth and darkening of body hair.

↑↑ = increase, ↑ = slight increase, ↔ = no change, ↓ = slight decrease, ↓↓ = decrease, CHF = congestive heart failure.

TABLE 4–7. Angiotensin Converting Enzyme (ACE) Inhibitors

| DRUGS | PHARMACOLOGIC EFFECTS | | | | | INDICATIONS | | ADVERSE REACTIONS (CAN OCCUR WITH ANY OF THESE DRUGS) |
	PERIPHERAL VASCULAR RESISTANCE	CARDIAC OUTPUT	HEART RATE	PLASMA VOLUME	PLASMA RENIN ACTIVITY	HTN	CHF	
Benzepril (Lotensin)	↓↓	↔↑	↔		↑↑	✓		General: First-dose effect, hypotension, chronic cough, headache, dizziness, fatigue, angina, gastrointestinal upset, dyspnea, asthenia. A symptom complex has occurred and may include: positive antinuclear antibodies, ↑ erythrocyte sedimentation rate, arthralgia, arthritis, myalgia, fever, interstitial nephritis, vasculitis, rash, eosinophilia, and photosensitivity.
Captopril (Capoten)	↓↓	↔↑	↔	↑	↑↑	✓	✓	
Enalapril (Vasotec)	↓↓	↑↑	↔	↔↑	↑↑	✓	✓	
Fosinopril (Monopril)	↓↓	↔↑	↔		↑↑	✓		
Lisinopril (Prinivil, Zestril)	↓↓	↔↑	↔		↑↑	✓	✓	
Quinapril (Accupril)	↓↓	↔↑	↔		↑↑	✓	✓	
Ramipril (Altace)	↓↓	↔↑	↔		↑↑	✓	✓	

↑↑ = increase, ↑ = slight increase, ↔ = no change, ↓ = slight decrease, ↓↓ = decrease, ✓ = indicated, ↔↑ = slight increase to no change, CHF = congestive heart failure, HTN = hypertension.

TABLE 4-8. Calcium Channel Blocking Agents

DRUGS	PHARMACOLOGIC EFFECTS				INDICATIONS			
	PERIPHERAL VASCULAR RESISTANCE	CARDIAC OUTPUT	HEART RATE	MYOCARDIAL CONTRACTILITY	ANGINA	CHF	HTN	ARRHYTHMIAS
Amlodipine (Norvasc)	↓↓	↑	↑↔	↔	✓		✓	
Felodipine (Plendil)	↓↓	↑	↑	↔			✓	
Isradipine (Dynacirc)	↓↓	↑	↑↔	↔↑			✓	
Nicardipine (Cardene)	↓↓	↑↑	↑	↔↑	✓		✓	
Nifedipine (Procardia, Adalat)	↓↓	↑↑	↑↔	↔→	✓	✓	✓	
Diltiazem (Cardizem, Dilacor)	↓	↔↑	↓↔↑	↔↓	✓	✓	✓	
Verapamil (Calan, Isoptin, Verelan)	↓↓	↑↓	↑↓	↓↓	✓		✓	✓
Bepridil (Vascor)	↓	↔	↓	↓				✓

↑↑ = increase, ↑ = slight increase, ↔ = no change, ↓ = slight decrease, ↓↓ = decrease, ✓ = indicated, ↔↑ = no change or increase, ↓↔ = no change or decrease, ↑↓ = either increase or decrease, CHF = congestive heart failure, HTN = hypertension.

- If the patient has a third heart sound or an enlarged heart with a low ejection fraction, digitalis should be used.
- Most patients with CHF, especially those with dilated hearts and mitral or aortic insufficiency, should be placed on an ACE inhibitor.
- The agents used in treating CHF, their indications, and adverse reactions appear in Table 4–9.

CARDIAC GLYCOSIDES

The cardiac glycosides include digoxin, deslanoside, and digitoxin. Although these glycosides differ pharmacokinetically, their therapeutic effects on the heart are qualitatively similar. The influence of the digitalis glycosides on the myocardium is dose-related and involves both a direct action on the cardiac muscle and the specialized conduction system and indirect actions on the cardiovascular system, which are mediated by the autonomic nervous system. These indirect actions involve a vagomimetic action, which is responsible for depression of the sinoatrial (SA) node and prolonged conduction

to the atrioventricular (AV) node (see Tables 4–10 and 4–11 and "Antiarrhythmic Drugs," page 125).

- Direct effects of digitalis include increasing the force and velocity of myocardial contraction (positive inotropic action), prolonging the refractory period of the AV node, and raising total peripheral resistance (TPR).
- In higher doses digitalis increases sympathetic outflow from the CNS to both cardiac and peripheral sympathetic nerves, which may be an important factor in digitalis cardiac toxicity.
- The cardiac manifestations of digitalis intoxication are cardiac arrhythmias, including conduction defects (AV block) and enhanced automaticity. Extra cardiac manifestations of digitalis toxicity are mediated through the CNS and include gastrointestinal (anorexia, nausea, and vomiting), neurologic (headache, drowsiness, and confusion), and visual (blurred or yellow vision) symptoms. The incidence of toxicity has decreased with the introduction of the digitalis serum assay.

TABLE 4–9. Drugs Used in the Treatment of Congestive Heart Failure

DRUG	MODE OF ACTION	INDICATIONS	ADVERSE REACTIONS
Cardiac glycosides Digoxin, (Lanoxin, Lanoxicaps) Deslanoside (Cedilanid-D) Digitoxin (Crystodigin)	Direct action on cardiac muscle and conduction system leads to ↑ force and velocity of systolic contraction and ↑ TPR. Also act indirectly through the CNS.	CHF, all degrees, most effective in low-output failure. ↑ cardiac output leads to ↑ diuresis and improvement of failure.	Cardiac toxicity, gastrointestinal effects (which mimic CHF) and CNS effects; headache, weakness, and visual disturbances.
Amrinone (Inocor)	Positive inotropic agent with vasodilator activity.	CHF for those not responding adequately to digitalis, diuretics, and vasodilators.	Thrombocytopenia, nausea, hypotension, arrhythmias.
Milrinone (Primacor)	Inotropic/vasodilator agent; little chronotropic activity.	CHF; can use concurrently with digitalis, diuretics.	Arrhythmias, hypotension, headache, ↓ potassium.
ACE inhibitors (see Table 4–7) Diuretics (see Table 4–2)			

ACE = angiotensin converting enzyme, CHF = congestive heart failure, CNS = central nervous system, TPR = total peripheral resistance.

POSITIVE INOTROPIC AGENTS

Amrinone and milrinone are both positive inotropic agents with vasodilator activity. However, these agents are indicated only for short-term management of CHF and only in patients who have not responded adequately to digitalis, diuretics, or vasodilators and can be closely monitored. The primary adverse reactions of both drugs are cardiac arrhythmias and hypotension.

ACE INHIBITORS

In patients with CHF, captopril and enalapril significantly decrease peripheral resistance, BP (afterload), pulmonary capillary wedge pressure (preload), pulmonary vascular resistance, and heart size, thereby increasing cardiac output and exercise tolerance. Quinapril reduces TPR and renal vascular resistance with little or no change in heart rate or cardiac index (see Table 4–7).

DIURETICS

Diuretics are generally recommended for CHF patients with edema and are effective alone in managing many cases. Diuretics are indicated to promote loss of salt and water in fluid-retaining states and to control BP. In patients with CHF, diuretic-induced fluid loss can increase cardiac output, improve the function of fluid-congested organs, and decrease uncomfortable peripheral edema. The therapeutic potency of a diuretic is closely paralleled by side effects. Electrolyte imbalance or dehydration, serious arrhythmias and marked decreases in cardiac output can develop. Listed in Tables 4–1 and 4–2 are the diuretic agents in use and their specific pharmacologic actions.

4.3 ANTIARRHYTHMIC DRUGS

Optimal therapy of cardiac arrhythmias requires documentation, accurate diagnosis, modification of precipitating causes, and if indicated, proper selection and use of antiarrhythmic drugs. These drugs are classified according to their effects on the action potential of cardiac cells and their presumed mechanism of action

TABLE 4–10. Currently Available Antiarrhythmic Agents, and Mechanism of Action

GENERIC AND TRADE NAMES

Class I: local anesthetics or membrane stabilizing agents that depress phase 0
  Subclass IA: depress phase 0 and prolong action potential duration
    Disopyramide (Norpace)
    Procainamide (Pronestyl, Procan SR)
    Quinidine (Quinora, Quinidex Extentabs, Quinaglute Duratabs, Cardioquin)
  Subclass IB: depress phase 0 slightly and may shorten action potential duration
    Lidocaine (Xylocaine, Lidopen)
    Mexiletine (Mexitil)
    Phenytoin (Dilantin)
    Tocainide (Tonocard)
  Subclass IC: marked depression of phase 0, slight effect on repolarization, and profound slowing of conduction
    Encainide (Encaid)
    Flecainide (Tambocor)
    Moricizine† (Ethmozine)
    Propafenone (Rhythmol)

Class II: β-blockers‡ that depress phase 4 depolarization
    Acebutolol (Sectral)
    Esmolol (Brevibloc)
    Propanolol (Inderal, Inderal LA)
    Sotalol§ (Betapace)

Class III: Prolongation of phase 3 (repolarization)
    Amiodarone‖ (Cordarone)
    Bretylium (Bretylol)
    Sotalol (Betapace)

Class IV: Calcium channel blockers that depress phase 4 depolarization and lengthen phases 1 and 2 of repolarization
    Diltiazem (Cardizem, Cardizem CD, Dilacor SR)
    Verapamil (Calan, Isoptin, Verelan)

Digoxin: Causes a decrease in maximal diastolic potential and action potential duration and an increase in the slope of phase 4 depolarization

*Was voluntarily withdrawn from market but is available on a limited basis.
†Class I antiarrhythmic that shares characteristics of group IA, IB, and IC agents.
‡Antiarrhythmic effects occur in concentrations associated with β-blockade.
§Has both Class II and III properties; class III properties occur at doses >160 mg.
‖Exhibits all properties of class III plus noncompetitive α- and β-adrenergic blockade.

TABLE 4-11. Electrophysiologic Effects and Indications of Antiarrhythmic Agents

GROUP	DRUG	ELECTROPHYSIOLOGIC EFFECTS — AUTOMATICITY	CONDUCTION VELOCITY	REFRACTORY PERIOD	INDICATIONS — PREMATURE ATRIAL CONTRACTIONS	PAROXYSMAL ATRIAL TACHYCARDIA	ATRIAL FLUTTER	ATRIAL FIBRILLATION	JUNCTIONAL PREMATURE CONTRACTIONS AND TACHYCARDIA	PREMATURE VENTRICULAR CONTRACTIONS	VENTRICULAR TACHYCARDIA	DIGITALIS-INDUCED ARRHYTHMIAS	ADVERSE REACTIONS
IA	Quinidine	↓	↓	↑	✓	✓	✓	✓	✓	✓	✓		Proarrhythmic, gastrointestinal upset is most common, CHF, and hypotension are most serious; lupus erythematosis may develop.
	Procainamide	↓	↓	↑							✓		
	Disopyramide	↓	↓	↑		✓*					✓		
IB	Lidocaine	↓	↔	↓						✓	✓		Primarily CNS reactions (ataxia, dizziness, gastrointestinal upset, hypotension).
	Phenytoin	↓	↔	↓						✓	✓	✓	
	Tocainide	↓	↔	↓						✓	✓		
	Mexitil	↓	↔	↓						✓			
IC	Flecainide	↓	↓↓	↑			✓	✓		✓	✓		Proarrhythmic, CNS reactions (dizziness, gastrointestinal upset), CHF.
	Propafenone	↓	↓↓	↑		✓	✓	✓		✓	✓		
	Encainide	↓	↓↓	↑					✓	✓	✓		
	Moricizine	↓	↓	↔						✓	✓		Proarrhythmic, CHF, palpitations, syncope, gastrointestinal upset, fatigue, shortness of breath.

	Drug										Adverse Effects
II†	Acebutolol	↓	↓	←					✓	✓	Primarily mild and transient; bradycardia, dizziness, hypotension, fatigue, gastrointestinal upset, sexual dysfunction.
	Esmolol	↓	↓	←				✓	✓	✓	
	Propanolol	↓	↓	←				✓	✓		
III	Sotalol	↓	↓	↑↑					✓		Proarrhythmic, hypotension, dizziness, ↑ digitalis toxicity, ↓ potassium, CHF.
	Bretylium	←	↔→	↓↑‡		✓	✓		✓		
	Amiodarone§	↓	→	←		✓		✓	✓		
IV	Verapamil	↓	↓	←	✓	✓	✓	✓	✓		Dizziness, gastrointestinal upset, headache, do not use within 2 hours of IV β-blockers.
	Diltiazem	→	→	↔→↑	✓	✓	✓	✓	✓		
	Digoxin	↓	↓	↑	✓	✓	✓				Cardiac toxicity, gastrointestinal upset, visual disturbances.

CHF = congestive heart failure, CNS = central nervous system.
*Unlabeled use includes paroxysmal atrial tachycardia.
†Unlabeled uses of various beta blockers include ventricular arrhythmias (atenolol, metoprolol, timolol, and pindolol) and supraventricular tachycardias (bisoprolol).
‡Because of a complex balance of direct and indirect autonomic effects.
§Unlabeled uses include paroxysmal atrial tachycardia, atrial flutter, and atrial fibrillation.

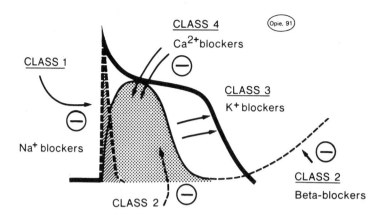

FIGURE 4-1. The action potential and its phases of activation of the excitable cell with the sites of intervention of the four classic types of antiarrhythmic agents. Class I agents decrease phase zero of the rapid depolarization of the action potential (rapid sodium channel). Class II agents, β-blocking drugs, have complex actions including inhibition of spontaneous depolarization (phase 4) and indirect closure of calcium channels, which are less likely to be in the "open" state when not phyosphorylated by cyclic AMP. Class III agents block the outward potassium channels to prolong the action potential duration and hence refractoriness. Class IV agents, verapamil and diltiazem, and the indirect calcium antagonist adenosine, inhibit the inward calcium channel, which is most prominent in nodal tissue, particularly the atrioventricular node. Most antiarrhythmic drugs have more than one action. (From Opie LH (ed.): *Drugs for the Heart,* 3rd Ed. Philadelphia, W. B. Saunders Co., 1991, p. 182.)

(see Fig. 4–1 and Tables 4–10 and 4–11). Although drugs within the same group are similar, different agents may be more effective and/or safer in different individuals.

By their nature, antiarrhythmic agents have the potential to cause or aggravate arrhythmias. Such proarrhythmic effects range from an increased frequency of premature ventricular contractions (PVCs) to the development of ventricular tachycardia or ventricular fibrillation, which may have fatal consequences. It is often not possible to distinguish a drug's proarrhythmic effect from the patient's underlying rhythm disorder.

CLASS I AGENTS

Within class I, there are three subcategories, based on slightly different mechanisms of action. In addition, there is one drug (moricizine) that shares some of the characteristics of all three subclasses.

• In the usual therapeutic concentrations, the class IA agents (quinidine, procainamide, and disopyramide) lengthen the effective refractory period (ERP) by two different mechanisms: first, they inhibit the fast sodium current and the upstroke of the action potential; second, they prolong the action potential duration (mild class III effect). These drugs can cause proarrhythmic complications by prolonging the QT interval in predisposed individuals, or by depressing conduction and promoting reentry.

• The class IB agents (lidocaine, phenytoin, mexiletine, and tocainide) inhibit the fast sodium current (typical class I effect) while shortening the action potential duration. The former has the more powerful effect, whereas the latter might actually predispose the patient to arrhythmias but ensures that QT prolongation does not occur. The class IB agents act selectively on diseased or ischemic tissue, where they are thought to promote conduction block, thereby preventing reentry circuits. Possibly because of their affinity for binding with inactivated sodium channels with rapid onset-offset kinetics, these drugs are ineffective in treating atrial arrhythmias with the shortened action potential durations.

• The class IC agents (flecainide, propafenone, and encainide) have three major electrophysiologic effects. First, they are powerful inhibitors of the fast sodium channels causing marked depression of the upstroke of the cardiac action potential. Second, they have a marked inhibitory effect on His-Purkinje conduction with QRS widening. Third, they markedly shorten the action potential duration of the Purkinje fibers, leaving unaltered that of the surrounding myocardium. The class IC agents are all potent antiarrhythmics used mainly to control ventricular tachyarrhythmias resistant to other drugs.

- Moricizine, a class I antiarrhythmic agent with potent local anesthetic activity and myocardial membrane stabilizing effects, shares some of the characteristics of all three subcategories of the class I agents. Moricizine reduces the fast inward current carried by sodium ions and shortens phase 2 and 3 repolarization, decreasing the action potential duration and ERP. Moricizine is effective in treating ventricular arrhythmias in patients with and without organic heart disease and in those for whom other antiarrhythmics are ineffective, not tolerated, or contraindicated.

Class II Agents

The antiarrhythmic activity of the various β-blockers is reasonably uniform (see Tables 4–3 and 4–11). The critical property is that of β-adrenergic blockade with only minor, if any, effects on membrane depression (local anesthetic action), cardioselectivity, and intrinsic sympathomimetic activity. The only exception is the additional class III effect of sotalol. The β-blockers may be used to prevent and control supraventricular and ventricular arrhythmias and are especially useful when there is an added indication such as angina or HTN.

Class III Agents

Class III compounds (bretylium, amiodarone, and sotalol) act by lengthening the action potential duration, and hence the ERP, and must inevitably prolong the QT interval to be effective. By acting only on the repolarization phase of the action potential, class III agents should leave conduction unchanged. However, these drugs all have additional properties that modify conduction: amiodarone is a significant sodium channel inhibitor, sotalol is a β-blocker, and bretylium initially causes catecholamine release and blocks adrenergic neurons.

Class IV Agents

The calcium channel blockers verapamil and diltiazem inhibit slow channel-dependent conduction through the AV node. Pharmacologic effects on the cardiovascular system include depression of mechanical contraction of myocardial and smooth muscle and depression of both impulse formation (automaticity) and conduction velocity. These agents are particularly useful in treating supraventricular arrhythmias.

4.4 ANTIANGINAL AGENTS

Angina pectoris is a disease characterized by chest discomfort precipitated by myocardial ischemia (see page 70). Classic angina is typically precipitated by physical activity or emotional disturbance.

- Antianginal agents include rapid-acting nitrates used to relieve the pain of acute angina and long-acting preparations used for prophylaxis or to decrease the severity of angina.
- Dipyridamole, β-blocking agents, and calcium channel blockers are also used in the prophylaxis of chronic angina (Table 4–12).

Organic Nitrates

The nitrates are potent vasodilators of vascular smooth muscle and appear to exert their effects by reducing myocardial oxygen demand secondary to a reduction in preload and afterload. The nitrates also produce a vasodilator effect in segments of the coronary collateral channels and possibly the major coronary arteries.

- The effects of nitroglycerin are almost immediate in terms of pain relief and favorable alterations in the electrocardiographic patterns, but are short in duration (less than 30 minutes). In situations of increased demand where chest discomfort is likely (e.g., before physical therapy), nitroglycerine can be used prophylactically.
- A variety of longer acting nitrates have also been developed to provide prophylaxis of angina. The primary drug is isosorbide dinitrate, which is available in a variety of forms, including sublingual, chewable, and oral tablets. The sublingual tablets are shorter acting than the chewable tablets, which are shorter acting than the oral preparation.

TABLE 4-12. **Antianginal Agents**

		INDICATIONS			ADVERSE REACTIONS
DRUG	**DOSE FORM**	**ACUTE**	**PROPHYLACTIC**	**OTHER**	
Organic Nitrates					
Amylnitrate					
Aspirols	Inhalant	✓			General for or-
Vaporole	Inhalant	✓			ganic nitrates:
Nitroglycerin					Gastrointesti-
Tridil	IV	✓		HTN,	nal distur-
NitroBid	IV	✓		CHF	bances, head-
Nitrostat	Sublingual	✓	✓		ache, which
Nitrolingual	Translingual spray	✓	✓		may be severe
Nitrogard	Transmucosal tablet	✓	✓		and persistent,
Nitrong					apprehension,
Nitroglyn	Oral and oral		✓		vertigo, tachy-
Nitro-Bid	sustained release	✓	✓		cardia, hypo-
Minitron					tension, arth-
Nitro-Dur	Transdermal patch		✓		ralgia; adverse
Transderm-Nitro					reactions to ni-
Nitrol	Topical ointment	✓	✓		trates are usu-
Nitro-Bid					ally dose-
Isosorbide dinitrate					related and
Isordil	Sublingual, oral, and	✓	✓		secondary to
Sorbitrate	oral-sustained release				vasodilation.
Isosorbide mononitrate					
Ismo	Oral		✓		
Monoket	Oral		✓		
Erythrityl tetranitrate					
Cardilate	Sublingual, chewable,		✓		
	and oral				
Pentaerythritol tetranitrate					
Peritrate SA	Oral and oral		✓		
Duotrate	sustained release				
Others					
Dipyridamole	Oral		✓		Dizziness, gas-
Persantine					trointestinal
					upset, head-
					ache, rash
β-blockers†			✓		
Calcium channel					
blockers‡			✓		

CHF = congestive heart failure, HTN = hypertension.
*"Possible effective" for chronic angina; may decrease frequency of or eliminate anginal episodes.
†See Table 4–3. ‡See Table 4–8.

- The major adverse effects associated with nitroglycerin and other nitrates include headache, dizziness, weakness, palpitations, and occasionally syncope.
- Tolerance can develop with these drugs and intermittent dosing is often effective for achieving the desired effect.

β-ADRENERGIC BLOCKING AGENTS

The β-blocking drugs competitively inhibit the binding of catecholamines to their receptor sites and reduce sympathetic activity, thus decreasing the oxygen demands of the heart. In general, the β-blockers are effective in curtailing the number of angina attacks and improving exercise tolerance. However, there is a wide variety of activity and selectivity within the β-blocking drugs (see Table 4–3).

- The cardioselective agents (e.g., atenolol, betaxolol, metoprolol, and acebutolol) selectively block the β_1-receptors in the heart and generally have fewer effects on the β_2-receptors found in the smooth muscle (e.g., lungs).
- All β-blockers can cause bradycardia, hypotension, and dizziness.

CALCIUM CHANNEL BLOCKERS

The calcium channel blocking drugs are useful in the treatment of stable angina, unstable angina, and Prinzmetal's angina (i.e., coronary spasm). These drugs are potent dilators of the coronary arteries.

- The various drugs differ in the type of effects they produce. Nicardipine and nifedipine produce the greatest systemic vasodilation, whereas verapamil has the greatest negative inotropic effect. Nicardipine appears to produce the greatest increase in coronary blood flow.
- All the calcium channel blockers can cause hypotension. See Table 4–8 for the pharmacologic effects of and indications for the different calcium channel blockers.

4.5 VASOPRESSORS USED IN SHOCK

Shock is a state of inadequate tissue perfusion. It can be caused by (or cause) a decreased supply or an increased demand for oxygen and nutrients. The imbalance between supply and demand interferes with normal cellular function, which if widespread, can result in death. Inadequate tissue perfusion can occur even if cardiac output, peripheral resistance, and other factors that determine BP (e.g., blood volume) are normal or elevated. Therefore, hypotension need not be present for the patient to be in shock.

- Although the causes of shock are varied, advanced shock tends to follow a common clinical course. Yet identifying the underlying cause may assist in the selection of general supportive therapy and is essential for selecting specific therapy.

- Management of shock is aimed at providing basic life support (airway, breathing, and circulation) while attempting to correct the underlying cause(s).
  - Antibiotics, inotropic agents, hormones (e.g., insulin and thyroid hormones), and other drugs may be used to treat the underlying disease states in the shock patient.
  - However, initial pharmacologic interventions are primarily aimed at supporting the circulation.

FLUIDS

Relative or absolute volume depletion occurs in most shock states, especially in the early phase in which vasodilation is prominent. Adequate volume repletion is necessary to maintain cardiac output, urine flow, and the integrity of the microcirculation. Attempts to support the circulation with vasopressors or inotropes will be unsuccessful if the intravascular volume is depleted.

SYMPATHOMIMETIC AGENTS

Sympathomimetic agents are used in shock to treat hypoperfusion in normovolemic patients and in those unresponsive to whole blood or plasma volume expanders.

These vasopressor agents produce α-adrenergic stimulation (for vasoconstriction), β_1-adrenergic stimulation (for increased myocardial contractility, heart rate, automaticity, and AV conduction), and β_2-adrenergic activity (for peripheral vasodilation), as shown in Table 4–13. Dopamine also causes vasodilation of the renal, mesenteric, cerebral, and coronary beds by dopaminergic receptor activation. The relative activity and predominance of these actions result in a number of hemodynamic responses that may improve coronary and renal perfusion, cardiac output, TPR, and BP.

- The actual response of an individual patient will depend largely on clinical status at the time of administration.
- In cardiogenic shock or advanced shock from other causes associated with a low cardiac output, sympathomimetic agents may be combined with vasodilators (e.g., nitroprusside or nitroglycerin) to improve myocardial performance and maintain BP.

TABLE 4-13. Vasopressors Used in Shock

DRUG	SITES OF ACTION				HEMODYNAMIC RESPONSE				ADVERSE REACTIONS
	CONTRACTILITY INOTROPIC β_1	SA NODE RATE CHRONO-TROPIC β_2	VASOCON-STRICTION α	VASODI-LATION β_2	RENAL PERFUSION	CARDIAC OUTPUT	TOTAL PERIPHERAL RESISTANCE	BLOOD PRESSURE	
Isoproterenol (Isuprel)	+++	+++	0	+++	↑↓	↑	↓	↑↓	Tachycardia, palpitations, HTN, flushing, sweating, tremors, nausea.
Dobutamine (Dobutrex)	+++	0-+	0-+	+	0	↑	↓	↑	Tachycardia, HTN, nausea, angina, headache.
Dopamine (Intropin, Dopastat)	+++	+-++	+-+++	0-+	↑	↑	↓↑	0-↑	Ectopic beats, nausea, tachycardia, angina, palpitations, dyspnea, headache, hypotension.
Epinephrine (Adrenalin)	+++	+++	+++	++	↓	↑	↓	↑↓	Hemiplegia, anxiety, headache, palpitations, arrhythmias.
Norepinephrine (Levophed)	++	++	+++	0	↓	0-↓	↑	↑	Bradycardia, headache, sulfite sensitivity and other allergic reactions.
Ephedrine	++	++	+	0-+	↓	↑	↑↓	↑	Palpitations, tachycardia, headache, vertigo, respiratory difficulty, confusion.
Mephentermine (Wyamine)	+	+	+	++	↑↓	↑	0-↑	↑	Anxiety, arrhythmias, hypertension.
Metaraminol (Aramine)	+	+	++	0	↓	↓	↑	↑	Tachycardia, flushing, sweating, headache, dizziness, tremors, nausea.
Methoxamine (Vasoxyl)	0	0	+++	0	↓	0-↓	↑	↑	Hypertension, severe headache, sweating, gastrointestinal upset.
Phenylephrine (Neo-Synephrine)	0	0	+++	0	↓	↓	↑	↑	Bradycardia, excitability, restlessness, headache, arrhythmias.

+++ = pronounced effect, ++ = moderate effect, + = slight effect, 0 = no effect, ↑ = increase, ↓ = decrease, ↑↓ = either increase or decrease, HTN = hypertension.

4.6 HYPERLIPIDEMIC AGENTS

Studies indicate that higher blood concentrations of both total and low-density lipoprotein (LDL) cholesterol are associated with a greater risk for atherosclerotic cardiovascular disease. Currently, there is renewed emphasis on more intensive treatment regimens to lower high blood cholesterol, particularly LDL, as part of a comprehensive approach to reducing the known risk factors for the progression of this disease.

- Drug therapy is indicated after serious efforts with diet and exercise have failed to reduce LDL below 130 mg/dL.
  - The major drugs are those capable of substantial reductions in LDL and proven to be safe and effective with long-term use.
    — These include niacin, bile acid sequestrants, and hydroxymethylglutaryl-coenzyme A (HMG-CoA) reductase inhibitors, also known as statins.
    — These agents may be used singly, or bile acid sequestrants may be used in combination with either niacin or a HMG-CoA reductase inhibitor.
  - The minor drugs have only modest ability to lower LDL; these include fibric agents (gemfibrozil and clofibrate), probucol, and dextrothyroxine.
- When either diet or drug therapy is prescribed, the patient should have a follow-up LDL determination at 4 to 6 weeks and again at 3 months to evaluate effectiveness.
- The effects of lipid-modifying agents on lipid values, possible major adverse effects, and pharmacologic action appear in Table 4–14.

BILE ACID SEQUESTRANTS

Bile acid sequestrants are positively charged resins that bind the negatively charged bile acids in the intestines to form a complex that is excreted in the feces. This results in a compensatory increase in hepatic bile acid synthesis from cholesterol that ultimately leads to a decrease in serum LDL.

- Because bile acid sequestrants are not absorbed from the gastrointestinal tract, they do not produce systemic side effects. However, gastrointestinal side effects do occur, the most frequent and common of which is constipation.
- Bile acid sequestrants have the potential to interfere with absorption of medications from the gastrointestinal tract. To minimize any possible interference with absorption, patients should take other medications at least 1 to 2 hours before or 4 hours after the bile acid sequestrants.

HMG-CoA REDUCTASE INHIBITORS

The HMG-CoA reductase inhibitors suppress the conversion of HMG-CoA to mevalonic acid (the rate-limiting step in the hepatic production of cholesterol) by competitively inhibiting the enzyme HMG-CoA reductase. Ultimately, this action leads to increased activity of LDL receptors on hepatocytes, which pull LDL from the blood.

- Statins are well tolerated by most patients. Gastrointestinal side effects are the most common and occur in 5% or less of patients.
- Statins should be taken in the evening with food or milk for maximal reduction of LDL because the activity of HMG-CoA reductase is greatest in the late evening and early morning hours.

NICOTINIC ACID

Nicotinic acid (niacin, vitamin B_3) lowers cholesterol and triglycerides by altering their production in the liver.

- Niacin is associated with several side effects that make long-term compliance difficult.
  - The most bothersome side effect of niacin, particularly the regular release form, is a flushing reaction that may be accompanied by itching and tingling.
  - The more serious side effects of hepatitis and gastrointestinal upset occur more often with the sustained-release forms.
- Niacin should be avoided by diabetic persons because of increased serum glucose concentrations.
- Niacin can precipitate gout attacks by interfering with renal excretion of uric acid.

TABLE 4–14. **Hyperlipidemic Agents**

DRUG	MODE OF ACTION	PHARMACOLOGIC EFFECTS					ADVERSE REACTIONS
		LIPIDS		LIPOPROTEINS			
		CHOLESTEROL	TRIGLYCERIDES	VLDL	LDL	HDL	
Bile acid sequestrants							
Cholestyramine (Cholybar, Questran)	Resin binds bile acids in intestine and form insoluble complexes resulting in ↑ oxidation of cholesterol, a ↓ in LDL, and ↓ serum cholesterol.	↓	→↑	→↑	↓	→↑	Gastrointestinal upset, distention, abdominal pain; may cause malabsorption of fat-soluble vitamins.
Colestipol (Colestid)		↓	→↑	↑	↓	→↑	
HMG-CoA reductase inhibitors							
Lovastatin (Mevacor)	Inhibits enzyme (HMG-CoA) reductase, which catalyzes early step in cholesterol biosynthesis.	↓	↓	↓	↓	↑	Gastrointestinal upset, abdominal pain, myalgia, headache, fatigue.
Pravastatin (Pravachol)		↓	↓	↓	↓	↑	
Simvastatin (Zocor)		↓	↓	↓	↓	↑	
Probucol (Lorelco)	↑ LDL catabolism and ↓ cholesterol synthesis and slightly ↓ absorption of dietary cholesterol.	↓	→	↑↓	↓	↓	Syncope arrhythmias, dizziness, headache, palpitations.
Dextrothyroxine (Choloxin)	↑ Catabolism and excretion of cholesterol and its degradation products.	↓	→	→	↓	→	Angina, arrhythmias, insomnia, anxiety, and visual disturbances.
Clofibrate (Atromid-S)	↑ Catabolism of VLDL to LDL and ↓ hepatic synthesis of VLDL.	↓	↓	↓	→↓	→↑	Arrhythmia, myalgia, cholelithiasis, rash, gastrointestinal upset, fatigue.
Gemfibrozil (Lopid)	↓ Peripheral lipolysis, ↓ hepatic extraction of free fatty acids, ↓ triglyceride production, and ↓ VLDL production.	↓	↓	↓	→↑	↑	Gastrointestinal upset, fatigue, abdominal pain.
Nicotinic acid (Niacin, Slo-Niacin)	↓ Lipolysis in adipose tissue, ↓ esterification of triglyceride, and ↑ lipoprotein lipase activity.	↓	↓	↓	↓	↑	Flushing of face and upper body, headache, gastrointestinal upset, dizziness, hypertension.

↑ = increase, ↔ = no change, ↓ = decrease, →↑ = no change or increase, →↓ = no change or decrease, HDL = high-density lipoprotein, LDL = low-density lipoprotein, VLDL = very low-density lipoprotein.

4.7 RESPIRATORY DRUGS

The most commonly used drugs in the management of pulmonary disease are the bronchodilators. Antiinflammatory drugs are used both for the prophylaxis of bronchospasm and the treatment of acute inflammatory processes affecting the lungs. Oxygen, another frequently encountered drug, has already been discussed in Chapter 2 (see page 57). A variety of other medications, including mucolytic agents, decongestants, antihistamines, expectorants, and paralyzing agents, play more minor roles in the treatment of pulmonary disease and will only be briefly discussed.

A summary of the effects of various medications, including those used in lung disease, on exercise responses is provided in Table 4–15.

β-ADRENERGIC AGENTS

Bronchodilators are believed to act primarily by reversing the contraction of airway smooth muscle. β-adrenergic agonists (also called sympathomimetics) are the most effective bron-

TABLE 4–15. **Effects of Medications on Heart Rate, Blood Pressure, the Electrocardiogram (ECG), and Exercise Capacity**

MEDICATIONS	HEART RATE		BLOOD PRESSURE REST (R) AND EXERCISE (E)	ECG		EXERCISE CAPACITY
	REST	EXERCISE		REST	EXERCISE	
I. β-blockers (including labetalol)	↓*	↓	↓	↓HR*	↓Ischemia†	↑ In patients with angina; ↓ or ↔ in patients without angina
II. Nitrates	↑	↑ Or ↔	↓ (R) ↑ Or ↔ (E)	↑ HR	↑ Or ↔ HR ↓Ischemia†	↑ In patients with angina; ↔ in patients without angina; ↑ or ↔ in patients with CHF
III. Calcium channel blockers Felodipine Isradipine Nicardipine Nifedipine Bepridil						
	↑ Or ↔	↑ Or ↔	↓	↑ Or ↔ HR	↑ Or ↔ HR ↓ Ischemia† ↓ HR	↑ In patients with angina; ↔ in patients without angina
Diltiazem Verapamil	↓	↓	↓	↓ HR	↓ Ischemia†	↑ In patients with angina, ↔ in patients without angina
IV. Digitalis	↓ In patients w/atrial fibrillation and possibly CHF. Not significantly altered in patients w/sinus rhythm		↔	May produce nonspecific ST-T wave changes	May produce ST segment depression	Improved only in patients with atrial fibrillation or in patients with CHF
V. Diuretics	↔	↔	↔ Or ↓	↔	May cause PVCs and "false-positive" test results if hypokalemia occurs. May cause PVCs if hypomagnesemia occurs	↔, Except possibly in patients with CHF (where it may improve)
VI. Vasodilators, nonadrenergic vasodilators	↑ Or ↔	↑ Or ↔	↓	↑ Or ↔ HR	↑ Or ↔ HR	↔, Except ↑ or ↔ in patients with CHF
ACE inhibitors	↔	↔	↓	↔	↔	↔, Except ↑ or ↔ in patients with CHF
α-Adrenergic blockers	↔	↔	↓	↔	↔	↔
Antiadrenergic agents without selective blockade of peripheral receptors	↓ Or ↔	↓ Or ↔	↓	↓ Or ↔ HR	↓ Or ↔ HR	↔
VII. Antiarrhythmic agents				All antiarrhythmic agents may cause new or worsened arrythmias (proarrhythmic effect)		
Class I Quinidine Disopyramide	↑ Or ↔	↑ Or ↔	↑ Or ↔ (R) ↔ (E)	↑ Or ↔ HR May prolong QRS and QT intervals	Quinidine may result in "false negative" test results	↔

Continued on following page

TABLE **4–15.** **Effects of Medications on Heart Rate, Blood Pressure, the Electrocardiogram (ECG), and Exercise Capacity** *Continued*

MEDICATIONS	HEART RATE		BLOOD PRESSURE	ECG		EXERCISE CAPACITY
	REST	EXERCISE	REST (R) AND EXER-CISE (E)	REST	EXERCISE	
Procainamide	↔	↔	↔	May prolong QRS and QT intervals	May result in "false positive" test results	↔
Phenytoin Tocainide Mexiletine	↔	↔	↔	↔	↔	↔
Flecainide Moricizine	↔	↔	↔	May prolong QRS and QT	↔	↔
Propafenone	↓	↓ Or ↔	↔	↓ HR	↓ Or ↔ HR	↔
Class II β-Blockers (see I)						
Class III Amiodarone	↓	↓	↔	↓ HR	↔	↔
Class IV Calcium channel blockers (see III)						
VIII. Bronchodilators Anticholinergic agents	↔	↔	↔	↔	↔	Bronchodilators ↑ exercise capacity in patients limited by bronchospasm
Methylxanthines	↑ Or ↔	↓ Or ↔	↔	↑ Or ↔ HR May produce PVCs	↑ Or ↔ HR May produce PVCs	
Sympathomimetic agents	↑ Or ↔	↑ Or ↔	↑, ↔, Or↓	↑ Or ↔ HR	↑ Or ↔ HR	
Cromolyn sodium	↔	↔	↔	↔	↔	
Corticosteroids	↔	↔	↔	↔	↔	

IX. Hyperlipidemic agents
Clofibrate may provoke arrhythmias, angina in patients with prior myocardial infarction.
Dextrothyroxine may ↑ HR and BP at rest and during exercise, provoke arrhythmias and worsen myocardial ischemia and angina.
Nicotinic acid may ↓ BP.
Probucol may cause QT interval prolongation.
All other hyperlipidemic agents have no effect on HR, BP, and ECG.

MEDICATIONS	HEART RATE		BLOOD PRESSURE	ECG		EXERCISE CAPACITY
	REST	EXERCISE	REST (R) AND EXER-CISE (E)	REST	EXERCISE	
X. Psychotropic medication						↔
Minor tranquilizes	May ↑ HR and BP by controlling anxiety. No other effects					
Antidepressants	↑ Or ↔	↑ Or ↔	↓ Or ↔	Possible ↑ PR and QT intervals, ST-T changes	May cause "false positive" test results	
Major tranquilizers	↑ Or ↔	↑ Or ↔	↓ Or ↔	As above plus QRS widening	May cause "false positive" or "false negative" test results	

TABLE 4-15. **Effects of Medications on Heart Rate, Blood Pressure, the Electrocardiogram (ECG), and Exercise Capacity** *Continued*

MEDICATIONS	HEART RATE REST	HEART RATE EXERCISE	BLOOD PRESSURE REST (R) AND EXERCISE (E)	ECG REST	ECG EXERCISE	EXERCISE CAPACITY
Lithium	↔	↔	↔	May result in T wave changes and arrhythmias	May result in T wave changes and arrhythmias	
XI. Nicotine	↑ Or ↔	↑ Or ↔	↑	↑ Or ↔ HR; may provoke ischemia, arrhythmias	↑ Or ↔ HR; may provoke ischemia, arrhythmias	↔ Except ↓ or ↔ in patients with angina
XII. Antihistamines	↔	↔	↔	↔	↔	↔
XIII. Cold medications with sympathomimetic agents	Effects similar to those described in sympathomimetic agents, although magnitude of effects is usually smaller.					↔
XIV. Thyroid medications Only levothyroxine	↑	↑	↑	↑ HR May provoke arrhythmias ↑ ischemia	↑ HR May provoke arrhythmias ↑ ischemia	↔, Unless angina worsened
XV. Alcohol	↔	↔	Chronic use may have role in ↑ BP	May provoke arrhythmias	May provoke arrhythmias	↔
XVI. Hypoglycemia agents Insulin and oral agents	↔	↔	↔	↔	↔	↔
XVII. Dipyridamole	↔	↔	↔	↔	↔	↔
XVIII. Anticoagulants	↔	↔	↔	↔	↔	↔
XIX. Antigout medications	↔	↔	↔	↔	↔	↔
XX. Antiplatelet medications	↔	↔	↔	↔	↔	↔
XXI. Pentoxifylline	↔	↔	↔	↔	↔	↑ Or ↔ in patients limited by intermittent claudication
XXII. Caffeine	Variable effects depending upon previous usage Variable effects depending on exercise capacity May provoke arrhythmias					
XXIII. Diet pills	↑ Or ↔	↑ Or ↔	↑ Or ↔	↑ Or ↔ HR	↑ Or ↔ HR	Possible ↑ in endurance

From American College of Sports Medicine: *Resource Manual for Guidelines for Exercise Testing and Prescription,* 2nd Ed. Philadelphia, Lea & Febiger, pp. 200-202, 1993.
↑ = increase, ↔ = no effect, ↓ = decrease, BP = blood pressure, CHF = congestive heart failure, HR = heart rate, PVC = premature ventricular contraction.
*Beta-blockers with ISA lower resting HR only slightly
†May prevent or delay myocardial ischemia (see text)

chodilators in use. In terms of β-adrenergic receptors, the airway smooth muscle has only the β_2-subtype so that selective stimulation of these receptors will result in bronchial relaxation. The β-adrenergic receptors on mast cells are also of the β_2-subtype. Therefore, there is no indication for the administration of nonselective β-adrenergic agonists, such as isoproterenol, which are associated with a high incidence of cardiovascular side effects even when administered by inhalation.

- Inhaled selective β_2-adrenergic agonists have a rapid onset of action (within minutes) and are indicated for short-term relief of bronchoconstriction and prevention of bronchoconstriction precipitated by exercise and other stimuli.
- Table 4–16 lists the β-adrenergic agonists commonly used. With the exception of isoproterenol and epinephrine, these agents are considered β_2-selective. However, clinically, albuterol, terbutaline, bitolterol, and salmeterol are the preferred β_2-selective agents utilized in respiratory distress and prophylaxis. Terbutaline is also available for subcutaneous injection where respiratory administration is difficult or not possible.
- Table 4–17 lists the types of drugs, their modes of action, the route of administration, and the most common adverse reactions.
- Unwanted side effects are uncommon when β-adrenergic agonists are given by inhalation but occur more commonly when administered by nebulizers or orally.

α-ADRENERGIC BLOCKING AGENTS

The α-adrenergic blockers (also called sympatholytics) inhibit the vasoconstriction and bronchoconstriction produced by α-sympathetic stimulation. Phentolamine, an α-adrenergic blocking agent, blocks presynaptic (α_2) and post-synaptic (α_2) α-adrenergic receptors. It is a competitive antagonist of endogenous and exogenous α-active agents. As a result, phentolamine is used to prevent or control respiratory depression.

The primary adverse reaction of phentolamine is acute and prolonged hypotension causing dizziness, which limits its clinical use. In ad-

TABLE 4–16. Common Respiratory Drugs Currently Available

GENERIC DRUGS	TRADE NAMES
α-Adrenergic blocking agent	
Phentolamine	Regitine
Anticholinergics	
Atropine*	Dey-Dose Atropine
Impratropium	Atrovent
β-Adrenergic agonists†	
Albuterol	Proventil, Ventolin
Bitolerol	Tornalate
Epinephrine‡	Adrenalin, Sus-phrine
Isoetharine	Bronkosol, Bronkometer
Isoproterenol	Isuprel
Metaproterenol	Alupent, Metaprel
Salmeterol xinafoate§	Serevent
Terbutaline	Brethine, Bricanyl
Cromolyn sodium	
Cromolyn sodium	Intal, Gastrocrom, Nasalcrom
Glucocorticoids	
Beclomethasone	Beclovent, Vanceril
Dexamethasone	Decadron Turbinaire
Flunisolide	Aerobid
Triamcinolone	Azmacort
Methylxanthines	
Aminophylline	—
Diphylline	Lufyllin
Theophylline	Theolair, Theo-Dur, Slo-Phyllin

*Withdrawn from market.
†All agents have minor β_1-activity.
‡Also has α-adrenergic blocking activity.
§Long-acting at the β_2-receptor site.

dition, it is only available for intravenous or intramuscular injection.

ANTICHOLINERGIC AGENTS

Anticholinergic agents (also known as parasympatholytic agents) block muscarinic receptors in airway smooth muscle and thus inhibit vagal cholinergic tone and prevent bronchoconstriction. These drugs only inhibit the component of bronchoconstriction due to cholinergic nerves; they have no action against the direct effects of mediators on airway smooth muscle, in contrast to β-adrenergic agonists, which inhibit bronchoconstriction irrespective of the precipitating agent. Anticholinergics are usually used in combination with other bronchodilators. The currently available anticholinergics include, but are not limited to, atropine and ipratropium (Atrovent). Atropine for inhalation has been taken off of the market because of its adverse side effects, but it is still available for intravenous use in serious, acute respiratory distress.

- The onset of action of inhaled anticholinergics (e.g., ipratropium) is slower than that of the b-adrenergic agonists (peaking at 1 hour), but their action is more prolonged, lasting up to 8 hours.
- Systemic adverse reactions (anticholinergic effects) do not occur with ipratropium because it is poorly absorbed systemically.

METHYLXANTHINES

The methylxanthines (theophylline and its soluble salts and derivatives) are less effective bronchodilators than are β-adrenergic agonists but may have a synergistic effect. Initially, theophylline was thought to cause bronchodilation by inhibiting the production of phosphodiesterase. However, other mechanisms of action have now been proposed: antagonism of adenosine receptors, inhibition of the intracellular release of calcium, and stimulation of catecholamine release. Unlike the β-adrenergic agonists, theophylline inhibits the late response to allergens, suggesting that it has an antiinflammatory action; however, it does not inhibit the release of mediators from eosinophils.

TABLE 4–17. **Common Respiratory Drugs**

DRUG CLASS	MODE OF ACTION	ROUTE OF ADMINISTRATION	ADVERSE REACTIONS
α-Adrenergic blocking agents	Blocks presynatpic (α_2) and postsynaptic (α_1) receptors; causes vasodilation and cardiac stimulation	IV, IM	Weakness, dizziness, hypertension, flushing, tachycardia, gastrointestinal upset, anxiety.
Anticholinergic agents	Produces bronchodilation by a local, site-specific effect by competitive inhibition of acetylcholine at muscarinic receptors.	INH, IV	Gastrointestinal upset, cough, dry mouth, headache, dizziness, nervousness.
β-adrenergic agonists*	β_1-adrenergic stimulation (vasoconstriction and pressor effects) and β_2-adrenergic stimulation (bronchial dilation and vasodilation)	PO, SL, INH, IV, SQ	Nervousness, tremor, palpitations, tachycardia, vertigo, hyperactivity, headache, gastrointestinal upset, bronchospasm.
Cromolyn sodium	Stabilizes mast cell membranes, inhibiting the release of histamine and slow-reacting substances of anaphylaxis.	PO, INH, nasal spray	Bronchospasm, cough, throat irritation, bad taste, gastrointestinal upset.
Glucocorticoids	May ↓ number and activity of inflammatory cells, ↑ effect of β-adrenergic drugs, ↓ bronchoconstrictor mechanisms, or produce direct smooth muscle relaxation.	PO, INH, IV	Throat irritation, cough, dry mouth, rash, fungal infections, adrenal insufficiency.
Methylxanthines	Directly relaxes the smooth muscle of the bronchi and pulmonary blood vessel.	PO, IV, SUPP	Gastrointestinal upset, irritability, insomnia, headache, muscle twitching, palpitations.

IM = intramuscular injection, IHN, = inhaled, IV = intravenous, PO = oral, SL = sublingual, SQ. = subcutaneous, SUPP = rectal suppository.
*β₂-selective agents provide greatest benefit with minimal side effects.

- Theophylline is not available for inhalation and must be administered either orally, intravenously, or via intramuscular injection (aminophylline). The systemic administration of these medications is responsible for the relatively high incidence of unwanted side effects. The common side effects are nausea and headache, but more serious problems, such as cardiac arrhythmias and seizures, may occur when plasma drug concentrations are high ($\geq$20 mg/mL).

CROMOLYN

Cromolyn is an antiasthmatic and antiallergic agent and mast cell stabilizer, which prevents the immediate hypersensitivity reaction. It has no intrinsic bronchodilator, antihistaminic, anticholinergic, vasoconstrictor, or antiinflammatory activity. Cromolyn acts locally on the lungs via inhalation and is undoubtedly capable of preventing bronchoconstriction, although it is less effective than steroids given by inhalation.

- Cromolyn protects against various indirect bronchoconstrictor stimuli such as exercise.
- Cromolyn is the antiasthmatic drug of choice in children because it has few side effects; steroids given by inhalation are preferred in adults because they are considerably more effective.
- The major adverse reactions to cromolyn inhalation are dry mouth and throat and airway irritation, which can cause bronchospasm in some individuals.

GLUCOCORTICOIDS

Glucocorticoids do not have a rapid bronchodilator effect, must be given on a long-term basis, and should be regarded as prophylactic. Steroids given by inhalation are more effective than orally administered steroids in reducing bronchoconstriction, suggesting an action on cells close to the lumen of the airways. The precise mechanism of action of the aerosolized drug in the lung is unknown. Glucocorticoids may decrease the number and activity of inflammatory cells, enhance the effect of β-adrenergic drugs inhibiting bronchosconstriction mechanisms, or produce direct smooth muscle relaxation.

- Use of the inhaler makes it possible to provide effective local steroid activity with minimal systemic effects. Naturally occurring adrenal cortical steroids (e.g., hydrocortisone) and synthetic steroid compounds (e.g., prednisolone, dexamethasone, and betamethasone) are available for intravenous or oral administration for the treatment of acute respiratory distress due to various causes. The lowest possible dose should always be used since adverse reactions and complications are very likely with systemic administration.
- Side effects of inhaled steroids include oropharyngeal candidiasis and dysphonia. Orally administered steroids can produce osteoporosis, weight gain, and HTN, among others.

METERED-DOSE INHALERS

Metered-dose inhalers (MDIs) are small portable devices that deliver medication in an aerosol form so it can be inhaled. The medication is dissolved or suspended in a liquid in a small canister. The canister fits into a plastic device with mouthpiece that releases a set amount of medication, a metered dose.

- Inhalation is more successful because the drug is delivered directly to the lungs. This permits lower doses of medicine, more rapid onset of action, and fewer side effects.
- The recommended closed-mouth technique for MDIs is described in Table 4–18.
- The open-mouth technique involves the same procedure, only with a modification of step 4. Instead of placing the mouthpiece between the lips, the mouthpiece is held about 1½ inches in front of the wide-open mouth. Follow the rest of the procedure.
- If the patient has difficulty coordinating the squirt of the inhaler and taking a breath, a spacer can facilitate MDI use. The spacer is used as a holding chamber for the medication. The dose of medicine is squirted into one end of the spacer, and the patient inhales at the opposite end. Spacers have been shown to increase the amount of medication in the lungs and to decrease the amount of medicine left in the back of the mouth.

TABLE 4–18. **Recommended Technique for Closed-Mouth Use of Metered Dose Inhalers (MDIs)**

1. Remove the cap and shake the inhaler before each use.
2. Breathe out fully.
3. Hold the inhaler in an upright position.
4. Based on the physician's recommendation, place the mouthpiece of the inhaler between the lips, keeping the tongue and teeth from blocking the mouthpiece.
5. With the head upright, begin to inhale slowly and deeply, and press down on the canister once.
6. Continue to breathe in slowly and deeply through the mouth for as long as possible.
7. Hold breath for at least 5 to 10 seconds or for as long as possible.
8. Breathe out slowly through pursed lips or through the nose.
9. If the doctor has prescribed two puffs, wait 2 minutes and repeat the procedure.
10. Clean the plastic mouthpiece thoroughly with soap and water after each use.

ANCILLARY PULMONARY MEDICATIONS

Although the major drugs used in treating pulmonary disease are the bronchodilators and antiinflammatory steroids, there are several other groups of ancillary agents that are frequently used, including decongestants, antihistamines, antitussives, expectorants, mucolytics, and paralyzing agents.

- Decongestants are used to treat the upper airway mucosal edema and discharge that produce the typical runny nose and stuffy head of the common cold and seasonal allergies. The most common agents are α-sympathetic agonists (e.g., pseudoephedrine hydrochloride and phenylpropanolamine), which stimulate vasoconstriction of the blood vessels in the mucosal lining of the upper airway, reducing congestion. Because of their sympathetic activity, their primary side effects consist of headache, dizziness, nervousness, nausea, elevated BP, and palpitations.
- Antihistamines are used to block histamine-mediated reactions associated with seasonal allergies. They reduce mucosal congestion, irritation, and discharge caused by inhaled allergens and are frequently combined with decongestants. The most common side effects associated with antihistamines include sedation, fatigue, dizziness, blurred vision, and loss of coordination. In addition, their anticholinergic effects may cause drying of secretions and lead to further airway obstruction in some patients.
- Antitussives suppress the cough reflex and are used to treat the irritating, dry, hacking cough associated with minor throat irritations and the common cold. They are not indicated for coughs due to increased secretions. Two main classifications of drugs provide antitussive effects: nonnarcotic, over-the-counter, cough suppressants (e.g., dextromethorphan and benzonatate), and narcotics (e.g., codeine). The most common adverse side effect is sedation, although some may also cause dizziness and gastrointestinal distress.
- Expectorants may help loosen phlegm and thin bronchial secretions to facilitate the mobilization and clearance of mucus. However, there is some controversy regarding their effectiveness. Among the many drugs available are guaifenesin, potassium iodide, and ammonium chloride. In patients with chronic obstructive lung disease, bronchodilators may additionally facilitate expectoration.
- Mucolytics decrease the viscosity of pulmonary mucous secretions and promote expectoration. Acetylcysteine (Mucomyst), which may improve clearance and disrupt and loosen impacted mucous plugs, is most frequently seen in the management of cystic fibrosis. Its problematic side effects include mucosal irritation, coughing, bronchospasm, and nausea.
- Paralyzing agents, or nondepolarizing neuromuscular agents, help to facilitate the management of patients undergoing mechanical ventilation or to facilitate tracheal intubation. The most frequent adverse reactions are an extension of the pharmacologic actions and can vary from skeletal muscle weakness to profound and prolonged skeletal muscle relaxation, resulting in respiratory insufficiency or apnea.

4.8 DRUGS USED WITH ORGAN TRANSPLANTATION

The fate of transplanted organs, including cardiac and pulmonary organ transplants, depends on a number of factors, but the recipient's immune response to the transplanted organ(s) is the central event. When histocompatability differences exist between donor and recipient, it is necessary to modify or suppress the immune response in order to prevent graft rejection. Immunosuppressive therapy in general suppresses all immune responses, including those to various infections.

- Glucocorticoids modify the body's immune response to diverse stimuli and are routinely utilized in conjunction with immunosuppressant agents because of their potent antiinflammatory activity. Therapy initially is administered parenterally, and as soon as possible is switched to the oral form, most commonly prednisone. As with all steroid therapies, it is extremely important to maintain the patient on the lowest possible dose to minimize the various adverse reactions associated with chronic administration.
- The currently available immunosuppressant agents include azathioprine (Imuran), cyclosporine (Sandimmune), tacrolimus (Prograf), and muromonab-CD3 (Orthoclone)
- With the exception of muromonab-CD3, these preparations are available for oral administration
- The specific mechanism of action for these agents is somewhat obscure, but the effects are similar. These agents suppress some humoral immunity and to a greater extent, cell-mediated reactions, such as allograft rejection. This action is due to specific and reversible inhibition of immunocompetent lymphocytes, preferentially inhibiting T lymphocytes.
  - Currently, tacrolimus is approved for liver transplantation only, but the principles of immunosuppression remain constant; it is anticipated that further experience with the drug will result in its approval for use in other organ transplantation also.
- The principal adverse reactions associated with immunosuppressive agents are renal dysfunction, tremor, hypertension, and gastrointestinal effects. One of the most serious consequences of sustained immunosuppressive therapy is the development of lymphomas. Their occurrence is related to the intensity and duration of therapy rather than the use of specific agents.

4.9 DRUGS USED TO TREAT DIABETES MELLITUS

The current diagnostic criteria for diabetes mellitus (DM), regardless of causes, require that one of the following must exist: (1) A random plasma glucose level of 200 mg/dL or greater plus classic signs and symptoms of diabetes, including polydypsia, polyuria, and weight loss, or (2) a fasting plasma glucose level of 140 mg/dL or greater on at least two occasions. The pharmacologic management of DM includes insulin and oral hypoglycemic agents. The major goal of

TABLE 4–19. **Insulin Preparations and Their Properties**

TYPE	ONSET	PEAK EFFECT (HR)	DURATION (HR)
Rapid-acting insulin			
Regular, crystalline (CZI)	30–60 min	2–4	6–8
Semilente	60–90 min	2–6	6–8
Intermediate-acting insulin			
Neutral protamine (NPH), isophane	60–90 min	6–12	18–24
Lente	60–90 min	6–12	18–24
Long-acting insulin			
Protaminezine (PZI)	4–8 hr	14–24	36
Ultralente	4–8 hr	18–24	36

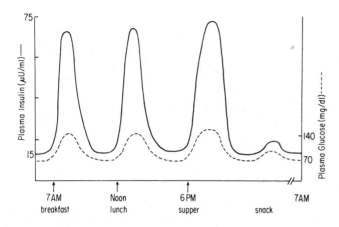

FIGURE **4-2**. Normal insulin-glucose interrelationships throughout the day. Grey line, plasma insulin level; black line, plasma glucose level. (Reproduced with permission from Kozak GP: *Clinical Diabetes Mellitus.* Philadelphia, W. B. Saunders Co., 1982, p. 77.)

treatment is to control hyperglycemia and thus prevent acute metabolic derangements and minimize the morbidity and mortality associated with DM (see Chapter 3, page 102). In general, it is reasonable to attempt to control each patient as tightly as possible without producing hypoglycemia. The commonly used plasma glucose targets are fasting plasma levels ranging from 120 to 150 mg/dL; postprandial glucose values (1 to 2 hours after a meal) are between 150 and 200 mg/dL.

- Individuals with type I, or insulin-dependent, DM are required to take insulin, which is available in a variety of forms.
  - The most common form of therapy is daily injection of insulin preparations, listed in Table 4–19. By using some combination of short-, intermediate-, and long-acting insulin, an attempt is made to mimic the normal endogenous physiologic insulin profile, with basal levels in between meals and at night and sharp peaks at meal times (Figs. 4-2 and 4-3).
  - Intensive insulin therapy, which allows for adjustment of insulin dose throughout the day based on the results of frequent blood glucose monitoring, achieves the most normal physiologic levels of insulin but requires maximal patient participation and cooperation. It involves multiple daily injections or the use of continuous subcutaneous insulin infusion via an open loop pump. Insulin doses are adjusted according to the pattern of need, size of impending meal, and antici-

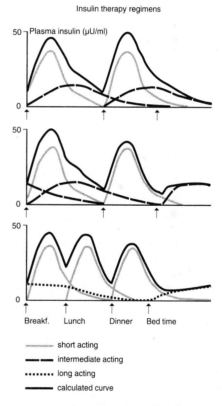

FIGURE **4-3**. Some common insulin therapy regimens and the insulin levels they produce. The calculated curve is the sum of the plasma insulin levels derived from the combined insulin dosages. (Reproduced with permission from Krall LP (ed.): *World Book of Diabetes in Practice*, Vol. 3. Amsterdam, Elsevier, 1988, p. 157.)

TABLE 4–20. **Oral Hypoglycemic Agents and Their Properties**

GENERIC DRUG (TRADE NAME)	DURATION OF ACTION (HR)	USUAL DAILY DOSE (RANGE) (MG)
Tolbutamide (Orinase, Oramide)	6–12	2000 (500–3000)
Chlorpropamide (Diabinese)	24–72	250–500 (100–750)
Acetohexamide (Dymelor)	12–24	500–1000 (250–1500)
Tolazamide (Ronase, Tolinase)	10–24	250–500 (100–1000)
Glyburide (Micronase, DiaBeta)	10–30	2.5–10.0 (2.5–30.0)
Glipizide (Glucotrol)	10–30	15–25 (5–40)

pated activity level. Implantable pumps are also available but their size and limited programmability limit their practicality at this time.

- In type II, or noninsulin-dependent, DM, treatment with diet and exercise is recommended initially, especially for the control of obesity, which is seen in 70% to 90% of individuals.
  - For patients who fail to achieve adequate glycemic control, oral hypoglycemic agents are prescribed (Table 4–20). The second-generation sulfonylurea agents (glipizide, glyburide) are associated with fewer side effects compared with the first-generation agents (e.g., chlorpropramide, tolbutamide, tolazamide, and acetohexamide). When the agent is selected, it is important to begin with the lowest possible dose and titrate the dose slowly upward, as necessary.
  - Some individuals, who continue to be hyperglycemic despite treatment with diet, exercise, and oral hypoglycemic agents, benefit from the addition of insulin; usually only one or two doses of intermediate-acting insulin are required each day. Insulin may also be required during acute illness or stress situations, such as infection, myocardial infarction, trauma, and general anesthesia.
- The primary problem encountered with oral hypoglycemics and insulin therapy is the predisposition to hypoglycemia, especially during exercise. Signs of mild hypoglycemia include weakness, diaphoresis, mental confusion, and muscle rigidity, which can occur during or up to 24 hours following exercise. Since exercise decreases insulin requirements, hypoglycemia

can be prevented or treated by taking a supplemental carbohydrate source approximately 1 hour before beginning exercise or at the first signs of hypoglycemia.

REFERENCES

1. Braunwald E: *Heart Disease: A Textbook of Cardiovascular Medicine*, 3rd Ed. Philadelphia, W. B. Saunders Co., 1988.
2. Ciccone C: *Pharmacology in Rehabilitation*, 4th Ed. Philadelphia, F. A. Davis, 1990.
3. Dipiro JT: *Pharmacotherapy*, 2nd Ed. New York, Elsevier, 1993.
4. Echt DS, Liebson PR, Mitchell LB, et al.: Mortality and morbidity in patients receiving encainide, flecainide, or placebo. The cardiac arrhythmia suppression trial. *N. Engl. J. Med.* 324:781–788, 1991.
5. Ferguson G, Cherniack RM: Management of chronic obstructive pulmonary disease. *N. Engl. J. Med.* 328:1017–1022, 1993.
6. Gerber JG, Nies AS: Antihypertensive agents and the drug therapy of hypertension. *In* Goodman and Gilman: *The Pharmacologic Basis of Therapeutics.* Tarrytown, NY, Pergamon Press, 1990.
7. Herfindal ET: *Clinical Pharmacy and Therapeutics*, 5th Ed. Baltimore, Williams & Wilkins Co., 1992.
8. Hume AL, Barbour MM, Lapane KL, Willey CJ, Assaf AR, Charleton RA: Changing trends in antihypertensive drug therapy in two southeastern New England communities during the 1980s. *Pharmacotherapy* 13:244–251, 1993.
9. Hunningmake DB: Drug treatment of dislipoproteinemia. *Endocrinol. Metabol. Clin. North Am.* 19(2):345–360, 1990.
10. Johnson G: *Essentials of Drug Therapy.* Philadelphia, W. B. Saunders Co., 1991.

11. Joint National Committee on Detection, Evaluation, and Treatment of Hypertension: The fifth report of the Joint National Committee on Detection, Evaluation, and Treatment of Hypertension. *Arch. Intern. Med.* 153:154–183, 1993.

12. Kaplan NM: Calcium entry blocker in the treatment of hypertension. Current status and future prospects. *JAMA* 262:817–823, 1989.

13. Nelson HS: Adrenergic therapy of bronchial asthma. *J. Allergy Clin. Immunol.* 77:771–785, 1986.

14. Opie L: *Drugs for the Heart,* 3rd Ed. Philadelphia, W. B. Saunders Co., 1991.

15. Rodgers, K: CHF: Current strategies, future developments. *Drug Topics* 138:20–28, 1994.

16. Saunders E, Weir MR, Kong BW, et al.: A comparison of the efficacy and safety of a beta-blocker, a calcium channel blocker, and a converting enyzme inhibitor in hypertensive blacks. *Arch. Intern. Med.* 150:1707–1713, 1990.

17. Snyder S: Comparison of cholesterol-lowering regimens. *American Family Physician* 42:761–768, 1990.

18. Steiner A, Weisser B, Vetter W: A comparative review of the adverse effects of treatments for hyperlipidemia. *Drug Safety* 6(2):118–130, 1991.

5

CARDIOPULMONARY ASSESSMENT

Because cardiopulmonary disease is so prevalent in our society, it is likely that a significant portion of the patients referred for physical therapy have some form of disease or dysfunction related to these systems, even though many have never been diagnosed (e.g., although 75% of patients with cerebrovascular disease have been documented to have coronary artery disease by angiography, only 25% to 48% have a history of it).[7,12] Therefore, assessment of the cardiopulmonary systems is important to include in the physical therapy evaluations of all patients over 40 years of age and younger patients with coronary risk factors, possible cardiopulmonary symptomatology, or diseases or disorders that can affect the cardiopulmonary systems.

This chapter includes descriptions of the various components of a cardiopulmonary assessment for physical therapists: the medical chart review, patient/family interview, physical assessment, including an activity and endurance evaluation, as well as important "red flags" (i.e., precautions and contraindications). Some of these components become more or less valuable, depending on their availability and the setting in which the therapist is working. When one component is more difficult to obtain or accomplish, the remaining components become even more critical. For example, the therapist working in the outpatient or home care setting usually does not have access to the patient's medical record and may be given minimal information regarding the patient's medical history other than the diagnosis for which treatment is requested; thus, the patient/family interview and physical assessments take on additional importance.

5.1 MEDICAL CHART REVIEW

When the patient is in the hospital, a careful review of the physician and nursing admission and progress notes, as well as physician orders and results of various diagnostic tests, can provide the therapist with valuable information about the patient's medical status and possible treatment needs even before the therapist meets the patient. Important findings that may influence the therapist are presented below according to their location in the medical chart.

ADMISSION NOTES

The physician and nursing admission notes usually offer the most complete summary of the patient's medical history and physical examination.

- Specific medical information that may be of particular value to the therapist include the admitting diagnosis, the date of admission, the patient's symptoms or medical complaints, the patient's past medical and surgical history, and medications being taken at the time of admission. Important considerations for each of these are presented in Table 5–1.
- The level of disability of cardiac patients is often described according to the NYHA functional classifications, which are characterized in Table 5–2.
- Also commonly found in the admission notes are the patient's coronary risk factors and social history, and sometimes, occupation, home environment and family situation. Some of the questions that should be considered include:
  - Does the patient smoke? What (cigarettes, cigars, pipe)? Has the patient ever smoked?

TABLE 5-1. **Important Medical Information Found in a Patient's Medical Chart**

INFORMATION	IMPORTANT CONSIDERATIONS
Admitting diagnosis	Is the diagnosis cardiopulmonary in nature?
	Does the diagnosis have any cardiac or pulmonary complications associated with it? (See pages 100–101.)
Admission date	How long has the patient been in the hospital? (The longer the hospitalization, the greater the likelihood of major medical problems or complications.)
Patient symptoms or complaints	What were the patient's complaints prompting admission?
	Does the patient have any symptoms that can be attributed to cardiac disease (e.g., chest discomfort, shortness of breath, palpitations, lightheadedness, as on page 8) or lung disease (e.g., dyspnea, wheezing, cough, sputum production, as on page 42)?
	Specific descriptors offered by the patient are particularly helpful, since they provide medical personnel with vocabulary that is meaningful to the patient (e.g., "chest tightness" might not be considered to be "chest pain" by the patient).
Past medical and surgical history	Does the patient have any past history of cardiovascular or pulmonary problems, or other diseases with possible cardiopulmonary complications, whether or not related to the admission diagnosis (e.g., HTN or DM)?
	Will other medical problems limit the patient's ability to exercise (e.g., arthritis, neurologic or neuromuscular disease)?
Medications	Was the patient taking any medications on a regular basis before admission?
	Do any of the previously prescribed medications indicate possible cardiovascular or pulmonary disease (e.g., HTN, angina, heart failure, bronchospasm)?
	What medications is the patient currently taking?
	Will any of the currently prescribed medications alter the patient's physiologic responses to physical therapy interventions, such as exercise or hubbard tank? (See pages 135–137)
	Is the patient receiving oxygen therapy? What amount and by what method (e.g., 3 L/min by nasal cannula, 60% by face mask)?

DM = diabetes mellitus, HTN = hypertension.

How many pack years (number of packs per day times the number of years)?
- Does the patient have any other risk factors for coronary disease (e.g., hypertension, family history, elevated cholesterol, obesity) or pulmonary disease (e.g., occupational exposure to known irritants, recurrent infections, immunosuppression)?
- What is the patient's history of alcohol use? High intake is associated with an increased incidence of hypertension, cardiac disease, and aspiration pneumonia.
- Does the patient use any illicit drugs? Marijuana use can result in chronic obstructive pulmonary disease (COPD); cocaine use is associated with coronary spasm and arrhythmias.
- Is the patient's lifestyle active or predominantly sedentary?
- What social support systems are available for patient? Are there people who can provide help if needed? Will the patient require home health services?
- Will the lifestyle habits of those close to the patient support or interfere with recommended changes for the patient?
- What is the patient's occupation? What are the physical requirements of the job? Will the patient be able to return to that job or will a change need to be made?

- Where does the patient live? With whom? Are there physical barriers that may be a problem?
  - Who is the patient's medical insurance provider? Will the insurance provider cover continued therapy after discharge? How many treatments?
- The relevant data from the patient's physical examination (often listed as review of systems [ROS]) include the general observations, chest, cardiovascular system, abdomen, extremities, and others, which are described in Table 5–3.
- Analytes measured during clinical laboratory testing that may indicate cardiopulmonary dysfunction include arterial blood gases, myocardial enzymes (e.g., creatine phosphokinase [CPK], lactate dehydrogenase [LDH], and serum aspartate aminotransferase [AST]), white blood cell count, and renal function tests.
  - Patterns of abnormalities seen in cardiac or pulmonary disease include:
    — Increased white blood cell count, sedimentation rate, myocardial enzymes (CPK, LDH, AST) in acute myocardial infarction
    — Possible hypoxemia, hypercapnia, respiratory acidosis, increased white blood cell count and bacteremia in acute pulmonary disease
    — Increased sedimentation rate, white

blood cell count, and streptolysin O titers in acute rheumatic fever
— Increased blood urea nitrogen, proteinuria, and granular casts in cardiac failure
— Possible polycythemia, hypoxemia, hypercapnia, compensated respiratory acidosis in chronic pulmonary disease
— Increased cholesterol and triglyceride levels, as well as possible glucose intolerance, in coronary artery disease
— Increased serum creatinine and blood urea nitrogen, decreased creatinine clearance, and proteinuria in renal insufficiency, plus anemia in renal failure
- Abnormalities that might result in cardiopulmonary dysfunction or decreased exercise tolerance:
  — Increased K^+ (especially if decreased Ca^+), decreased K^+, decreased Mg^+, and toxic digitalis levels (which may be potentiated by decreased K^+ or Mg^+) may cause arrhythmias.
  — Anemia (decreased hematocrit, hemoglobin) can result in fatigue and dyspnea.
  — Severely decreased phosphorous may depress myocardial function.
  — Metabolic acidosis (e.g., diabetic ketoacidosis) elicits hyperventilation, whereas metabolic alkalosis (e.g., excess sodium bicarbonate during cardiopulmonary resuscitation) results in hypoventilation.

TABLE 5-2. **NYHA Functional Classification of Heart Disease, with Relationship to Exercise Tolerance**

FUNCTIONAL CLASSIFICATION	DESCRIPTION	EXERCISE TOLERANCE
I	Patient with cardiac disease but without any resulting limitations of physical activity; ordinary physical activity does not cause undue fatigue, palpitations, dyspnea, or anginal pain.	6–10 METs
II	Slight limitations of physical activity; comfortable at rest, but ordinary physical activity results in fatigue, palpitations, dyspnea, or anginal pain.	4–6 METs
III	Marked limitation of physical activity; comfortable at rest, but less than ordinary physical activity causes symptoms, as above.	2–3 METs
IV	Unable to carry out any physical activity without discomfort; symptoms of cardiac insufficiency or of angina may be present even at rest; if exertion is undertaken, discomfort increases.	<2 METs

MET = metabolic equivalent of energy expenditure (1 MET = approximately 3.5 ml O_2/kg/min).

TABLE 5-3. **Important Information Obtained from a Review of the Patient's Physical Examination**

SYSTEM	IMPORTANT CONSIDERATIONS
	Are there any findings that might suggest cardiovascular or pulmonary disease or result in increased workload on these systems?
General appearance	Obesity, cachexia, barrel-shaped chest, signs of distress (e.g., tachypnea, use of accessory muscles of respiration, intercostal retractions)
Vital signs	↓ Or ↑ heart rate, blood pressure or respiratory rate; presence of fever
Skin	Cold and clammy in low–cardiac output states; pale, blue, and cold if peripheral vasoconstriction; cyanosis if marked arterial hypoxemia; or xanthomas in familial hypercholesterolemia
Head, eyes, ears, nose, and throat (HEENT)	Abnormal funduscopic eye examination (e.g., retinal arteriolar changes in HTN and DM)
	Abnormal neck examination (e.g., jugular venous distension in right or biventricular heart failure, exaggerated venous pulse waves in pulmonary HTN or right-sided valvular disease, or prominent carotid pulsations in aortic incompetence)
	Signs of upper respiratory infection (which might be seeding lower respiratory tract)
Chest, lungs	Abnormal chest examination (e.g., ↓ chest or diaphragmatic excursions in chronic obstructive pulmonary disease, prominent pulsations in cardiac hypertrophy, thrills in valve disease)
	Abnormal breath sounds (e.g., decreased, bronchial, or adventitious breath sounds, see page 161)
Cardiovascular	Abnormal heart sounds (e.g., murmurs in valvulvar disease, third and/or fourth heart sounds if diastolic dysfunction or reduced ventricular compliance, friction rubs in pericarditis, see page 163)
	Abnormal peripheral pulses (e.g., decreased if atherosclerotic disease or aortic stenosis, bounding in aortic incompetence)
Abdomen	Enlarged liver and spleen, ascites in right heart failure
Extremities	Abnormal extremity exam (e.g., peripheral edema, digital clubbing)

↓ = decreased, ↑ = increased, HTN = hypertension, DM = diabetes mellitus.

• Finally, the results of any diagnostic tests and procedures performed before or at the time of admission are usually described in the admission note. The most common cardiopulmonary studies and important considerations are listed in Table 5–4.

PROGRESS NOTES

Within the physician and nursing progress notes are the details of the patient's hospital course, ongoing clinical laboratory data, the results of diagnostic tests and procedures, and therapeutic interventions (e.g., surgical procedures, changes in medications, electrolyte replacement, nutritional support). In addition, the patient's actual diagnosis may not be determined until a few days of hospitalization have passed.

More importantly, any complications that develop or secondary diagnoses that are identified are documented in these pages. These may have important implications for physical therapy intervention. Some common examples are discussed below:

• Fever is a common postoperative occurrence for all kinds of surgery and is often due to acute pulmonary complications; all therapists should request the patient to cough (while therapist splints the incision if necessary) after any change of position or rehabilitation activity, and encourage the patient to deep breathe, cough, and move as much as allowed.
• Large discrepancies between fluid intake and output, resulting in either fluid overload

TABLE 5-4. **Important Cardiopulmonary Considerations from Common Diagnostic Tests and Procedures**

DIAGNOSTIC TEST/PROCEDURE	IMPORTANT CARDIOPULMONARY CONSIDERATIONS
Arterial blood gases (ABGs)	Is oxygenation normal (P_{O_2} >80 with O_2 saturation >97%) or adequate (P_{O_2} >60 with O_2 saturation >90%)? If O_2 saturation <85%, exercise is contraindicated. Are P_{CO_2} and pH within normal limits (35–45 mm Hg and 7.35–7.45, respectively)? Are alterations acute or chronic (see page 269)? Was the patient receiving supplemental oxygen when ABGs were drawn? Does the patient need oxygen during treatment?
Bronchoscopy	What were the findings and conclusions? If there was mucous plugging, more aggressive bronchial hygiene is indicated.
Cardiac catheterization	Were the chamber and vessel pressures normal (see page 23)? Were there any gradients across the valves? Was ventricular performance normal (see RNA below)? Were there any obstructions in the coronary arteries? If so, how many, in which vessels, and to what degree?

Chest radiography (CXR)	Are there any abnormalities?
	     Infiltrates, atelectasis, consolidation, air bronchogram, interstitial markings and nodules, pleural effusion, or masses may be visualized in acute pulmonary disease.
	     Flattened diaphragms and hyperinflated chest are seen in COPD, plus possible blebs and bullae in emphysema; possible peribronchial thickening.
	     Pulmonary fibrosis (e.g., reticular markings, honeycomb shadowing) or pleural thickening may be seen in RLD with ↓ lung compliance.
	     ↑ Chamber or heart size, ↑ pulmonary vascular markings, infiltrates, and/or pleural effusions are commonly observed in cardiac disease, particularly if LV failure is present.

Echocardiography (Echo)	Are chamber sizes and wall thicknesses normal (see page 16)? Are all cardiac valves functioning normally? What is the ejection fraction (at least 40–50%)? Are there areas of abnormal wall motion (e.g., hypokinesis, akinesis, or dyskinesis)?
Electrocardiography (ECG)	Is there evidence of acute, evolving, or old MI? Any chamber enlargement or hypertrophy? Any arrhythmias or conduction disturbances? Do they improve over time or with therapeutic interventions? Are there any other abnormalities (see pages 9–10)?
Exercise testing	How well did the patient perform (e.g., how many minutes on what protocol)? Why did the patient stop (i.e., what limited performance)? Were the patient's responses to exercise normal (see pages 174 and 186)? Were there any abnormalities? What was the maximal MET level achieved?

Pulmonary function tests (PFTs)	Are there abnormalities that indicate obstructive or restrictive dysfunction?
	     In COPD: ↑ vital capacity and total lung capacity, mostly due to ↑ residual volume and functional residual capacity, and ↓ expiratory flow rates.
	     In RLD: ↓ lung volumes and capacities and ↓ diffusing capacity.
	 How do the current results compare with previous PFTs, if available?

Radionuclide angiography/ ventriculography (RNA or RNV)	What is the ejection fraction (at least 40–50%)? Does it increase during exercise? Are there areas of abnormal wall motion?

Continued on following page

TABLE 5-4. **Important Cardiopulmonary Considerations from Common Diagnostic Tests and Procedures**—*Continued*

DIAGNOSTIC TEST/PROCEDURE	IMPORTANT CARDIOPULMONARY CONSIDERATIONS
Thallium scan	Were there any perfusion defects following exercise?
	Was there reperfusion during the resting scan or were the defects fixed?
Ventilation-perfusion scan	Were there any defects in either scan?
	What was the diagnostic conclusion?

$\downarrow$ = decreased, $\uparrow$ = increased, COPD = chronic obstructive pulmonary disease, LV = left ventricular, MET = metabolic equivalent of energy expenditure, MI = myocardial infarction, RLD = restrictive lung dysfunction.

(another common postoperative finding) or dehydration, will impair the patient's tolerance for activity.

- It is important for therapists to recognize a complicated course following acute myocardial infarction (e.g., ventricular tachycardia or fibrillation, atrial flutter or fibrillation, second or third degree atrioventricular [AV] block, persistent sinus tachycardia or systolic hypotension, pulmonary edema, cardiogenic shock, or postinfarction angina or extension of infarction), for these patients have a higher risk of serious morbidity and mortality than those with an uncomplicated course.

PHYSICIAN ORDERS

A running chronicle of the prescribed and discontinued medications and their doses, as well as any ordered tests and procedures and prescribed activity level, can be found in the physician orders. When the specific decisions regarding patient management are not clearly defined in the physician progress notes, the order sheets will disclose them. In addition, a list of the patient's prescribed medications will be found on the nurses' medication cart.

OTHER REPORTS

The remaining sections of the patient's medical chart usually contain the records of vital signs and intake and output (if ordered), reports of diagnostic tests and procedures, surgical reports, physician consultation reports, and the evaluation and treatment notes of allied health professionals, such as physical, occupational, speech, and respiratory therapists. Usually there are also copies of any electrocardiograms (ECGs) ob-

tained since admission, which can be examined; even when the therapist is not formally trained in the interpretation of 12-lead ECG, repeated review of the recordings along with the printed reports, especially if obtained serially, and asking questions of friendly nurses and physicians often results in increasing recognition of a number of abnormalities and an appreciation for any changes over time.

5.2 PATIENT/FAMILY INTERVIEW

Following review of the medical chart, the therapist has some impression of the patient's medical status and major problems and is ready to meet the patient and family. The purpose of the interview with the patient and family is to clarify the information obtained from the medical chart and fill in any missing information so that an appropriate evaluation can be performed and suitable treatment goals and plan can be developed. Of particular concern are any symptoms the patient might reveal and their possible causes, which are presented in Table 5–5. Notably, sometimes the patient/family interview provides a completely different picture of the patient's status than the impression created by the medical chart review. Other important benefits of the interview include establishing rapport with the patient and family, discerning their level of understanding of the medical problem(s), and ascertaining their goals and expectations for rehabilitation.

Typically, questions should be open ended and straightforward. For example:

- What prompted you to come to the hospital?

TABLE 5-5. **Common Patient Complaints and Possible Causes**

COMPLAINT	POSSIBLE CAUSES
Chest pain/discomfort	Cardiac disease
	Myocardial ischemia
	Pericarditis
	Myocarditis or endocarditis
	LV outflow obstruction
	Pulmonary disease
	Pleurisy
	Pulmonary embolism
	Other causes
	Musculoskeletal (e.g., cervical, sternocostal)
	Dissecting aortic aneurysm
	Referred pain from the esophagus
	"Heart burn"/indigestion
	Herpes zoster infections
Dyspnea, shortness of breath	Cardiac dysfunction
	Impaired LV filling (i.e., diastolic dysfunction)
	Reduced LV systolic function
	Pulmonary disease
	Chronic obstructive pulmonary disease
	Restrictive lung dysfunction
	Mixed obstructive-restricted defects
	Other causes
	Anemia
	$\uparrow$ Demand for oxygen (e.g., exercise, sepsis)
	Peripheral arterial disease
	Metabolic acidosis
	Deconditioning
	Psychogenic
Edema, swelling	RV or biventrentricular failure (e.g., CAD, valvular disease, cardiomyopathy, pulmonary HTN, cor pulmonale)
	Fluid overload (e.g., kidney disease, postoperative state)
	Venous disease (venous valve incompetence, venous obstruction)
	Lympathic incompetence
	Other (e.g., medications, cirrhosis, inflammation, trauma)
Fatigue	Poor LV function
	CAD
	Cardiac valve disease
	Cardiomyopathy of any type
	Hypertensive heart disease
	Myocarditis
	Arrhythmias
	Paroxysmal supraventricular tachycardia
	Frequent ventricular ectopy
	Multiple other causes
	Illness/disease (e.g., anemia; dehydration: diarrhea, vomiting, fever; hypothroidism, hypoxemia, hyperglycemia, hypocalcemia)
	Inadequate nutrition
	Medications (e.g., β-blockers)
	Treatment interventions (e.g., radiation therapy)
	Depression
	Deconditioning

Continued on following page

TABLE 5–5.   **Common Patient Complaints and Possible Causes**—*Continued*

COMPLAINT	POSSIBLE CAUSES

Lightheadedness, dizziness	Hypotension
	  Decreased cardiac output (see "Fatigue," above)
	  Excessive peripheral vasodilation
	Cerebral ischemia
	Hyperventilation
	Hypoglycemia

Leg pain	Peripheral vascular disease (e.g., intermittent claudication, venous stasis ulcer, gangrene) Joint disease (e.g., arthritis, gout) Shin splints (e.g., muscle fiber microtears, stress fracture) Nerve irritation (e.g., sciatica) Anterior compartment syndrome Peripheral neuropathy (e.g., diabetes mellitus)

Pallor or cyanosis	Inadequate cardiac output (see "Fatigue," above)
	Hypoxemia
	  Pulmonary disease
	  Congenital heart disease with right-to-left shunting
	Anemia

Palpitations	Premature atrial contractions (PACs) Premature ventricular contractions (PVCs) Paroxysmal atrial/supraventricular tachycardia (PAT, PSVT) Atrial fibrillation (a-fib) or flutter Ventricular tachycardia (v-tach, VT)

Syncope, near syncope	Dangerous arrhythmias
	  Profound bradycardia
	  Second- or third-degree AV block, vasovagal reaction
	  Asystole
	  Rapid tachycardia of any type
	  Ventricular fibrillation
	LV outlet obstruction
	  Aortic stenosis
	  Obstructive hypertrophic cardiomyopathy
	Orthostatic hypotension
	Cardiac tamponade
	Acute pulmonary embolus
	Seizure
	Hypoglycemia

AV = atrioventricular, CAD = coronary artery disease, HTN = hypertension, LV = left ventricular, RV = right ventricular.

- Do you ever have problems with shortness of breath, chest pain or discomfort of any kind, lightheadedness or dizziness, getting tired easily, palpitations, etc.?
- Can you describe your symptoms for me?
- What brings on your symptoms?
- How long have you had these symptoms?
- Do the symptoms interfere with things you would like to do? Such as?
- Have you discovered any ways to relieve the symptoms?
- What has your doctor told you about your problem?
- What would you say your major difficulty is right now?
- What would you like us to work on before you go home?
- What are your goals for your recovery?

5.3 RED FLAGS

Based on the information obtained from the medical chart review and/or the patient/family interview, the therapist might identify some potential problems related to patient evaluation and treatment planning. Diagnoses and situations that require caution are presented in Table 5–6. Depending on the circumstances and the therapist's experience and comfort level, the therapist may decide to proceed slowly with careful monitoring of the patient's responses to position changes and minimal activities. If these results are normal or nearly normal, the therapist may decide to proceed with the activity evaluation; otherwise, it will be deferred to another day. However, certain circumstances present absolute or relative contraindications to exertion of any kind, as explained in Table 5–7.

5.4 PHYSICAL THERAPY EXAMINATION

The physical therapy examination has many of the same cardiopulmonary components as that done by the physician and nurse: inspection, palpation, percussion, and auscultation. However, the physical therapy assessment usually contains one element not typically found in the examinations of others: an evaluation of exercise responses. Furthermore, each time the therapist sees the patient, the patient's status is reassessed both before and after the treatment session so appropriate modifications in the treatment plan can be made.

INSPECTION

Although objective observations of a patient's appearance are an essential component of all physical therapy evaluations, they are especially valuable in patients with possible cardiopulmonary dysfunction because subtle changes often represent important variations in a patient's clinical status.

- Cardiopulmonary inspection typically involves observation of the patient and the patient's status. Important components and specific observations include:
  - General appearance
    — Level of consciousness (e.g., alert, automatic, confused, delirious, stuporous, semicomatose, comatose)
    — Body type (e.g., obese, normal, cachectic)
    — Level of distress (e.g., cardiac: chest discomfort, dyspnea, lightheadedness, or dizziness; pulmonary: use of accessory muscles, nasal flaring, pursed-lip breathing, speech interrupted to take breaths, decreased breath control; general: facial expression, anxiety)
    — Any monitoring or support equipment in use (e.g., supplemental oxygen, cardiac monitor, oxygen saturation monitor, arterial line, central or pulmonary arterial line(s), mechanical ventilation)
    — Presence of incisions, wounds, dressings, casts, etc.
    — Other (e.g., pallor, cyanosis, edema, jugular distension, digital clubbing)
  - Chest
    — Position of trachea (e.g., midline versus deviated to one side)
    — Configuration (e.g., normal is symmetric thorax with rib angles <90° and vertebral attachment at ~45°, and anteroposterior diameter that is approximately one half of the transverse diameter)
    — Nonrespiratory movements (e.g., pulsations)
  - Breathing pattern
    — Inspiratory muscles employed (e.g., normal is relaxed breathing with abdominal rise followed by symmetric expansion of the lateral ribs without recruitment of any accessory muscles)
    — Characteristics of expiration (e.g., normal is passive, approximately twice the duration of inspiration)
  - Cough
    — Characteristics (e.g., strength/force, depth, length, dry- versus full-sounding)
    — Production of secretions (e.g., dry versus productive, quantity, color, smell, consistency of sputum)
  - Posture
    — Presence of any structural abnormalities (e.g., scoliosis, kyphosis)
    — Position of choice (e.g., leaning forward with arms supported seen in COPD)
  - Range of motion
    — Presence of any gross limitations of spine, shoulders, and neck

TABLE 5–6. **Patient Diagnoses or Situations That Require Caution**

DIAGNOSIS	IMPORTANT CONSIDERATIONS
Acute MI within past 2–3 months	Area of infarction is still undergoing remodeling with scar formation, so vigorous activities should be avoided.
Alcoholic hangover	The patient is clearly not functioning normally and may be dehydrated. The patient's physiologic responses to activity may be exaggerated.
h/o Angina, especially if recent	There is potential for myocardial ischemia, particularly on exertion; therefore, monitoring of vital signs and symptoms is important.
Recurrent angina following an MI	Additional myocardium is at risk for infarction.
Arrhythmias	The patient's BP should be taken to determine whether an arrhythmia is hemodynamically significant. For other considerations see page 75.
Cardiac valve disease	Most defects are tolerated well for decades, but some can cause major problems if patient overexerts. Lack of symptoms plus normal BP responses during exertion indicate safety to proceed.
Cerebral dysfunction: dizziness, vertigo	The patient runs an increased risk of falling. Cause could be related to cardiovascular dysfunction (see Table 5–5).
Drug intake	Decongestants, bronchodilators, and diet pills increase the work of the heart, usually through ↑ HR, and may ↑ the HR response to activity.
Emotional turmoil	The patient is already under the influence of increased sympathetic nervous system stimulation with elevated demands on the cardiovascular and respiratory systems.
Environmental extremes: weather, air pollution	Workload on the heart is increased even at rest; exercise responses may be exaggerated.
Evidence of end-organ damage in HTN: retinopathy, renal impairment, LV hypertrophy	BP must be controlled at rest and during exercise to avoid further end-organ damage.
Mural thrombus	RV thrombus creates potential for pulmonary emboli; LV thrombus may result in cerebral or peripheral emboli.
Positive exercise test following acute MI	Additional myocardium is at risk for infarction.
Overindulgence: heavy meal within 2 hours, caffeine	Workload on the heart is increased even at rest; exercise responses may be exaggerated.
Recent pericarditis or myocarditis	During recovery from cardiac inflammation, activity should be low level and physiologic monitoring of exercise responses should be performed in order to determine how much the patient can do safely.
h/o Pulmonary edema, CHF	Careful monitoring of vital signs and symptoms is indicated to prevent overexertion.
Sodium retention: edema, weight gain	Sodium retention could indicate onset of RV or biventricular heart failure.
Severe sunburn	Fluid shifts to the peripheral tissues (i.e., edema) and pain increase the workload of the heart at rest.

↑ = increased, BP = blood pressure, CHF = congestive heart failure, h/o = history of, HR = heart rate, HTN = hypertension, LV = left ventricular, MI = myocardial infarction, RV = right ventricular.

- Strength
  — Functional level as opposed to specific manual muscle testing
  — Presence of respiratory weakness or dyscoordination, especially in patients with neurologic or neuromuscular impairment (e.g., via gross assessment of inspiratory muscle strength and cough force)
- Mobility

TABLE 5-7. **Contraindications to Exercise or Exertion**

CONTRAINDICATIONS	IMPORTANT CONSIDERATIONS
Unstable or rest angina, or change in symptoms in past 24 hours	Myocardial oxygen demand exceeds supply during minimal exertion or even at rest; therefore, patient will probably not tolerate much physical therapy.
Dissecting aneurysm	Increasing BP, as with exertion, places additional stress on an already weakened arterial wall, which could rupture.
Severe aortic stenosis or obstructive hypertrophic cardiomyopathy	There is an ↑ risk of exercise-induced syncope and sudden death.
Dangerous arrhythmias: supraventricular tachycardia, ventricular tachycardia or fibrillation, second- or third-degree heart block	Exercise demands ↑ cardiac output that can not be ejected when the heart is not pumping effectively, as in hemodynamically significant arrhythmias.
Symptomatic CHF/pulmonary edema	The heart is unable to pump adequate cardiac output to meet current demands, let alone those of physical therapy.
Uncontrolled diabetes mellitus	When blood sugar is >250–300 mg/dL, an insulin deficiency impairs glucose uptake by exercising muscles so that ↑ hepatic glucose production exceeds peripheral utilization, so exertion results in even more marked hyperglycemia.
Uncontrolled HTN: Resting SBP > 200 mm Hg Resting DBP > 105–110 mm Hg	LV and arterial wall tensions are already extremely high at rest and will increase further during exertion. In addition, if any end-organ damage exists, there is risk of ↑ morbidity.
Persistent hypotension following MI (SBP <90 mm Hg)	This is an indication of very poor LV function at rest and poor ability to tolerate demands of exertion.
Acute infection or fever	With acute illness, the heart and the immune system have increased demands, so exercise is not recommended.
Active pericarditis or myocarditis	Increasing the demands on an inflamed heart is not advised.

↑ = increased, BP = blood pressure, CHF = congestive heart failure, DBP = diastolic blood pressure, HTN = hypertension, LV= left ventricular, MI = myocardial infarction, SBP = systolic blood pressure.

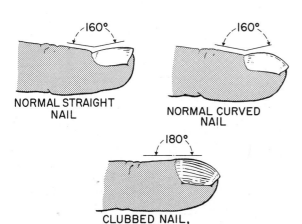

FIGURE 5-1. Digital clubbing compared with a normal finger with a straight nail or a curved nail. Note the base angle of ≥180°. Clubbing becomes more pronounced as lung disease progresses. (From Cherniack RM, Cherniack L: *Respiration in Health and Disease,* 3rd Ed. Philadelphia, W.B. Saunders Co., p. 189, 1983.)

TABLE 5-8. **Terminology Used for Common Breathing Patterns**

BREATHING PATTERN	CHARACTERISTIC FEATURES
Eupnea	Normal rate, depth, and rhythm of breathing
Apnea	Cessation of breathing following expiration, interrupted by eventual inspiration or becomes fatal
Tachypnea	Increased breathing rate, usually shallow with regular rhythm (as in restrictive lung dysfunction)
Bradypnea	Slow rate, shallow or normal depth, regular rhythm (as in drug overdose)
Hyperpnea	Increased breathing due to increased depth, but usually not increased rate
Cheyne-Stokes (periodic) respiration	Cyclic waxing and waning of depth of breathing with periods of apnea interspersed between cycles (seen in severe CNS lesions)
Apneustic breathing	Cessation of breathing following inspiration, interrupted by periodic expiration (seen in brainstem disorders)
Biot's breathing	Irregular breathing with slow, shallow breaths and periods of apnea (seen in meningitis)
Cluster breathing	Clusters of normal breaths separated by irregular pauses (seen in high medullary or low pontine lesions)
Hyperventilation	Fast, deep breathing so that ventilation exceeds metabolic needs (e.g., anxiety attack)
Kussmaul breathing	Marked continuous hyperventilation with increased rate and depth of breathing in order to eliminate excess carbon dioxide (e.g., diabetic ketoacidosis)
Doorstop respirations	Normal breathing rate and rhythm but with abrupt cessation of inspiration, usually due to pain (seen in pleurisy)
Prolonged expiration	Breathing marked by fast inspiration and slow, prolonged expiration so that normal rate, depth, and rhythm is maintained (seen in COPD)
Pursed-lip breathing	Use of almost-closed (pursed) lips during expiration to maintain positive pressure within the bronchioles and thus prevent premature collapse of the weakened airways; seen in patients with emphysema
Paradoxical breathing	Two types: Inward motion of the abdomen with expansion of the rib cage on inspiration (seen in diaphragmatic fatigue or isolated paralysis with intact accessory muscles) Strong contraction of the diaphragm so that abdomen rises with collapse of upper chest on inspiration (seen in strong diaphragm but absence of intercostal spaces; e.g., C_5 or lower quadriplegia)
Respiratory alternans	Cyclic alternation between a series of diaphragmatic breaths (i.e., solely abdominal rise) and a series of predominantly accessory muscle breaths (i.e., mostly rib cage movements); seen in respiratory muscle fatigue

CNS = central nervous system, COPD = chronic obstructive pulmonary disease.

— Functional mobility (e.g., in bed, transfers, gait): level of independence, use of any assistive devices
- Digital clubbing is illustrated in Figure 5–1.
- Terminology used for common breathing patterns is explained in Table 5–8; some of these patterns are depicted in Figure 5–2.
- The clinical manifestations of hypoxemia and respiratory muscle fatigue are presented in Chapter 3 (see page 89).

AUSCULTATION

Auscultation entails listening to the patient's chest with a stethoscope. To accurately identify a patient's lung or heart sounds, the therapist should have a stethoscope with properly fitting earpieces, adequate but not excessive tubing without cracks, and both a diaphragm and a bell. In addition, the room should be quiet and the patient should be positioned properly.

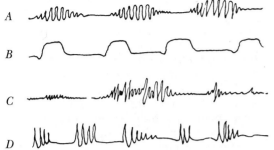

FIGURE 5-2. Abnormal neurogenic breathing patterns. *(A)*, Cheyne-Stokes respiration. *(B)*, Apneustic breathing. *(C)*, Biot's breathing. *(D)*, Cluster breathing. (From Prakash UBS: Neurologic diseases. *In* Baum GL, Wolinsky E (eds.): *Textbook of Pulmonary Diseases*, 4th Ed. Boston, Little, Brown & Co., 1989. Used with permission.)

LUNG SOUNDS

Even therapists who do not routinely auscultate a patient's lungs can learn to understand the descriptions of normal and abnormal lung sounds from the physical examination notes in a patient's chart. Therapists are encouraged to learn auscultation of breath sounds, which can be achieved easily by asking a friendly nurse or physician for a few minutes of tutoring for several days.

- The areas to auscultate are illustrated in Figure 5–3.
- The proper techniques used to auscultate lung sounds include the following steps:
  - Ideally, the patient should be in a sitting position with bare skin exposed and should breathe deeply but slowly through an open mouth.
  - Using the bell of the stethoscope, systematically listen to the entire lung space (anterior then posterior, or vice versa) with at least one breath per bronchopulmonary segment, comparing right and left sides for intensity, pitch, and quality while moving from upper to lower chest.
  - If breath sounds are difficult to auscultate, remind the patient to take slow deep breaths with an open mouth.
  - Specific precaution should be taken, as indicated:

- Patients who are weak or have poor balance or orthostatic intolerance are at risk for falling; therefore, additional support must be provided in the sitting position.
- Patients may become dizzy as a result of hyperventilation if deep breaths are performed too rapidly; the therapist should move slowly from one pulmonary segment to the next.
- Females may feel embarrassed by a bare chest; therefore, appropriate draping should be maintained during auscultation.

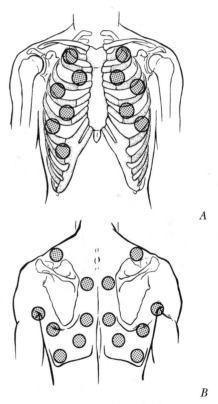

FIGURE 5-3. Areas to auscultate for breath sounds. *(A)*, Anterior chest. *(B)*, Posterior thorax. At least one breath should be taken per bronchopulmonary segment, comparing right and left sides while moving from upper to lower chest. (From Buckingham EB: *A Primer of Clinical Diagnosis*, 2nd Ed. New York, Harper & Row, 1979. Used with permission.)

- The topographic relationships between the chest wall and the pulmonary segments are depicted in Figure 5–4.
- Common errors in auscultating lung sounds include:
  - Listening to breath sounds through the patient's gown (the stethoscope should be placed directly against the patient's chest wall).
  - Allowing tubing to rub against bed rails or patient's gown (tubing should be kept free from contact with any objects during auscultation).

- Attempting to auscultate in a noisy room (television or radio should be turned off, other people in the room should be asked to be more quiet or to leave the room).
- Interpreting chest hair sounds as adventitious lung sounds (chest hair can be wetted before auscultation if thick).
- Auscultating only the "convenient" areas (alert patients should sit up; comatose patients should be rolled onto side to auscultate posterior lobes).
- Lung sounds are divided into breath sounds and added, or adventitious, sounds.

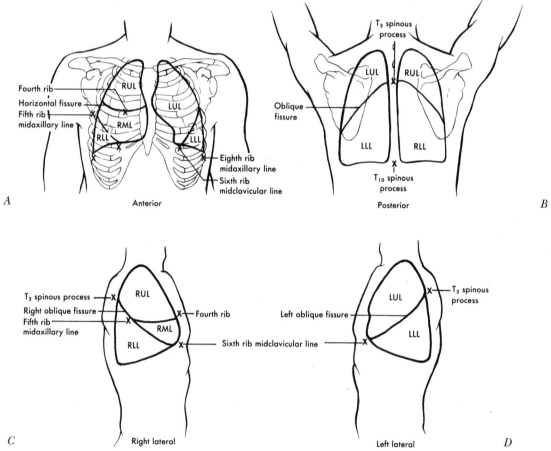

FIGURE 5–4. The topographic relationships between the chest wall and the pulmonary segments. *(A)*, Anterior. *(B)*, Posterior. *(C)* and *(D)*, Right and left lateral, respectively. (From Andreoli KG, Fowkes VK, Zipes DP, Wallace AG (eds.): *Comprehensive Cardiac Care—A Textbook for Nurses, Physicians, and Other Health Practitioners,* 6th Ed. St. Louis, The CV Mosby Co., p. 50, 1987. Used with permission.)

TABLE 5-9. **Lung Sounds and Their Descriptions**

TYPE OF SOUND	DESCRIPTION
Breath Sounds	
Normal or vesicular	Soft, low-pitched sounds heard throughout inspiration and the first third of expiration over most lung areas.
Bronchovesicular	Medium intensity and medium-pitched sounds with equal inspiratory and expiratory components without an intervening pause, which are heard over the carina and largest bronchi.
Decreased	Lower intensity than normal, vesicular sounds; heard in hyperinflation (e.g., COPD) or hypoinflation (e.g., atelectasis, pneumothorax, and pleural effusion).
Absent	Lack of breath sounds; due to interference with transmission (e.g., large pleural effusion, pneumothorax, severe hyperinflation, obesity).
Bronchial	Loud, somewhat harsh, high-pitched, "tubular" sounds with equal inspiratory and expiratory components and an intervening pause; heard over areas of consolidation.
Added Sounds	
Crackles	Discontinuous, nonmusical, crackling sounds (similar to the sound caused by rubbing several hairs together) heard most often on inspiration, which may result from the sudden opening of closed airways (e.g., atelectasis, fibrosis, pulmonary edema, or compression by pleural effusion) or the movement of secretions in the airways during inspiration and expiration; also called rales.
Wheezes	Continuous, musical sounds of variable pitch and duration, which can be monophonic or polyphonic and heard on either inspiration, expiration (most common), or both; polyphonic wheezes occur when there is diffuse airway narrowing (as by bronchospasm or secretions), whereas monophonic wheezes are heard when there is localized stenosis; low-pitched wheezes are sometimes called rhonchi.
Pleural rub	Inspiratory and expiratory grating, creaking sounds, like two pieces of sandpaper or leather being rubbed together, which are heard over the lower lateral lung areas and indicate pleural inflammation or reaction.
Vocal Sounds	
Normal	Soft, muffled, and indistinct sounds
Decreased	Weaker or softer than normal sounds; heard over pleural effusion, pneumothorax, and atelectasis, as well as fibrosis and airway obstruction.
Absent	Lack of transmission of any vocal sounds; occurs over pleural effusion, pneumothorax, atelectasis, and obstructed airway.
Increased	Louder, distinct voice transmission; heard over areas of consolidated lung tissue and pulmonary fibrosis.
Bronchophony	Occurs when a patient is asked to say "99" and the words are transmitted clearly.
Egophony	Demonstrated when a patient is asked to say "E" and it is heard as "A."
Whispered pectoriloquy	Evident when a patient is asked to whisper, and the words are distinctly heard using a stethoscope.

COPD = chronic obstructive pulmonary disease.

- Over most lung areas, breath sounds are soft and rustling and are termed normal or vesicular. However, breath sounds over the area of the main stem and segmental bronchi (upper intrascapular area) are somewhat more intense and higher in frequency and are called bronchovesicular.
- Abnormal conditions of the lungs can result in decreased, absent, or bronchial breath sounds, as described in Table 5-9.

- In addition, there may be adventitious sounds, such as crackles and wheezes, superimposed on normal or abnormal breath sounds.
- Vocal sounds are also transmitted through the lungs.
- Lung sounds should be evaluated both before and after treatment.
  - With appropriate treatment, the pathologic process may improve or resolve, and thus, the posttreatment auscultative findings may differ from those noted before treatment.
  - On the other hand, it is possible, on rare occasions, that the treatment procedures can result in a new acute pulmonary complication (e.g., bronchospasm, pneumothorax), which would be revealed during the reassessment.
  - Overexertion in a patient with cardiac dysfunction may be manifested as the development of crackles or rales at the lung bases, heard on auscultation following activity but not present before. The cause is poor left ventricular (LV) function with increasing filling pressures during activity so that pulmonary pressure increases and fluid begins to exude from the pulmonary capillaries into the interstitial space and possibly into some of the alveoli.

HEART SOUNDS

Auscultation of the heart can provide valuable information for the clinician regarding a patient's cardiac anatomy and function. Even if a physical therapist is not skilled in auscultating heart sounds, the therapist should be able to interpret the physician's observations in a patient's medical chart. The clinician listens to the individual heart sounds, their intensity, and timing and notes any additional sounds that are present, as well as their qualities and timing in the cardiac cycle.

- The techniques for listening to heart sounds consist of the following steps:
  - The diaphragm of the stethoscope is used to auscultate the entire chest, particularly the high-pitched sounds, whereas the bell is used to accentuate lower frequency sounds.
  - The patient should be lying in the supine position, with bare chest exposed, and should breathe quietly through the nose.

- The clinician listens to five main topographic areas (Fig. 5–5):
  — The *aortic area* is located near the second intercostal space just to the right of the sternum.
  — The *pulmonic area* is auscultated best at the second intercostal space to the left of the sternum.
  — The *third left intercostal space* can reveal murmurs of either aortic or pulmonary origin.
  — The *tricuspid area* is found at the lower left sternal border around the fourth or fifth intercostal space.
  — The *mitral area* is located at the apex of the heart, usually in the fifth left intercostal space, medial to the midclavicular line.
- Auscultation should be performed systematically so that each area is included, and attention is directed to both the intensity and timing, as well as any splitting, of the first and second heart sounds, and to any extra sounds and murmurs that may be present.
- The various heart sounds are described in Table 5–10, along with the most common causes of abnormalities.
- Although many cardiac sounds may change with the increased demands of physical activity, they are not typically auscultated during

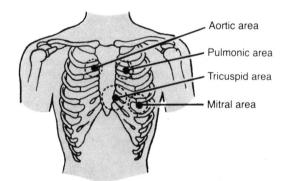

FIGURE 5–5. Areas to auscultate for sounds generated from the aortic, pulmonic, tricuspid, and mitral valves. In the normal heart, the mitral area is the apical pulse point and the point of maximal impulse (PMI). (From Guyton AC: *Textbook of Medical Physiology*. Philadelphia, W.B. Saunders Co., 1991. Used with permission.)

TABLE 5-10. **Heart Sounds and Causes of Abnormalities**

HEART SOUND	COMMENTS
S₁ (first heart sound)	Associated with mitral and tricuspid closure and corresponds with the onset of ventricular systole. Heard best at the apex or the tricuspid area. ↑: mitral stenosis with mobile leaflets, LA myxoma, MV prolapse, short PR interval, any condition causing tachycardia and vigorous ventricular contraction. ↓: prolonged PR interval, fibrotic or calcified MV, severe LV dysfunction, left bundle branch block, mitral regurgitation, ↓ sound conduction through chest wall.
S₂ (second heart sound)	Associated with aortic and pulmonary valve closure and corresponds with the start of ventricular diastole. Heard loudest in the aortic and pulmonic areas and is often split into two components, aortic (A₂) followed by pulmonic (P₂), with ↑ splitting on inspiration and ↓ splitting on expiration. ↑ A₂: systemic HTN, congenital defects with the aorta arising anteriorly (e.g., transposition of the great arteries), aortic dilatation. ↑ P₂: pulmonary HTN, thin-chested individuals. ↓ A₂: aortic stenosis. ↓ P₂: pulmonic stenosis.
Fixed splitting	Delayed P₂ or early A₂: Acute pulmonary embolus, right bundle branch block, atrial septal defect, pulmonic stenosis.
Wider splitting	Delayed PV closure: Proximal right bundle branch block, LV paced or ectopic beats, acute massive pulmonary embolus, RV failure, and some congenital heart defects. Early AoV closure: Mitral regurgitation, ventricular septal defect.
Parodoxical splitting	Delayed aortic closure: Left bundle branch block, RV paced or ectopic beats, LV outflow tract obstruction (e.g., aortic stenosis, obstructive hypertrophic cardiomyopathy), hypertensive heart disease, CAD, peripheral vasodilation, poststenotic dilation of the aorta, patent ductus arteriosus.
S₃ (third heart sound) "ventricular gallop"	Associated with early rapid diastolic filling of the ventricles. A low-pitched sound best heard with the patient lying on the left side so the apex of the heart is closest to the chest wall. May be heard in children and adults <40 years, in which case it is termed *physiologic.* Also commonly heard if: Impaired LV function of any cause with ↑ end-systolic volume (e.g., congenital heart disease, valvular disease, systemic or pulmonary HTN, ischemic heart disease, cardiomyopathy). Constrictive pericarditis. Hyperdynamic states (e.g., severe anemia, liver disease, thyrotoxicosis, systemic arteriovenous fistula, pregnancy).
S₄ (fourth heart sound) "atrial gallop"	Associated with ventricular filling due to atrial contraction. A low-pitched sound heard late in diastole just before S₁. Commonly heard if: LV or RV hypertrophy (e.g., outflow tract obstruction, systemic or pulmonary HTN, hypertrophic cardiomyopathy). Ischemic heart disease (e.g., acute myocardial ischemia or infarction, coronary artery bypass surgery). Hyperdynamic states (see S₃ above).

Continued on following page

TABLE 5-10. **Heart Sounds and Causes of Abnormalities**—*Continued*

HEART SOUND	COMMENTS
S$_4$ (fourth heart sound) "atrial gallop"—cont'd	Acute valvular regurgitation (e.g., MV, AoV, TV). Arrhythmia (e.g., heart block, atrial flutter).
Summation gallop	Fusion of S$_3$ and S$_4$ and implies volume overload and need for more vigorous atrial contraction (e.g., dilated cardiomyopathy), especially with tachycardia.
Ejection sounds	Associated with the opening of a stenotic semilunar valve or ejection of blood into a dilated aorta or pulmonary artery.
Midsystolic clicks	Associated with maximal excursion of prolapsed valve leaflets and elongated chordae tendinae (e.g., MV prolapse).
Opening snaps	Diastolic sound associated with the opening of stenotic atrioventricular valves (e.g., mitral or tricuspid stenosis); occur before the S$_3$, if present.

↑ = increased intensity, ↓ = decreased intensity, AoV = aortic valve, CAD = coronary artery disease, HTN = hypertension, LA = left atrial, LV = left ventricular, MV = mitral valve, PV = pulmonary valve, RV = right ventricular, TV = tricuspid valve.

activity. However, it is important to reassess the cardiac sounds following exercise.

• The most significant change is the onset of a third heart sound, S$_3$, as a result of activity; this finding indicates the development of diastolic dysfunction with reduced ventricular compliance because of delayed or impaired myocardial relaxation. There are a number of possible causes for the development of diastolic dysfunction during activity (e.g., myocardial ischemia, hypertension, cardiomyopathy, valvular disease, congenital heart disease), but all involve the same common mechanism: less effective ventricular performance during exertion. If pulmonary pressures become elevated as a result, new crackles may also be auscultated following exertion, as described previously (see page 162).

• Another significant finding is the onset of a new murmur following exertion.

HEART MURMURS

Heart murmurs are vibrations of longer duration than the heart sounds and frequently represent turbulent flow across abnormal valves caused by congenital or acquired cardiac defects.

• The principal heart murmurs are presented in Figure 5–6.
• Heart murmurs are graded according to their intensity:

• Grade 1: murmur is barely audible with special effort.
• Grade 2: murmur is faint but easily heard.
• Grade 3: murmur is moderately loud.
• Grade 4: murmur is very loud; there may be a thrill.
• Grade 5: murmur is extremely loud; one edge of stethoscope must be on the chest to hear.
• Grade 6: murmur is exceptionally loud, audible with stethoscope just above the chest.

PALPATION

Abnormalities identified through the medical chart review, inspection, and auscultation can be further assessed using palpation. Through touch, the clinician can determine the position of the trachea, the presence of subcutaneous emphysema or unstable rib fractures, the extent and symmetry of chest expansion and what muscles are active, the transmission of voice sounds as vibrations to the chest wall (i.e., vocal fremitus), the presence of chest wall pain, the location of the cardiac apical pulse (i.e., the point of maximal impulse), and the status of the peripheral pulses.

• Tracheal position is evaluated to determine the presence of mediastinal shift, which occurs because of differences in intrathoracic pressure or lung volumes between the two sides of the thorax.

- The techniques for palpation of tracheal position are as follows:
  — The patient is sitting upright with the neck slightly flexed to relax the sternocleidomastoid muscles and the chin in midline.
  — The examiner inserts the tip of a fully extended index finger into the suprasternal notch, just medial to one sternoclavicular joint, and presses inward toward the cervical spine.
  — Then the same technique is repeated on the other side.
- Deviation occurs toward the side of the lesion when there is loss of lung volume on one side (e.g., atelectasis, fibrosis, or surgical excision of lung tissue).
- Deviation is away from the side of the abnormality when there is an increase in lung volume on one side of the thorax (e.g., tension pneumothorax, pleural effusion).
- The mediastinum may normally be shifted to the right in older patients as a result of an elongated atherosclerotic aortic arch.
- Palpation of chest motion is illustrated in Figure 5–7.
  - Upper lobes
    — With the patient sitting or lying facing the examiner, the examiner places his/her palms anteriorly over the first four ribs with the finger tips extended over the trapezius muscles.

— The skin is stretched downward until the palms are in the infraclavicular areas and then drawn medially until the tips of the extended thumbs meet in the midline.
— With the elbows and shoulders maintained in a relaxed position, the examiner asks the patient to take a deep inspiration and allows his/her hands to reflect the movement of the underlying lung.
- Right middle lobe and lingular segment
  — The examiner places his/her widely outstretched fingers of both hands over the posterior axillary folds and his/her palms over the anterior chest wall.
  — The skin is then drawn medially until the tips of the extended thumbs meet in the midline.
  — Again, with the elbows and shoulders maintained in a relaxed position, the examiner asks the patient to take a deep inspiration and allows his/her hands to reflect the movement of the underlying lung.
- Lower lobes
  — With the patient sitting with his/her back to the examiner, the examiner places both hands high up in the axilla with outstretched fingers over the axillary folds.
  — Then the skin is drawn medially until the extended thumbs meet in the midline.

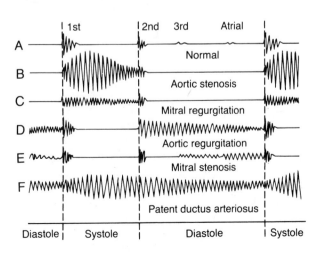

FIGURE 5-6. Phonocardiograms from normal and abnormal heart sounds. (From Guyton AC: *Textbook of Medical Physiology*. Philadelphia, W.B. Saunders Co., p. 256, 1991. Used with permission.)

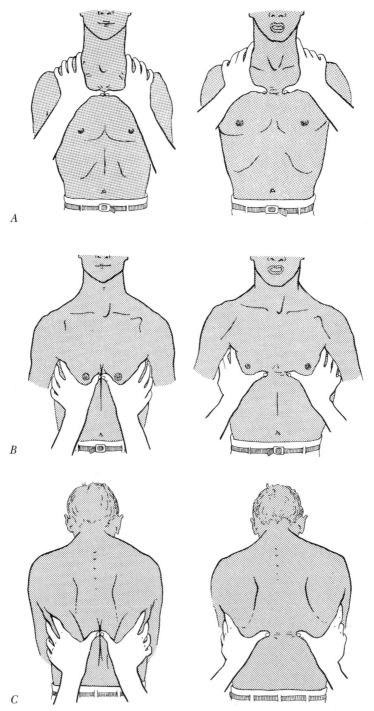

FIGURE 5-7. The techniques for palpating the expansion of the upper lobes *(A)*, right middle lobe and left lingula *(B)*, and the lower lobes *(C)*. (Modified from Cherniack RM, Cherniack L: *Respiration in Health and Disease*, 3rd Ed. Philadelphia, W.B. Saunders Co., 1983.)

— Again, with the elbows and shoulders maintained in a relaxed position, the examiner asks the patient to take a deep inspiration and allows his/her hands to reflect the movement of the underlying lung.

- Normally, the lungs should expand equally, and thus the examiner's thumbs and hands will move with equal timing the same distance from each other during both quiet and deep breathing.
  — Diminished or delayed movement of one side often provides the earliest evidence of reduced distensibility of a portion of the lung.
  — Reduced movement of one lobe together with ipsilateral tracheal deviation suggests that there is either ipsilateral loss of volume in that lobe or contralateral volume gain.

- Palpation of the apical impulse of the heart is also included in the chest examination.
  - The techniques involved in palpation of the apical impulse of the heart are listed below:
    — With the patient sitting up and leaning forward or lying on the left side, the examiner uses the pads of his/her fingers to explore the third to sixth intercostal spaces from the left midaxillary line to the middle of the sternum.
    — The most lateral point where a definite localized systolic pulsation is felt identifies the apex of the heart, or the point of maximal impulse (PMI).
    — The intensity of the apical impulse can be assessed using the palm of the hand.
  - The apical impulse is normally located in the fourth or fifth left intercostal space near the midclavicular line and consists of a brief, localized, early systolic outward thrust of moderate intensity; it may be exaggerated in thin, young individuals and when the patient is lying on the left side.
    — The apical impulse will shift according to tracheal deviation when there is mediastinal shift due to lung disease (see above).
    — Lateral displacement of the apical impulse without tracheal deviation most likely indicates LV hypertrophy.

— The apical impulse will be hyperkinetic when there is increased LV stroke volume (e.g., aortic or mitral regurgitation, severe anemia, anxiety, exercise).
— The apical impulse will be sustained (i.e., lasting past the first half of systole) but normal in location when there is concentric hypertrophy and normal chamber size (e.g., hypertension, aortic stenosis); it will be laterally displaced and sustained with LV enlargement with decreased LV function.
— The most common causes of a hypokinetic apical impulse are chest configuration and lung disease, although it is also seen in obesity, pericardial effusion or constriction, and shock.
— Right ventricular (RV) hypertrophy is present when a sustained outward movement at the left sternal edge is palpated in the third or fourth intercostal space.

- Other palpation techniques are also used during chest assessment.
  - Vocal fremitus
    — The examiner places either the palms or the hypothenar eminences of his/her hands lightly on symmetric areas of the chest wall. Then the patient is instructed to say "99," and the intensity of the vibrations detected in each hand are compared as the examiner moves his/her hands over several areas of the chest, including apical, anterior, lateral, and posterior.
    — Under normal conditions, equal vibrations of moderate intensity are perceived during speech, but not during quiet breathing.
      – Increased fremitus is noted when there is increased density of the underlying lung tissue (e.g., consolidation).
      – Fremitus is decreased or absent when there is fluid or air in the pleural space or when there is atelectasis due to bronchial obstruction.
      – When vibrations are detected during quiet breathing, it is termed *rhoncal fremitus*.
  - Respiratory muscle activity
    — Scalene muscles

– With the patient sitting and facing away, the examiner places his/her hands on the upper trapezius muscles so the fingers rest on the clavicles and the thumbs meet near the midline posteriorly. Activity of the scalene muscles is assessed as the patient takes at least two quiet breaths.

– Normally, the scalene muscles are inactive during quiet breathing. Active scalene contraction indicates that the tertiary muscles of inspiration are being recruited, and therefore the work of breathing is increased.

— Diaphragm (Fig. 5–8).

– With the patient lying supine and flat, the examiner places both hands lightly over the anterior chest with thumbs over costal margins so that their tips almost meet at the xiphoid. The patient is instructed to take a deep inspiration while the examiner's hands are allowed to move with chest expansion.

– Because of its dome shape, contraction of the diaphragm causes descent of the central tendon and elevation and outward rotation of the lower ribs. Therefore, normal diaphragmatic function results in equal upward motion of each costal margin. Inward motion of the costal margins during inspiration occurs when the diaphragm is no longer dome-shaped, as in hyperinflation (e.g., COPD), or when there is fluid or air in the pleural space (i.e., pleural effusion or pneumothorax).

• Chest pain

— After obtaining a description of the patient's pain (e.g., type, extent, location, precipitating factors, and mechanisms of relief), the examiner asks the patient to outline the borders of the painful area(s). Starting well away from this area, the examiner then palpates the ribs and intercostal spaces by pressing firmly downward. In addition, the effects of deep breathing, coughing, breath holding, and ipsilateral arm motion on the pain are determined.

— Chest pain can result from numerous cardiac, pulmonary, and other causes (see Table 5–6).

– A localized area of intense pain accompanied by a grating sensation with expiration is indicative of a rib fracture.

– Localized intercostal tenderness may represent fibrositis of an intercostal muscle.

– Pain due to subluxation of a costal cartilage can be reproduced by squeezing the ribs on either side of the dislocation.

– Pleuritic pain, which is usually due to bacterial pneumonia, is sharp, usually localized, and aggravated by inspiration and coughing.

– Chest wall pain due to musculoskeletal dysfunction is usually nonsegmental, localized to the anterior chest, and ag-

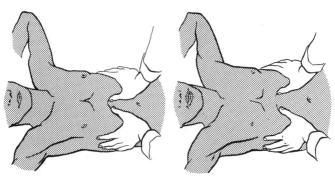

A   *B*

FIGURE 5–8.   Palpation of diaphragmatic motion. *(A)*, At rest. *(B)*, At the end of a deep inspiration. (From Cherniack RM, Cherniack L: *Respiration in Health and Disease*, 3rd Ed. Philadelphia, W.B. Saunders Co., 1983.)

gravated by deep inspiration but unrelated to exercise.
- Chest pain due to nerve root irritation radiates segmentally according to dermatonal distribution.
- Subcutaneous emphysema and unstable rib fractures
  — During palpation of chest expansion, vocal fremitus, or chest wall pain, other abnormalities are sometimes identified:
    - Subcutaneous air, or emphysema, is perceived as a crackling sensation that can be heard, as well as felt, and results from intrapulmonary rupture of air spaces (e.g., chest trauma, acute asthma, surgical incision)
    - Unstable rib fractures can be detected by "popping" of the segment during inspiration and coughing.

PERCUSSION

The final component of the chest wall examination is percussion, which allows the clinician to further evaluate any abnormal findings in terms of their relationship to changes in lung density. The pitch of the sound produced by percussion is determined by the ratio of air-containing tissue to solid tissue in the area underlying the percussing finger. Thus, areas of altered density can be identified, and the extent of the abnormality can be defined. In addition, percussion can be used to demonstrate the level of the diaphragm and its maximal excursion from end-expiratory to end-inspiratory positions.

- Percussion is most commonly performed indirectly using the mediate percussion technique, which is illustrated in Figure 5–9. However, it can also be performed using direct, or immediate, percussion, where the middle finger taps directly on the chest wall.
- The proper techniques for mediate percussion are as follows:
  - Lung density
    — Lightly position the pad of the middle finger of the nondominant hand along the intercostal space over the area in question while all other fingers are held away from the chest wall.
    — Position the other hand with the wrist in dorsiflexion; then using the wrist as

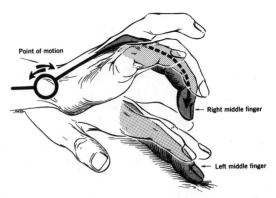

FIGURE 5–9. Hand position for performing mediate percussion. (From Buckingham EB: *A Primer of Clinical Diagnosis,* 2nd Ed. New York, Harper & Row, 1979. Used with permission.)

the fulcrum, strike the middle finger of the nondominant hand repeatedly with the tip of the middle finger of the dominant hand, recoiling instantly after each tap.
    — Systematically percuss from side to side along each intercostal space from apex to base of the lungs, both anteriorly and posteriorly, comparing the pitch, intensity and duration of the sound produced.
  - Diaphragmatic excursion
    — With the patient sitting, the examiner performs percussion down the chest until dullness is encountered.
    — The patient is then asked to exhale completely while the examiner defines the limit of diaphragmatic ascent.
    — After the patient then takes a deep breath, the examiner tracks diaphragmatic motion and identifies the extent of descent.
- Well-aerated lung tissue produces a low-pitched, resonant sound that is similar to a muffled drum, whereas more dense organs like the heart, liver, and subcostal abdominal viscera yield a duller sound, and less dense organs like the stomach produce a more tympanic sound.
  - A higher pitched, dull-to-flat note (i.e., a "thud") denotes an area of increased density, as in atelectasis, consolidation, or pleural effusion.

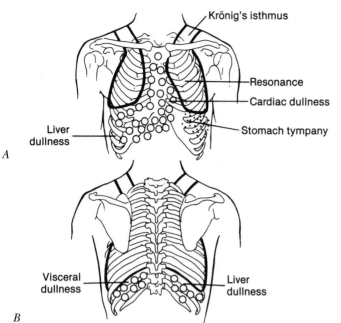

Krönig's isthmus

Resonance

Cardiac dullness

Liver
dullness

Stomach tympany

A

Visceral
dullness

Liver
dullness

B

FIGURE 5-10. Normal resonance pattern of the chest. *(A)*, Anteriorly. *(B)*, Posteriorly. Circles = areas of dullness; small dots = tympanic, or hyperresonant, areas. (From Humberstone N: Respiratory assessment and treatment. *In* Irwin S, Tecklin JS: *Cardiopulmonary Physical Therapy*, 2nd Ed. St. Louis, The C.V. Mosby Co., p. 294, 1990.)

- A loud, long, and hollow hyperresonant, or tympanic, note indicates decreased density (i.e., the presence of more air), as in pneumothorax or hyperinflated lungs.
- Diaphragmatic excursion is the distance between maximal expiration and maximal inspiration, which is normally 3 to 5 cm.
  - Diaphragmatic excursion is reduced bilaterally in COPD.
  - If there is unilateral diaphragmatic paralysis, it may be fixed in an elevated position or move paradoxically, rising above its resting level when a deep inspiration is made.
- The normal resonance pattern of the chest is depicted in Figure 5–10.

5.5 ACTIVITY AND ENDURANCE EVALUATION

Following completion of the resting assessment, the therapist is ready to perform an activity or endurance evaluation, as described in Table 5–11.

- In patients with known heart disease where activity is restricted, this initial evaluation is designed to document the patient's hemodynamic responses to increasing activity in order to design an appropriate treatment plan. Vital

signs (e.g., heart rate and rhythm and blood pressure), as well as signs and symptoms, are monitored with the patient supine, sitting, standing, performing some type of activity of daily living or range of motion exercises, and ambulating.
- In patients with other types of cardiac disease and other diagnoses where activity tolerance may be limited but is not necessarily restricted, a similar assessment of exercise responses is performed except that the ambulation distance and intensity are increased more aggressively, within patient tolerance, so that an exercise prescription to improve endurance can be immediately developed.
- Rating of perceived exertion is often used as an indication of perceived intensity of the various workloads during the endurance evaluation (Table 5–12) and can then be used to monitor exercise intensity when formulating an exercise prescription.
- Ask patients to pay close attention to how hard they feel they are working.
  - This should be the total inner feeling of exertion and fatigue rather than one specific factor, such as leg discomfort or shortness of breath.
- In order to quantify the distance and/or speed of ambulation, the patient can be timed

TABLE 5-11. **Activity and Endurance Evaluation**

PROCEDURE	COMMENTS
Activity Evaluation	
Monitor the patient's HR and rhythm, BP, and any signs and symptoms while supine, then sitting, and finally standing.	There are a number of methods of monitoring a patient's physiologic responses to activity.
Auscultate the patient's lungs and heart before and following activity.	Heart rate: HR can be measured by palpation, usually of the radial pulse, by auscultation of the heart apex, via the digital display of an ECG or oxygen saturation monitor, or directly from an ECG rhythm strip.
Monitor the patient's physiologic responses while the patient performs some simple ROM exercises or during some activity of daily living, such as dressing, combing or brushing hair, or brushing teeth.	Heart rhythm: The most accurate means of monitoring cardiac rhythm is by watching an ECG monitor and printing out rhythm strips.
Sometimes, the patient's responses to a Valsalva maneuver or hyperventilation are also assessed.	Alternatively, if ECG equipment is not available, the pulse can be palpated or the heart can be auscultated for 30–60 seconds.
Record and interpret all responses throughout the entire evaluation.	Blood pressure: BP is usually monitored using an arm cuff and a sphygmomanometer or an automatic BP monitor.
Terminate the evaluation any time responses are identified that indicate continued activity would be inappropriate or unsafe.	In critical care units, patient's often have an indwelling arterial line with a digital display of systolic, diastolic, and mean arterial pressure, which can be used to monitor BP responses.
Endurance Evaluation	
If the patient's responses to the activity evaluation (above) are determined to be safe and appropriate, the evaluation may continue by having the patient perform progressive ambulation in the hallway or some other form of graded aerobic activity (e.g., stationary cycling, treadmill walking).	Inpatients are usually evaluated during ambulation initially, since this is convenient and permits assessment of the patient's balance and coordination, level of independence, and functional efficiency (i.e., speed and distance).
Starting at a comfortable, relaxed pace, have the patient ambulate for 2–3 minutes and then measure the patient's responses while the patient continues to exercise	Ideally, the endurance evaluation should be structured so that the patient can perform at least two different intensities of exercise before fatigue sets in.
Include a RPE (see Fig. 5–7).	Be certain to take physiologic measurements while the patient is still walking or at least marching in place since the values will drop rapidly when activity is terminated.
Ask the patient to increase exercise intensity (i.e., walking pace or cycling resistance) and continue for another 2–3 minutes when responses are again measured.	To quantify the distance and speed of ambulation for hallway ambulation, the distances of various "loops" can be measured and charts can be created to plot the number of loops or distance walked in so many minutes (see Figs. 5–11 through 5–13).
Repeat this procedure until the patient reaches a RPE of "somewhat hard" (13 on scale of 6–20) or "somewhat strong" (4 on scale of 1–10).	The total walking time completed and the ending pace can be used to create an endurance exercise prescription for the patient.
Continue at this pace until the patient begins to feel fatigued. Note the total exercise time.	

BP = blood pressure, ECG = electrocardiography, HR = heart rate, ROM = range of motion, RPE = rating of perceived exertion.

TABLE 5–12. **Rating of Perceived Exertion (RPE) Scales**

CATEGORY RPE SCALE	CATEGORY-RATIO RPE SCALE	
6	0	Nothing at all
7 Very, very light	0.5	Very, very weak
8	1	Very weak
9 Very light	2	Weak
10	3	Moderate
11 Fairly light	4	Somewhat strong
12	5	Strong
13 Somewhat hard	6	
14	7	Very strong
15 Hard	8	
16	9	
17 Very hard	10	Very, very strong
18	•	Maximal
19 Very, very hard		
20		

Original scale (6–20) on left and revised scale (1–10) on right.
From Borg GA: Psychophysical basis of perceived exertion. *Med Sci Sports Exerc* 14:377–387, 1982.

and the distances can be calculated. The author routinely designs maps of various "loops" used for hallway ambulation in the different treatment areas (e.g., physical therapy department, patient floors) and their distances and creates charts that can be used to determine walking pace and total distance covered, as demonstrated in Figures 5–11 to 5–13.

CLINICAL MONITORING

In order for the data obtained from the activity and endurance evaluation to be meaningful, patient monitoring must be performed accurately. The proper techniques for patient monitoring are presented for heart rate and rhythm, blood pressure, and respiratory rate. In addition, ECG monitoring is described for therapists who have access to the required equipment. (NOTE: Most hospitals have functional, but older ECG monitoring equipment hidden away in storage that could be resurrected for monitoring exercise. Ideally, the first choice would be a telemetry unit; however, hard wiring is perfectly acceptable for monitoring activities using little space, such as treadmill walking and stationary cycling.) Finally, normal resting values and responses to activity are characterized.

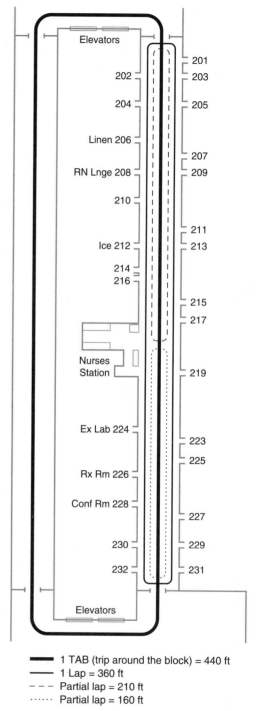

FIGURE 5–11. Example of a walking map posted on a hospital unit or in a rehabilitation department, which maps out various loops for ambulation and their distances.

# Laps	Distance (in feet)	Miles	Time (in min.) for specific distance (will indicate speed)				
			1.0 mph	1.5 mph	2.0 mph	2.5 mph	3.0 mph
1	360	.07	4.1	2.7	2.0	1.6	1.4
2	720	.14	8.2	5.5	4.1	3.3	2.7
3	1080	.20 (⅕)	12.3	8.2	6.1	4.9	4.1
4	1440	.27 (~¼)	16.4	10.9	8.2	6.5	5.5
5	1800	.34 (⅓)	20.5	13.6	10.2	8.2	6.8
6	2160	.41	24.5	16.4	12.3	9.8	8.2
7	2520	.48 (~½)	28.6	19.1	14.3	11.5	9.5
8	2880	.55	32.7	21.8	16.4	13.1	10.9
9	3240	.61	36.8	24.5	18.4	14.7	12.3
10	3600	.68 (~⅔)	40.9	27.3	20.5	16.4	13.6
11	3960	.75 (¾)	45.0	30.0	22.5	18.0	15.0
12	4320	.82 (~⅘)	49.1	32.7	24.5	19.6	16.4
13	4680	.89	53.2	35.5	26.6	21.3	17.7
14	5040	.95	57.3	38.2	28.6	22.9	19.1

FIGURE 5-12. A chart showing the distance walked along a hospital ward corridor according to the number of laps (see Fig. 5–11). Walking pace can also be determined by locating the time it took to complete the distance walked and looking up to the top of the column to find the corresponding speed. For example, if an individual walks 2 laps (720 feet) and it takes 6 minutes, the walking speed can be determined by looking to the right of 2 laps to find the time closest to 6 minutes, which is 5.5 minutes; since the walk actually took a little longer than 5.5 minutes, the individual was walking at a pace a little slower than 1.5 miles per hour (mph).

# TABs	Distance (in feet)	Miles	Time (in minutes) for specific distance (will indicate speed)				
			1.0 mph	1.5 mph	2.0 mph	2.5 mph	3.0 mph
1.0	440	.08 (1/12)	5.0	3.3	2.5	2.0	1.7
1.5	660	.13 (⅛)	7.5	5.0	3.8	3.0	2.5
2.0	880	.17 (⅙)	10.0	6.7	5.0	4.0	3.3
2.5	1080	.20 (⅕)	12.3	8.2	6.1	4.9	4.1
3.0	1320	.25 (¼)	15.0	10.0	7.5	6.0	5.0
4.0	1760	.33 (⅓)	20.0	13.3	10.0	8.0	6.7
6.0	2640	.50 (½)	30.0	20.0	15.0	12.0	10.0
8.0	3520	.67 (⅔)	40.0	26.7	20.0	16.0	13.3
9.0	3960	.75 (¾)	45.0	30.0	22.5	18.0	15.0
12.0	5280	1.00	60.0	40.0	30.0	24.0	20.0

FIGURE 5-13. A chart showing the distance walked around a hospital area according to the number of "trips around the block" (TABs) (see Fig. 5–11). Walking pace can also be determined according to the procedures described in Figure 5–12.

HEART RATE

For therapists working in cardiac rehabilitation or one of the critical care areas, the availability of bedside or telemetry ECG allows for simple accurate heart rate (HR) monitoring. In addition, some rehabilitation departments have their own portable ECG equipment or at least one of the simple HR monitoring devices, usually consisting of a chest strap containing two sensing electrodes and a watch-like display. Some patients in the acute care setting have bedside pulse oximetry for monitoring oxygen saturation, which usually displays a digital read out of HR as well, and this can be used by the therapist instead of palpation. In all other situations the therapist must depend on palpation, usually of the radial pulse, to monitor HR.

- Some specific suggestions to increase the accuracy of pulse monitoring include:
  - If HR can be counted while the patient continues to exercise, it should be palpated for 15 to 30 seconds.

- If the pulse is difficult to palpate while the patient is exercising, try counting it while the patient marches in place; using auscultation of the heart; or, as a last resort, obtaining a count during the first 15 seconds of recovery. (NOTE: HR begins to fall almost immediately on cessation of exercise.)
- If the pulse rate becomes increasingly irregular, all the impulses may not be peripherally palpable, and auscultation of the heart may provide a more accurate rate when compared with an ECG strip; however, the peripherally palpated rate may give a more accurate indication of the actual effective heart rate.
- If the digital display of an ECG or oxygen saturation monitor is being used to monitor HR responses, the therapist should be aware of the possibility of inaccuracies resulting from movement artifact during activity.
- The normal resting HR and the responses to activity are described in Table 5–13.

TABLE 5-13 Heart Rate: Normal Values and Responses to Exercise

NORMAL	COMMENTS
Resting: 50–100 bpm	Varies with age, health status, fitness level, balance of sympathetic and parasympathetic nervous system activity, circulating catecholamine levels, level of hydration, effects of any medications being taken, and other factors.
	More fit individuals tend to have lower resting HRs than sedentary individuals, probably due to ↓ sympathetic activity and ↑ ventricular filling resulting in ↑ cardiac efficiency.
	↑ resting HR means the heart is working harder (i.e., faster) in order to eject normal cardiac output.
Dynamic exercise: HR gradually increases, proportional to workload	Response is blunted in regular aerobic exercisers, because of training.
	Abnormal HR responses:
	Tachycardic (HR rises more rapidly than expected): usually seen in the severely deconditioned and those who have cardiovascular disease with limited ability to ↑ stroke volume; therefore, must ↑ HR to ↑ cardiac output.
	Bradycardic (very flat HR response despite increasing intensity): seen most commonly in patients taking β-adrenergic blockers or verapamil; occasionally, a true bradycardic response is observed in individuals not taking any medications, which is considered very ominous for severe CAD.
	Instances where palpable HR seems to ↓ during exertion, but ECG monitoring usually reveals increasing arrhythmias, some of which are not perceived peripherally (due to peripheral resistance).
Static/isometric exercise: less pronounced ↑ than with dynamic exercise	Caused by lower cardiac output requirements and associated with higher BP responses (due to peripheral resistance).

↓ = decreased, ↑ = increased, BP = blood pressure, bpm = beats per minute, ECG = electrocardiographic, HR = heart rate.

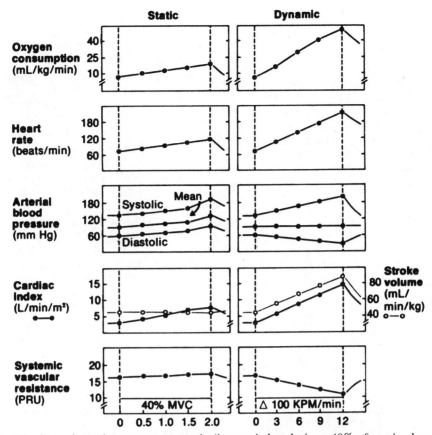

FIGURE 5–14. The hemodynamic responses to static (isometric handgrip at 40% of maximal contraction) versus progressive dynamic exercise (stationary cycling with 100 kpm/min increase in workload). (From Longhurst LC, Mitchell JH: *J. Cardiovasc. Med.* 8:227, 1983. Reprinted with permission from Physicians World Communication Group.)

- Most activities included in the typical activity evaluation are low in intensity, requiring an increase in metabolic rate of less than three to four times the resting rate (i.e., <3 to 4 METs, as explained on page 201). Therefore, the rise in HR in response to these activities should be fairly minimal, <20 to 30 beats per minute (bpm).
- The hemodynamic responses to static versus dynamic exercise are illustrated in Figure 5–14.

HEART RHYTHM

Using palpation, it is only possible to detect regularity versus irregularity of the rhythm and to state whether the irregularities occur in a regular or irregular pattern. Interpreting what arrhythmias the irregularities actually represent is not possible without an ECG. Therefore, ECG monitoring is strongly advised, at least for screening, for any patient with a history of arrhythmias and those who exhibit irregularities of pulse and any abnormal signs or symptoms during activity.

- Heart rhythm is normally regular or with only occasional asymptomatic irregularities.
- During exertion, there should be little change in rhythm.
- Abnormal rhythm responses include the onset of arrhythmias during or immediately following exertion or an increase in frequency or change in type of arrhythmia with an increase in activity.

- Occasionally, a patient will have arrythmias at rest that decrease or resolve with increasing heart rates, as with exertion.

ECG MONITORING

The availability of ECG monitoring markedly simplifies the task of performing a monitored patient evaluation, for it allows the therapist to concentrate on taking accurate blood pressure measurements and noting signs and symptoms while the ECG recorder prints out the heart rate and rhythm responses. The therapist merely needs to mark each ECG strip with the activity being monitored.

- Typically, a single lead is monitored and rhythm strips are printed out. The lead systems commonly used to monitor patients during activity are illustrated in Figure 5–15. The

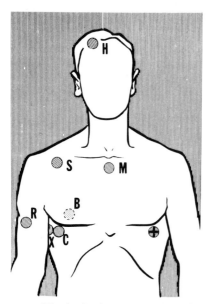

FIGURE 5-15. Bipolar lead systems commonly used in bedside or rehabilitation ECG monitoring. The positive electrode is placed in the V_5 position (fifth intercostal space at the midclavicular line), and the negative electrode is placed in any of the areas indicated by lettered spots. The leads can be named according to the two electrodes: CH_5, CS_5, CM_5, CR_5, CX_5, CC_5, and CB_5. (From Wilson PK, et al.: *Cardiac Rehabilitation, Adult Fitness, and Exercise Testing*. Philadelphia, Lea & Febiger, p. 259, 1981. © Williams & Wilkins 1981. Used with permission.)

challenge is placing the electrodes so they are not right over exercising muscle, which produces a great deal of artifact.

- Generally, any lead with a tall upright ventricular voltage (i.e., R wave) is acceptable for most patients; an exception is the patient with known myocardial ischemia, in whom the area of possible ischemia should be monitored. This can be accomplished by using one of the standard leads or creating a different one where the vector from the negative to the positive electrodes points to the area in question; (the ground electrode, if present, can be placed anywhere).

- Caution is warranted when interpreting ST segment changes obtained from ECG telemetry units. Most modern units contain special filters and amplifiers that dampen muscle artifact and provide a cleaner rhythm strip; these units do not accurately portray ST segment changes (i.e., 1 mm of ST segment depression on a rhythm strip does not necessarily mean 1 mV of depression; in actuality, it could be more or it could be less). Only units without special filters (often called "diagnostic" telemetry units) and similar hard-wire units can be used for valid ST segment interpretation.

ECG Waveforms and Intervals

To interpret a rhythm strip, one must be able to recognize a normal ECG pattern, as well as abnormal variations. The normal ECG waveforms and intervals are shown in Figure 5–16.

Analyzing rhythm strips is relatively straightforward if a systematic approach is used, as described in Table 5–14. Heart rate can be measured by using an ECG ruler, which involves placing the reference arrow on an R wave and then counting 2 to 3 R to R intervals (depending on the design of the specific ruler) and reading the corresponding rate. Alternatively, the rate can be calculated according to either of the methods illustrated in Figure 5–17. The characteristics of the various rhythms and arrhythmias are described below.

Sinus Node Rhythms and Arrhythmias

- Normal sinus rhythm (Fig. 5–18).
  - Rate: 60 to 100 bpm
  - P waves: identical, each followed by a QRS
  - PR interval: normal (0.12 to 0.20 seconds)
  - QRS: normal (0.04 to 0.10 seconds)

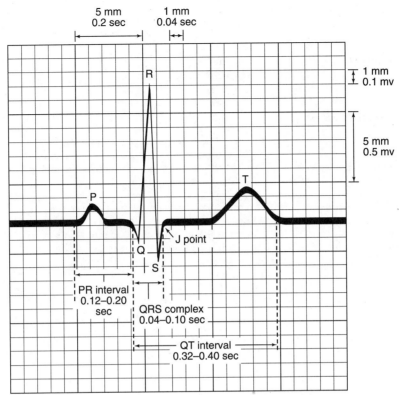

FIGURE 5–16. The ECG waveforms and intervals. The normal ranges of the different intervals are also included.

- Sinus tachycardia (see Fig. 5–19)
  - Rate: 100 to 150 bpm, otherwise same as normal sinus rhythm
  - Causes: compensatory mechanism of body to increase cardiac output under stressful situations (exercise, fear, fever, pain, etc.) and in congestive heart failure (CHF); various drugs (e.g., xanthine derivatives: theophylline, aminophylline)
  - Significance: minor, except as a signal of other underlying disorders; may have hemodynamic consequences if the patient has heart disease combined with an inability to handle increased workload created by faster HR
- Sinus bradycardia (Fig. 5–19)
  - Rate: less than 50 to 60 bpm, otherwise same as normal sinus rhythm
  - Causes: seen in many healthy individuals, especially athletes, during rest or sleep; increased vagal stimulation (gagging, vomit-

ing, tracheal suctioning, massage of carotid sinus); myocardial ischemia, medications (e.g., β-blockers, verapamil), pain, severe body anoxia, increased intracranial pressure, digitalis therapy
  - Significance: generally harmless, except as a sign of underlying disorders; if pronounced bradycardia, cardiac output will decrease and the patient may feel dizzy or faint; if myocardial ischemia or any signs and symptoms of cardiac and/or cerebral hypoxia develop, it is considered a medical emergency; also irritable ectopic sites may have time to take over as pacemaker.
- Sinus arrhythmia (Fig. 5–19)
  - Definition: phasic quickening and slowing of impulse formation, generally coordinated with respiration (increased on inspiration and decreased on expiration)
  - P waves: present and all identical

TABLE 5-14. **Systematic Approach for Analyzing ECG Rhythm Strips**

PROCEDURE	IMPORTANT OBSERVATIONS
Scan rhythm strip to obtain initial impression.	Is the rate unusually slow or fast? Is the rhythm fairly regular? Are any "funny beats" obvious?
Look at P waves to see if sinus node is pacemaker in command.	Are P waves present or absent? Are P waves all identical, smooth contoured, and upright in leads I, II, and III? Is each P wave followed by a QRS complex?
If P waves are present, measure PR interval to see if any delay in conduction through AV nodal region exists.	Is PR interval 0.12–0.20 sec in duration (i.e., 3.0–5.0 small boxes)? NOTE: PR interval varies inversely with the HR and is therefore normally lower in infants and children.
Examine QRS complexes to determine if conduction through ventricles is normal.	Are the QRS complexes 0.04–0.10 sec (i.e., 1.0 to 2.5 boxes) in duration? Are the QRS complexes all identical in shape?
Evaluate rhythm by comparing R to R intervals	Are all intervals equal or nearly equal (i.e., within 0.04 sec)? If irregularity is present, is there some kind of pattern or is it totally irregular?
Calculate heart rate using most appropriate method (see below).	If rhythm is regular, divide 300 by the number of large squares, including fractions of a square, between two consecutive R waves to get the ventricular rate. If every P wave is not followed by a QRS complex, follow the same process for P waves to obtain atrial rate. If rhythm is irregular, obtain ECG strip representing 6 sec (distance between 3 time marks at the top of many ECG papers), count the number of QRS complexes, and multiply by 10 to get the ventricular rate per minute. Follow the same process for P waves, if necessary.

AV = atrioventricular, ECG = electrocardiographic.

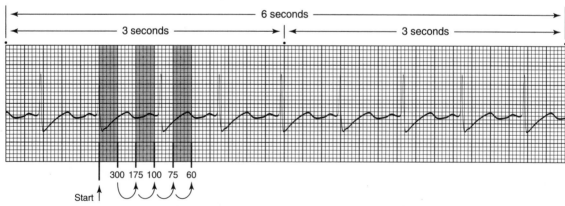

FIGURE 5-17. Heart rate can be calculated by counting the number of complexes in a 6-second strip and multiplying the result by 10 (particularly useful in very irregular rhythms) or by dividing 300 by the number of large squares between two R waves. To find the specific rate when the second R wave falls between two large squares, determine the difference between the two large squares on either side of the R wave (e.g., above, 100 − 75 = 25) and divide this number by 5 (the number of small boxes in a large square); then multiply the result by the number of small boxes between the lesser number and the R wave (e.g., above, 5 × 3 = 15) and add this result onto the value of the lesser of the two large squares.

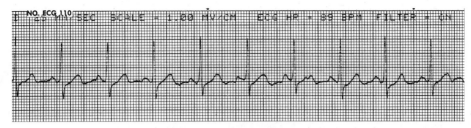

FIGURE 5-18. Normal sinus rhythm.

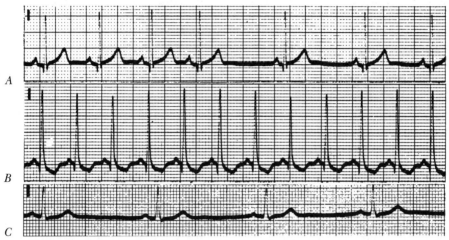

FIGURE 5-19. Various sinus rhythms: *(A)*, Sinus arrhythmia; *(B)*, sinus tachycardia; and *(C)*, sinus bradycardia. (From Marriott HJL: *Practical Electrocardiography,* 5th Ed. Baltimore, Williams & Wilkins, 1988. Used with permission.)

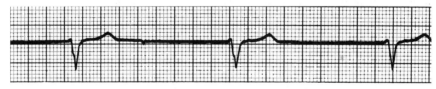

FIGURE 5-20. Sinus arrest. Also called sinus block or standstill. (From Patel JM, McGowan SG, Moody LA: *Arrhythmias—Detection, treatment, and cardiac drugs.* Philadelphia, WB Saunders, 1989. Used with permission.)

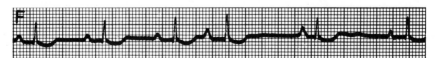

FIGURE 5-21. Premature atrial complex (PAC). The fourth beat is a PAC, and the remaining two beats are also initiated by atrial sites. (Note the different shapes of the P waves compared with the first three beats.) (From Marriott HJL: *Practical Electrocardiography,* 5th Ed. Baltimore, Williams & Wilkins, 1988. Used with permission.)

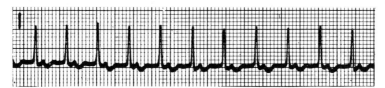

FIGURE 5-22. Atrial tachycardia with rate of 170. Upright P waves are seen immediately following QRS complex with a PR interval of 0.26 seconds (see first-degree AV block). (From Marriott HJL: *Practical Electrocardiography,* 5th Ed. Baltimore, Williams & Wilkins, 1988. Used with permission.)

- Causes: alterations in blood flow and pressures due to changes in intrathoracic pressure during respiration; commonly seen in very young and very old
- Significance: none, benign
- Sinus arrest or block (Fig. 5–20)
  - Definition: the sinoatrial (SA) node fails to initiate an impulse for one or more cycles
  - Characteristics: notably long P to P distance, complete absence of one or more waves or P-QRS complexes
  - Causes: frequently caused by digitalis toxicity, SA node disease, increased vagal influence
  - Significance: indicates failure of the SA node as pacemaker; if prolonged or frequent, cardiac output will drop and the patient will experience dizziness, fainting, or loss of consciousness.

Atrial Dysrrhythmias
- Premature atrial complexes (PACs, APCs) (Fig. 5–21)
  - Definition: an ectopic site in either atria initiates an impulse before the next impulse is initiated by the SA node.
  - Characteristics: a P-QRS-T complex occurs earlier than expected after the preceding P-QRS-T complex.
  - P wave: noticeably different than normal P waves (configuration depends on the site of impulse formation)
  - QRS: same as others from SA node
  - Causes: tobacco, coffee, alcohol, fatigue, apprehension, atrial irritation due to damage
  - Significance: generally benign; if very frequent, may result in decreased cardiac output; may progress to atrial tachycardia, flutter or fibrillation
- Atrial tachycardia (Fig. 5–22)
  - Definition: 3 or more PACs in a row
  - Rate: 150 to 200 bpm, frequently irregular
  - P waves: may be identical or different (unifocal versus multifocal)
  - QRS: usually the same as others from SA node, although aberrant conduction may occur.
  - Other: some degree of AV block is common at this rapid HR, so not every P wave may not be followed by a QRS complex.

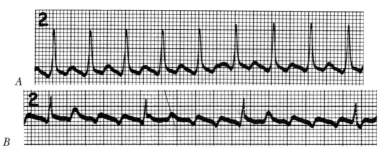

FIGURE 5-23. Atrial flutter. *(A),* With 2:1 block (most common ratio). *(B),* With 4:1 block (second most common ratio). (From Marriott HJL: *Practical Electrocardiography,* 5th Ed. Baltimore, Williams & Wilkins, 1988. Used with permission.)

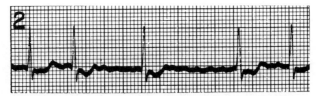

FIGURE 5-24. Atrial fibrillation (note typical, uneven, irregular "f" waves). (From Marriott HJL: *Practical Electrocardiography*, 5th Ed. Baltimore, Williams & Wilkins, 1988. Used with permission.)

- Causes: same as PACs
- Significance: may result in decreased ventricular filling and therefore decreased cardiac output
- Paroxysmal atrial or supraventricular tachycardia (PAT, PSVT)
  - Definition: sudden bursts of very rapid atrial or nodal tachycardia
  - Rate: 150 to 250 bpm, very regular
  - P waves: abnormal, usually merged with T wave
  - QRS: usually normal; may be some degree of block (see atrial tachycardia)
  - Other: begins and ends abruptly
  - Causes: digitalis toxicity; seen in coronary artery disease (CAD) and rheumatic heart disease; emotional stress, tobacco, coffee, alcohol; idiopathic
  - Significance: if rate is extremely rapid, ventricular filling may decrease, resulting in decreased cardiac output and decreased blood pressure; if poor ventricular function or CAD, the patient may develop chest discomfort, lightheadedness, and possibly CHF.
- Atrial flutter (Fig. 5–23)
  - Definition: very rapid atrial tachycardia
  - Rate: 250 to 350 bpm, absolutely regular
  - P waves: characteristic saw-tooth pattern in leads II, III, aVF
  - QRS: usually some blocked
  - Causes: organic heart disease (s/p cardiac

surgery, myocardial infarction, valve disease) or idiopathic
  - Significance: depends on ventricular rate (if very rapid rate cardiac output will decrease or CHF may develop); usually considered serious; may deteriorate into atrial fibrillation
- Atrial fibrillation (a-fib) (Fig. 5–24)
  - Definition: erratic quivering or twitching of the atrial muscle, called "f" waves
  - Rate: atrial rate is indeterminate; ventricular rate is highly variable and may be slow, fast, or normal; usually very irregular
  - P waves: absent; instead only chaotic baseline
  - QRS: typical for patient although they occur at irregular intervals
  - Causes: same as atrial flutter
  - Significance: depends on ventricular rate (if very fast or slow rate, cardiac output may drop or CHF may develop); if LV dysfunction, CHF is possible even at relatively normal rates in patients who are dependent on atrial contraction for adequate ventricular filling; stagnation of blood in atria may result in thrombus formation and embolization.

Nodal/Junctional Arrhythmias

- Premature nodal/junctional complexes (PNCs, PJCs) (Fig. 5–25)
  - Definition: premature impulses arising from the AV node or junctional tissue

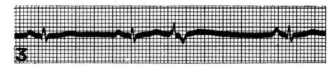

FIGURE 5-25. Premature nodal or junctional contraction. The third beat is a low nodal beat. (Note the inverted P wave following the QRS complex.) (From Marriott HJL: *Practical Electrocardiography*, 5th Ed. Baltimore, Williams & Wilkins, 1988. Used with permission.)

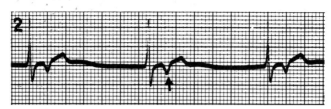

FIGURE 5–26. Nodal or junctional rhythm with a rate of 47. (Note inverted P waves following QRS complexes.) (From Marriott HJL: *Practical Electrocardiography*, 5th Ed. Baltimore, Williams & Wilkins, 1988. Used with permission.)

- P waves: abnormal; may occur before, during, or after the QRS segment, depending on the site of origin of the impulse
- QRS: same as from SA node
- Causes: decreased automaticity and conduction of the SA node or irritability of the junctional tissue
- Significance: generally benign
- Nodal or junctional rhythm (Fig. 5–26)
  - Definition: when the AV node or junctional tissue takes over as pacemaker of the heart
  - Rate: 40 to 60 bpm
  - P waves: same as PNCs (inverted II, III, aVF, if present)
  - QRS: same as SA node
  - Causes: same as PNCs/PJCs; trained athletes
  - Significance: generally well tolerated in normal individuals; in others, may reduce cardiac output or indicate failure of SA node; slow rate may allow ectopic foci to fire; in patients with ventricular dysfunction, lack of atrial "kick" may result in signs and symptoms of inadequate cardiac output or CHF; AV node is unreliable and may fail.
- Accelerated nodal/junctional rhythm (Fig. 5–27)
  - Definition: nodal/junctional rhythm with rate of 70 to 150 bpm, otherwise same as above
  - Causes: organic heart disease, digitalis toxicity, s/p cardiac surgery; idiopathic

- Significance: see preceding; also, hemodynamic impact depends upon rate (if very fast or slow, cardiac output may drop or CHF may develop)

Heart Blocks

- First-degree AV/heart block (see Fig. 5–28)
  - Definition: prolongation of PR interval >0.20 seconds
  - P waves: normal
  - QRS: same as SA node
  - Causes: digitalis toxicity, myocardial infarction damaging the AV node ischemia
  - Significance: generally well tolerated but may progress to more serious block
- Second-degree AV/heart block (Figs. 5–29 and 5–30)
  - Definition: nonconduction of some of the impulses through the AV node
  - Two types:
    — Mobitz I or Wenckebach: progressive prolongation of the PR interval until finally one impulse is not conducted (no QRS interval following a P wave); then the cycle repeats.
    — Mobitz II: nonconduction of an impulse without change in the PR interval
  - Causes: digitalis toxicity; myocardial infarction or ischemia involving the AV nodal region

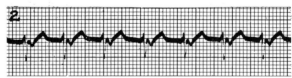

FIGURE 5–27. Accelerated nodal/junctional rhythm with rate of approximately 140. (Note P waves immediately following QRS complexes.) (From Marriott HJL: *Practical Electrocardiography*, 5th Ed. Baltimore, Williams & Wilkins, 1988. Used with permission.)

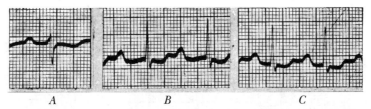

FIGURE 5-28. First-degree AV block. *(A)*, PR interval is 0.26 seconds. *(B)*, PR interval is 0.34 seconds because of digitalis. *(C)*, Effect of a maximal inspiration is an increase in heart rate and shortening of the PR interval to 0.22 seconds. (From Marriott HJL: *Practical Electrocardiography*, 5th Ed. Baltimore, Williams & Wilkins, 1988. Used with permission.)

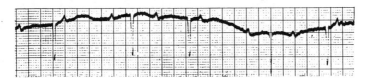

FIGURE 5-29. Second-degree AV block, Mobitz type I or Wenckebach phenomenon with an unusually long PR interval (shown in lead V_1). After the first QRS complex there is a blocked beat, then two conducted beats and a blocked beat. (From Marriott HJL: *Practical Electrocardiography*, 5th Ed. Baltimore, Williams & Wilkins, 1988. Used with permission.)

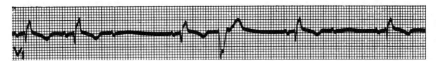

FIGURE 5-30. Second-degree AV block, Mobitz type II (lead V_1). Two consecutive PR intervals are unchanged before the dropped beat. The conducted beats show a normal PR interval and a right bundle-branch pattern; the fourth beat is a premature ventricular complex. (From Marriott HJL: *Practical Electrocardiography*, 5th Ed. Baltimore, Williams & Wilkins, 1988. Used with permission.)

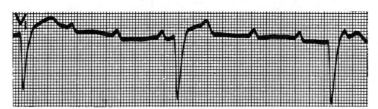

FIGURE 5-31. Third-degree, or complete, AV block. The P waves and QRS complexes are independent, at a ventricular rate of 28 and an atrial rate of 96. (From Marriott HJL: *Practical Electrocardiography*, 5th Ed. Baltimore, Williams & Wilkins, 1988. Used with permission.)

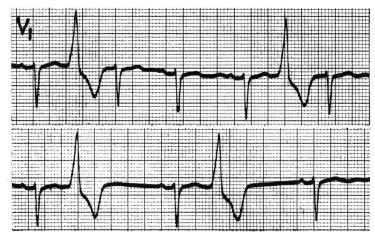

Figure 5-32. Premature ventricular complexes (PVCs). In the upper strip the PVCs are interpolated; in the lower strip the bigeminal PVCs are followed by a full compensatory pause. (From Marriott HJL: *Practical Electro-cardiography*, 5th Ed. Baltimore, Williams & Wilkins, 1988. Used with permission.)

- Significance: Mobitz I is generally benign; Mobitz II represents a more critical conduction defect; hemodynamic impact depends on ventricular rate; if ventricular rate is slow, cardiac output may fall; second-degree AV block may progress to third-degree heart block.
- Third-degree AV/heart block (Fig. 5–31)
  - Definition: all impulses are blocked at the AV node so that none of the impulses from the SA node or atria reach the ventricles; a separate pacemaker for the ventricles must be established.
  - Rate: separate atrial and ventricular rates; ventricular rate is usually 30 to 50 bpm.
  - P waves: usually present, but may be from SA node or atria; can have atrial fibrillation or flutter; no relationship to QRS complexes
  - QRS: may be either normal or abnormal
  - Causes: myocardial infarction or ischemia of the AV nodal region; other diseases of the AV node; digitalis toxicity
  - Significance: very unstable rhythm and considered a medical emergency; AV node is unreliable and may fail, so a pacemaker is indicated; if no ventricular pacemaker is established, the individual will die; if the ventricular rate is slow, cardiac output will fall.

Arrhythmias Originating from the Ventricles
- Premature ventricular complexes (PVCs, VPCs) (Figs. 5–32 and 5–33)

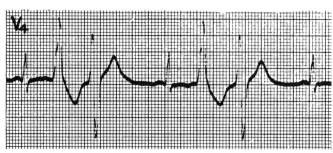

Figure 5-33. Paired multifocal premature ventricular complexes (PVCs). Each sinus beat is followed by a couplet of PVCs that have different morphologies, indicating different sites of origin. (From Marriott HJL: *Practical Electrocardiography*, 5th Ed. Baltimore, Williams & Wilkins, 1988. Used with permission.)

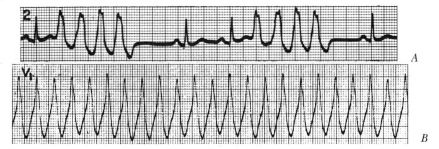

FIGURE 5–34. Ventricular tachycardia. *(A)*, Brief salvos of four beats each. *(B)*, A sustained run of rapid ventricular tachycardia, rate 204. No atrial activity is discernible. (From Marriott HJL: *Practical Electrocardiography*, 5th Ed. Baltimore, Williams & Wilkins, 1988. Used with permission.)

- Definition: when an ectopic site in the ventricles initiates an impulse before the SA node has a chance to fire
- P waves: usually not seen
- QRS: wide, bizarre looking, usually followed by a complete compensatory pause
- Other: can be isolated versus sequential, unifocal versus multifocal
- Causes: coffee, tobacco, alcohol, excitement; increased ventricular irritability due to cardiac disease, acid-base imbalance, electrolyte imbalance, or digitalis toxicity
- Significance: atrial "kick" is lacking and the diastolic period is reduced, leading to decreased ventricular filling and decreased stroke volume; increasing frequency of PVCs causes cardiac output to fall and may indicate increased irritability of the ventricular muscle; can progress to ventricular tachycardia or ventricular fibrillation
- Ventricular tachycardia (v-tach, VT) (Fig. 5–34)

- Definition: run of three or more PVCs
- P waves: not seen unless slow rate, then unrelated to QRS complex
- QRS: series of wide, bizarre QRS complexes
- Causes: acute myocardial infarction, atherosclerotic heart disease (ASHD), hypertensive heart disease, digitalis or quinidine toxicity; occasionally in athletes during exercise
- Significance: indicates very high ventricular irritability and is usually a medical emergency; lack of atrial contribution to ventricular filling plus rapid rate results in very low cardiac output and very low blood pressure and shock; frequently progresses to v-fib and death.
- Ventricular fibrillation (v-fib, VF) (Fig. 5–35)
  - Definition: erratic quivering of ventricular muscle
  - ECG: grossly irregular up-and-down fluctuations of the baseline; irregular zigzag pattern
  - Causes: same as v-tach, sequel to v-tach

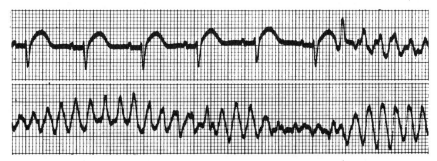

FIGURE 5–35. Ventricular fibrillation precipitated by an R-on-T phenomenon at the end of the upper strip. (From Marriott HJL: *Practical Electrocardiography*, 5th Ed. Baltimore, Williams & Wilkins, 1988. Used with permission.)

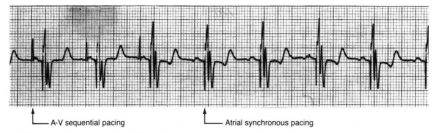

A-V sequential pacing | Atrial synchronous pacing

FIGURE 5–36. Electronic pacemaker bigeminy from a ventricular inhibited (VVI) pacemaker with an escape interval of 1.02 seconds, which inhibits activation unless the natural heart rate falls between 58 bpm. (From Phillips RE, Feeney MK: *The Cardiac Rhythms—A Systematic Approach to Interpretation,* 3rd Ed. Philadelphia, W.B. Saunders Co., 1990. With permission.)

• Significance: no effective pumping, no cardiac output, no pulse or BP; patient is clinically dead

Pacemaker Rhythms

• Multiprogrammable pacemakers may be activated with a variable degree of support depending on patient need (see pages 27 to 28).
• An electronic spike will immediately precede a paced beat.
• Different pacemaker modes are shown in Figures 5–36 and 5–37.

BLOOD PRESSURE

Of the physiologic measurements taken during activity, blood pressure (BP) is the most prone to error. Errors can occur because of either faulty equipment or technique. In addition, irregular cardiac rhythms can result in inaccuracies in BP because of the wide fluctuations they can create.

• Sphygmomanometers should be recalibrated at least once a year. Mercury manometers are the standard for BP measurement. If the level of the mercury is at zero, the glass column is clean and in good repair, and the rubber tubing is without cracks, the readings should be accurate. Aneroid manometers, which rely on a spring mechanism, are often out of calibration and require frequent checking against a mercury manometer to assure accuracy.
• The proper technique for obtaining BP measurements is as follows:
  · Place a properly sized cuff on the patient's arm, 2.5 cm above the antecubital space, with the bladder of the cuff centered over the palpated brachial artery. The width of the cuff should be approximately two thirds the distance between the axilla and the antecubital space, and the bladder of the cuff should be long enough to encircle ≥80% of the arm, as shown in Figure 5–38.
    — If the cuff is too short or too narrow, the reading will be erroneously high.
    — If the cuff is too wide or too long, it will be erroneously low.

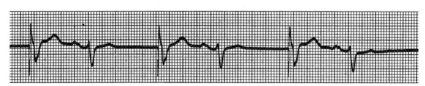

FIGURE 5–37. A DDD pacemaker exhibiting AV sequential and atrial synchronous modes. (From Phillips RE, Feeney MK: *The Cardiac Rhythms—A Systematic Approach to Interpretation,* 3rd Ed. Philadelphia, W.B. Saunders Co., 1990. With permission.)

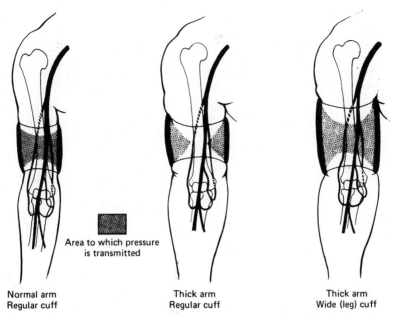

Area to which pressure
is transmitted

Normal arm   Thick arm   Thick arm
Regular cuff   Regular cuff   Wide (leg) cuff

FIGURE 5–38. Area of pressure transmission by various blood pressure cuffs. Note the inability of the regular, or standard-sized, cuff to transmit adequate pressure to occlude the brachial artery in a person with a thick arm. (From Sokolow M, McIlroy MB: *Clinical Cardiology*, 6th Ed. Los Altos, CA, Lange Medical Publications, 1993. Used with permission.)

— When a standard size cuff is two small for the upper arm and a larger cuff is not available, an alternative site for taking BP is on the forearm with auscultation over the radial artery in the wrist.

• BP is usually taken from the right arm unless: the pulse in that arm is significantly reduced, the patient has an IV line in that arm, the tone on that side is abnormal, or the reading is significantly higher on the left.

• Support the arm so that the cuff is at the level of the heart and while palpating the radial pulse, rapidly inflate the cuff 20 to 30 mm Hg past the point where the pulse disappears.

— If the patient's arm is not relaxed or is lower than his/her heart, both the systolic and diastolic values will be erroneously high.

— An auscultatory gap, where there is a temporary disappearance of pulsing sounds lasting up to 40 mm Hg after the initial systolic sounds, is common in patients with hypertension (Fig. 5–39). Therefore,

inflation past the point of radial pulse disappearance is crucial to avoid a false-low reading in these patients.

• Deflate the cuff slowly and note the reading at which the radial pulse is first palpated; then allow the cuff to deflate completely.

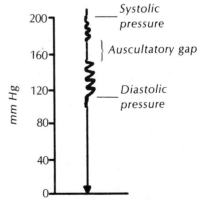

FIGURE 5–39. An auscultatory gap. (From Bates B: *A Guide to Physical Examination*, 5th Ed. Philadelphia, J.B. Lippincott, p. 283, 1991. Used with permission.)

- Place the diaphragm of the stethoscope over the brachial artery in the antecubital space and reinflate the cuff 20 to 30 mm Hg past the previously determined level.
- Deflate the cuff at a rate of 2 to 4 mm/beat while listening with the stethoscope over the brachial artery; the pressure level at which a sound is first heard (Korotkoff phase I) is noted as the systolic blood pressure (SBP).
- Continue slow deflation while listening to the sound increase in intensity, decrease, become muffled (phase IV), and finally disappear (phase V). Note the pressure levels for the last two phases. (There is disagreement about the use of phase IV versus phase V sounds as the diastolic blood pressure (DBP). When there is a significant discrepancy between the two values, both should be noted; otherwise use the phase V disappearance of sound as the DBP.)
  — Avoid keeping the cuff inflated for >30 to 60 seconds, as the discomfort from prolonged inflation will raise the BP.
  — Always deflate the cuff completely and wait for 30 to 60 seconds before reinflating it for another measurement.
- Record the measurements, noting the arm used and the patient's position.
- Once again, it is important that exercise values be measured while the patient is actually performing the activity, since BP falls as soon as exertion is stopped. If it is not possible to obtain an accurate reading during the activity or as the patient marches in place, the first three steps just described can be performed before the cessation of activity, and the fourth step can be completed as activity is stopping.
- Normal resting BP values are <140 mm Hg systolic (SBP) and <90 mm Hg diastolic (DBP) with a pulse pressure (SBP − DBP) of ≥20 mm Hg.
  - Increased SBP can be due to an increase in either cardiac output or peripheral vascular resistance (see pages 3–5).
  - Increased DBP is due to increased peripheral vascular resistance and results in an increased pressure load against which the LV must work to eject blood.
- Because BP is the product of cardiac output and peripheral vascular resistance, exercise re-

sults in different responses in the SBP and DBP, depending on the type of activity performed and the amount of muscle mass involved.
- Exertional BPs must be compared with the resting value obtained in the same position or posture (i.e., walking responses should be compared with the standing value and cycling responses should be compared with the sitting value).
- When exercise is dynamic and involves the large muscles of the body, vasodilation induced by local metabolic effects in the exercising muscles results in a drop in total peripheral resistance so that DBP usually drops slightly (a normal response is considered to be <10 mm Hg increase or decrease in DBP).
- When activity involves the smaller muscles of the body (e.g., upper extremities instead of lower extremities), the localized vasodilation is not sufficient to offset the generalized vasoconstriction caused by sympathetic nervous system stimulation, so peripheral vascular resistance increases and DBP rises. The smaller the exercising mass and the more intense the workload, the higher the DBP response will be.
- During static/isometric exercise, the strength of the muscle contraction directly affects the blood flow through the muscle and offsets the local metabolic effects so that there is a marked progressive increase in DBP.
- On the other hand, SBP always increases during activity because of the increase in cardiac output. In dynamic aerobic exercise, the rise in SBP is proportional to the workload (7 to 10 mm Hg per metabolic equivalent of energy expenditure (MET) increase in workload for exercise involving large muscles of body). With endurance exercise at the sustained submaximal workload, SBP rises slowly for first 2 to 3 minutes, then remains constant or may decrease slightly.
- In other forms of exercise, the increase in SBP due to higher cardiac output is superimposed on that caused by the elevated total peripheral resistance; thus, during isometric exercise there is a more marked progressive increase in SBP.
- Abnormal BP responses to activity consist of:

• *Hypertensive responses:* when SBP increases excessively for the workload (i.e., >10 mm Hg per MET increase), the exertional DBP increases >10 mm Hg compared with the resting value; the postexercise DBP remains elevated during recovery; or the SBP fails to level out when the body should be in steady-state condition during sustained submaximal exercise. Hypertensive responses are usually due to increased peripheral vascular resistance.

• *Hypotensive responses:* when the normal rise in SBP at lower level workloads is followed by a sudden progressive drop with increasing workloads, which is indicative of severe pathologic conditions (e.g., moderate to severe aortic stenosis, severe CAD, and/or poor LV function).

• *Blunted or flat BP responses:* when SBP increases minimally or negligibly with increased workloads (<7 mm Hg per MET increase); these are usually due to medications, especially β-blockers, although some individuals exhibit a truly blunted response in absence of medications (very ominous finding).

RESPIRATORY RATE

Measuring a patient's respiratory rate (RR) involves counting the number of breaths taken in a minute. Usually, patients are comfortable at rest with a normal RR of 12 to 20 breaths per minute, and the actual numbers of breaths is not necessarily measured by the therapist. However, when there are any signs of increased work of breathing (e.g., recruitment of accessory muscles of respiration, nasal flaring, pursed-lip breathing), the RR should be formally counted.

• Because RR frequently changes when a patient is aware of his/her breathing, the most accurate results are obtained when the patient is unaware of your measurement. This can best be done by observing from a distance or while pretending to attend to something else.

• The recommended time over which the RR is counted is a full minute, although a 30-second count will offer minimal error if the RR during that period is truly representative of the patient's status.

• During exertion the minute ventilation

($\dot{V}_E$) increases proportional to the workload because of increases in both tidal volume and RR.

• At lower intensities there is a greater relative increment in tidal volume than in RR; then closer to maximum, tidal volume levels off at its maximum, and further increases in $\dot{V}_E$ are due to higher RRs.

• When $\dot{V}_E$ exceeds 50 L, the energy cost of breathing becomes progressively greater, increasing from 1–4% of total oxygen consumption at lower $\dot{V}_E$s to ~30% when $\dot{V}_E$ is 70 L.

OXYGENATION STATUS

There are two ways to monitor a patient's oxygenation status: through direct sampling of the arterial blood and by indirect assessment of the oxygen saturation of the blood. Lacking either of these measures, the clinician has to rely on observation of the signs and symptoms of hypoxemia (see Table 3–5, page 89).

Arterial Blood Gases

Patients with pulmonary disease often have arterial blood gas (ABG) values in their charts. These values may be obtained to give an indication of the patient's baseline levels, to monitor the patient's status when acutely ill and document the efficacy of therapeutic interventions, as in critical care units, or to provide information about the patient's oxygenation status during exertion, as in exercise testing with ABG sampling. Regardless of the circumstances, the therapist should be able to interpret the results and alter the treatment plan if necessary.

To analyze ABG results, follow four simple steps (Fig. 5–40):

• *Look at pH to assess acid-base status.* Although the normal range is 7.35 to 7.45, for this purpose only 7.40 is considered normal:
  • pH <7.40 indicates acidosis.
  • pH >7.40 indicates alkalosis.
• *Look at the P_{CO_2}:*
  • First, as an indicator of ventilatory status:
    — P_{CO_2} = 35 to 45 mm Hg indicates adequate ventilation; no primary respiratory problem and no respiratory compensation for a metabolic problem.
    — P_{CO_2} <30 mm Hg indicates alveolar hyperventilation.

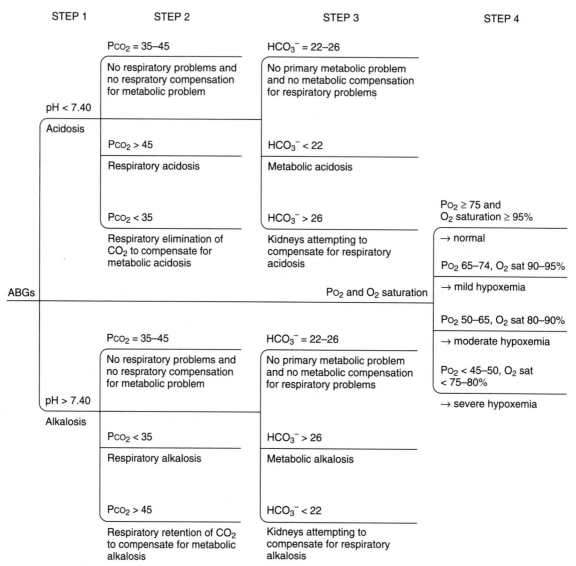

FIGURE 5-40. Steps involved in analyzing arterial blood gases (ABGs): (1) check pH, (2) check P_{CO_2} (mm Hg), (3) check HCO_3^- (mEq/L), and (4) check P_{O_2} (mm Hg) and O_2 saturation (O_2 sat, %).

— P_{CO_2} >50 mm Hg indicates alveolar hypoventilation, ventilatory failure.
• Next, to determine the cause of abnormal values, interpret levels in relation to pH:
  — P_{CO_2} >45 mm Hg and pH <7.40 indicate respiratory acidosis.
  — P_{CO_2} >45 mm Hg and pH >7.40 indicate respiratory retention of CO_2 to compen-

sate for metabolic alkalosis.
  — P_{CO_2} <35 mm Hg and pH >7.40 indicate respiratory alkalosis.
  — P_{CO_2} <35 mm Hg and pH <7.40 indicate respiratory elimination of CO_2 to compensate for metabolic acidosis.
• *Look at HCO_3^-:*
  • Normal HCO_3^- values (22 to 26 mEq/L)

indicate no primary metabolic problem and no metabolic compensation for a respiratory problem.

- Abnormal HCO_3^- values are interpreted in relation to pH:
  - HCO_3^- <22 mEq/L and pH <7.40 indicate metabolic acidosis.
  - HCO_3^- <22 mEq/L and pH >7.40 indicate renal compensation for respiratory alkalosis.
  - HCO_3^- >26 mEq/L and pH >7.40 indicate metabolic alkalosis.
  - HCO_3^- >26 mEq/L and pH <7.40 indicate renal compensation for respiratory acidosis.

- *Look at Po_2 and O_2 saturation (O_2 sat, SaO_2):*
  - Normal: 80 to 100 mm Hg at sea level with O_2 sat >95%.
  - Po_2 = 60 to 80 mm Hg indicates mild hypoxemia, O_2 sat will be 90% to 95% (if no shift in the oxyhemoglobin (HbO_2) curve).
  - Po_2 = 40 to 60 mm Hg indicates moderate hypoxemia, O_2 sat will be 60% to 90% (if no shift in the HbO_2 curve).
  - Po_2 <40 mm Hg indicates severe hypoxemia, O_2 sat will be ≤60% (if no shift in the HbO_2 curve).

Although ABGs provide the most accurate method of assessing a patient's oxygenation, current technology does not allow continuous monitoring of a patient's status.

Pulse Oximetry, Oxygen Saturation Monitor

Using a sensor attached to a finger or ear lobe or over the forehead, the pulse oximeter provides a digital readout of O_2 sat that is updated every few seconds and therefore is capable of providing immediate feedback regarding the effects of position change or activity on O_2 sat. Assessment of O_2 sat is strongly advised for all patients with forced expiratory volume in 1 second (FEV_1) of <50% of predicted or a diffusing capacity (DL_{CO}) of <60% of predicted, since these patients are likely to exhibit desaturation during activity. O_2 sat is normally >95%.

- O_2 sat values must be interpreted within the context of the patient's respiratory and metabolic status, since shifts of the HbO_2 curve will change the affinity of oxygen and hemoglobin (see Fig. 2–4, page 39).

- Because of the shape of the HbO_2 dissociation curve, small changes in O_2 sat from 96% to 90% represent large decreases in Po_2, as described in the previous section on ABGs, and should be considered significant. Then as O_2 sat drops below 90% and the curve gets steeper, larger decreases in O_2 sat are associated with an increasing rate of fall in Po_2.

- Activity should be terminated if O_2 sat drops to <90% in acutely ill patients or ≤85% in patients with chronic lung disease. Discussion with the physician is warranted regarding a trial or increased dose of oxygen therapy during activity.

SYMPTOMS AND OTHER SIGNS OF LIMITED EXERCISE TOLERANCE

In addition to the abnormal physiologic responses already discussed in this section, the patient's symptoms must always be considered, as well as some other signs that indicate limited exercise tolerance. Angina, dyspnea, and fatigue are the most common complaints during exertion. Subjective scales have been developed for angina (Table 5–15) and dyspnea (Table 5–16) to make assessment more meaningful. An alternative dyspnea scale that provides a more objective means of measuring the level of dyspnea is also valuable (Table 5–17). When the patient develops abnormal signs or symptoms, exercise intensity should be monitored closely and may need to be reduced during subsequent therapy sessions. The therapist should expect that the patient is likely to progress more slowly with the rehabilitation activities because of tolerance for only gradual increases in duration and intensity.

- Other signs and symptoms of limited exercise tolerance that develop during or immediately after exertion include:

Table 5–15. Angina Scale for Subjective Rating of Intensity

RATING	DESCRIPTION
1+	Light, barely noticeable
2+	Moderate, bothersome
3+	Severe, very uncomfortable
4+	Most severe pain ever experienced

From American College of Sports Medicine: *Guidelines for Exercise Testing and Prescription,* 4th Ed. Philadelphia, Lea & Febiger, 1991. Reprinted with permission.

TABLE 5-16. **Dyspnea Scale for Subjective Rating of Intensity**

RATING	DESCRIPTION
+1	Mild, noticeable to patient but not observer
+2	Mild, some difficulty, noticeable to observer
+3	Moderate difficulty, but can continue
+4	Severe difficulty, patient cannot continue

From American College of Sports Medicine: *Guidelines for Exercise Testing and Prescription,* 4th Ed. Philadelphia, Lea & Febiger, 1991. Reprinted with permission.

- Anginal discomfort
- Dyspnea
- Leg claudication
- Pallor
- Lightheadedness, dizziness
- Facial expression of distress
- Other signs and symptoms of limited exercise tolerance that develop later following exertion include:
  - Slow recovery from activity, especially persistent tachycardia >5 to 10 minutes after exertion
  - Excessive fatigue lasting >1 to 2 hours after exertion
  - Insomnia
  - Weight gain due to fluid retention

TABLE 5-17. **Dyspnea Levels**

LEVEL	DESCRIPTION
0	Able to count to 15 easily without taking an additional breath
1	Able to count to 15 but must take one additional breath
2	Must take two additional breaths to count to 15
3	Must take three additional breaths to count to 15
4	Unable to count

From Physical Therapy Management of Patients with Pulmonary Disease, Ranchos Los Amigos Medical Center, Physical Therapy Department, Downey, CA. Used with permission.
The patient is asked to inhale normally and then to count out loud to 15 over a 7.5- to 8-second period. Any shortness of breath can be graded by levels, as shown in the table.

5.6 ASSESSING YOUR FINDINGS

Throughout the patient evaluation, the therapist constantly assesses the patient's responses and decides how much activity the patient can safely perform versus when it is appropriate to stop. However, once the patient evaluation has been completed, all of the findings must be assessed to define appropriate treatment goals and develop the treatment plan. Although a single abnormal finding can indicate a life-threatening situation, this is generally not the case. Rather, it is the sum of all the clinical data that describes the patient's clinical status. Of particular importance are the heart rate, BP, O_2 sat, ECG (if available), patient complaints, and other signs of distress.

CHEST ASSESSMENT

The various abnormal findings that may be detected on chest assessment should be evaluated together and in relation to each other, for the pattern of abnormalities often reveals the anatomic disturbance responsible for them, as indicated in Table 5–18.

- By identifying the patient's pathologic condition through chest assessment, an appropriate treatment plan can be instituted.
- Following treatment, a brief reassessment is performed to document the effectiveness of treatment.

ACTIVITY AND ENDURANCE EVALUATION

In summary, many patients exhibit normal responses to increasing activity without any adverse signs and symptoms and therefore are safe to participate in unrestricted treatment programs. However, a significant percentage of patients have some form of diagnosed or undiagnosed cardiopulmonary dysfunction and exhibit abnormal responses to exertion, although these may not be recognized by the therapist if physiologic monitoring is not performed. Sometimes, the only abnormalities are related to orthostatic hypotension, with a drop in BP as the patient moves from supine to sitting to standing, which may result from deconditioning, antihypertension medications, or autonomic dysfunction.

TABLE 5–18. Physical Signs Observed in Various Disorders

CONDITION	BREATH SOUNDS	ADVENTITIOUS SOUNDS	VOICE SOUNDS	INSPECTION	TACTILE FREMITUS	PERCUSSION
Normal	Nl	None	Muffled, distant, indistinct	Trachea midline, symmetric chest expansion	Nl	Nl
Asthma, acute moderately severe attack	↓, Bronchial, prolonged expiration	Inspiratory plus expiratory wheezes	↓	↑ Use of accessory muscles, tachypnea	↓	Nl–↑
Atelectasis	↓ Or 0	Crackles	↓ Or 0	Trachea deviated to affected side	↓	↓–↓↓
Bronchiectasis	Nl	Crackles	Nl	↓ Expansion AS, tachypnea, clubbing	↑ Rhonchal fremitus	Nl
Bronchitis	Nl, possible prolonged expiration	Crackles, wheezes	Nl	Possible ↓ motion, occasional use of accessory muscles	↓ Bilaterally	↑ Bilaterally
COPD	↓↓, prolonged expiration	None versus crackles and wheezes	↓ Or 0 bilaterally	Barrel-shaped chest, moves as a unit, ↑ use of accessory muscles, ↓ chest expansion	↓ Bilaterally	↑ Bilaterally
Consolidation	Bronchial	Crackles	Whispered pectoriloquy	↓ Motion AS	↑	↓
Fibrosis						
Localized	↓	Crackles	↓	↓ Motion over area	↓ Or 0	↓
Generalized	↓	Crackles	↓	↓ Motion bilaterally	↓ Or 0	↓
Heart failure	Nl	Dependent crackles	Nl	Nl chest expansion, tachypnea	nl	nl
Pleural effusion (moderate to large)	↓ Or 0,* bronchial†	Possible pleural rub	↓* ↑†	↓ Motion AS, ↑ RR, trachea deviated to OS	↓ Or 0	↓–↓↓
Pneumothorax (>15%)	↓ Or 0	None	↓ Or 0	↓ Motion AS	↓ Or 0	↑

Nl = normal, ↓ = decreased, ↓↓ = very decreased, ↑ = increased, 0 = absent, AS = on affected side, COPD = chronic obstructive pulmonary disease, RR = respiratory rate, OS = opposite side.
*Over the effusion.
†Above the fluid.

Avoidance of quick changes of position is an important treatment modification for these patients. Other times, the abnormal signs and symptoms are extreme and imply exercise intolerance (see below), in which case the evaluation or treatment session should be terminated and consultation with the referring physician is probably indicated. Finally, the abnormalities may simply indicate a reduced level of physical fitness and the need to monitor intensity and the individual's responses to increasing activity and to progress slowly in the treatment program. Normative data for physical fitness levels according to age and activity level are shown in Table 5–19.

SIGNS AND SYMPTOMS OF EXERCISE INTOLERANCE

- Moderate dizziness or near syncope
- Syncope
- New onset angina, or level 2+/4+ angina (see Table 5–15)
- Nausea, vomiting
- Marked dyspnea (level 2+/4+) (see Table 5–15)
- Unusual or severe fatigue
- Ataxia, persistent unsteadiness, mental confusion
- Severe claudication (grade III/IV) or other pain
- Facial expression of severe distress
- Cyanosis or severe pallor
- Cold sweat
- Loss of sustained vigor of palpable pulse
- SBP >200 to 210 mm Hg
- DBP >110 mm Hg
- Increase in heart rate >50 bpm with low-level activity
- Drop in systolic BP >20 mm Hg
- Significant arrhythmias (complex PVCs, v-tach, second-degree or third-degree heart block, any arrhythmia accompanied by decreased BP)
- Onset of S_3, new or ↑ heart murmur
- Development of pulmonary crackles/rales

WARNING SIGNS AND SYMPTOMS OF LIMITED EXERCISE TOLERANCE

- Resting tachycardia
- Lack of heart rate or BP response to exertion
- Excessive heart rate or BP response to exertion
- Fall of systolic BP >10 mm Hg after initial increase

TABLE 5–19. Cardiorespiratory Fitness Classification

AGE (YRS)	WOMEN MAXIMAL OXYGEN UPTAKE (ML/KG/MIN)				
	LOW	FAIR	AVERAGE	GOOD	HIGH
20-29	<24	24-30	31-37	38-48	49+
30-39	<20	20-27	28-33	34-44	45+
40-49	<17	17-23	24-30	31-41	42+
50-59	<15	15-20	21-27	28-37	38+
60-69	<13	13-17	18-23	24-34	35+

AGE (YRS)	MEN MAXIMAL OXYGEN UPTAKE (ML/KG/MIN)				
	LOW	FAIR	AVERAGE	GOOD	HIGH
20-29	<25	25-33	34-42	43-52	53+
30-39	<23	23-30	31-38	39-48	49+
40-49	<20	20-26	27-35	36-44	45+
50-59	<18	18-24	25-33	34-42	43+
60-69	<16	16-22	23-30	31-40	41+

From American Heart Association, The Committee on Exercise: *Exercise Testing and Training of Apparently Healthy Individuals: A Handbook for Physicians.* American Heart Association, 1972. Used with permission.

- Increasing arrhythmias during or immediately following exertion
- Low anginal threshold
- Excessive dyspnea
- Leg claudication or other pain
- Pallor, facial expression of distress
- Lightheadedness, dizziness
- Slow recovery from activity
- Excessive fatigue lasting >1 to 2 hours after exertion

DEFINING THE PHYSICAL THERAPY PROBLEMS

The purpose of assessing all the evaluative findings is to define the physical therapy problems for each patient and thereby develop appropriate treatment goals and plans that directly address these problems.

- Patients with either cardiac or pulmonary dysfunction may have any of the following physical therapy problems:
  - Decreased exercise tolerance/deconditioning

- Abnormal physiologic responses to exertion
- Inability to meet the demands of daily living activities
- Increased coronary risk factors (e.g., sedentary lifestyle, obesity, hypertension, glucose intolerance)
- In addition, patients with pulmonary dysfunction may have any of the following physical therapy problems:
  - Impaired ventilation
    — Decreased chest expansion (e.g., due to decreased ventilatory muscle strength and/or endurance, restricted mobility, or reduced ventilatory drive)
    — Impaired lung compliance (e.g., due to pulmonary fibrosis, atelectasis, pneumonia)
  - Impaired oxygenation
    — Inadequate ventilation
    — Impaired secretion clearance
    — Increased airway resistance
    — Impaired perfusion
  - Impaired secretion clearance
    — Increased secretions
    — Impaired mucociliary action
    — Impaired cough
  - Impaired ability to protect airway
  - Increased work of breathing
    — Increased energy demands (resulting from any of the problems listed above)
    — Inefficient/abnormal breathing pattern
- The techniques commonly used to treat these problems and restore patients to better function are presented in Chapter 6.

REFERENCES

1. Bates DW: *Respiratory Function in Disease,* 3rd Ed. Philadelphia, W.B. Saunders Co., 1989.
2. Baum GL, Wolinsky E (eds.): *Textbook of Pulmonary Diseases,* 4th Ed. Boston, Little, Brown & Co., 1989.
3. Braunwald E (ed.): *Heart Disease—A Textbook of Cardiovascular Medicine.* Philadelphia, W.B. Saunders Co., 1992.
4. Brewis RAL, Gibson GJ, Geddes DM (eds.): *Respiratory Medicine.* London, Bailliére Tindall, 1990.
5. Burton GG, Hodgkin JE, Ward JJ (eds.): *Respiratory Care. A Guide to Clinical Practice,* 3rd Ed. Philadelphia, J.B. Lippincott Co., 1992.
6. Cherniack RM, Cherniack L: *Respiration in Health and Disease,* 3rd Ed. Philadelphia, W.B. Saunders Co., 1983.
7. Chimowitz MI, Mancini GBJ: Asymptomatic coronary artery disease in patients with stroke—Prevalence, prognosis, diagnosis, and treatment. *Curr. Concepts Cerebrovasc Dis Stroke* (American Heart Assoc) 26:23–27, 1991.
8. Chung EK (ed.): *Quick Reference to Cardiovascular Diseases,* 3rd Ed. Baltimore, Williams & Wilkins, 1987.
9. Cohen M, Michel TH: *Cardiopulmonary Symptoms in Physical Therapy Practice.* New York, Churchill Livingstone, 1988.
10. Farzan S: *A Concise Handbook of Respiratory Diseases,* 3rd Ed. Norwalk, CT, Appleton & Lange, 1992.
11. Flenley DC: *Respiratory Medicine,* 2nd Ed. London, Bailliére Tindall, 1990.
12. Herster NR, Young JR, Beven EG, et al.: Coronary angiography in 506 patients with extracranial cerebrovascular disease. *Arch. Int. Med.* 145:849–852, 1985.
13. Hillegass E: Cardiopulmonary assessment. *In* Hillegass EA, Sadowsky HS (Eds.): *Essentials of Cardiopulmonary Physical Therapy.* Philadelphia, W.B. Saunders Co., 1994.
14. Hobson L, Hammon WE: Chest assessment. *In* Frownfelter DL: *Chest Physical Therapy and Pulmonary Rehabilitation,* 2nd Ed. Chicago, Year Book Medical Publishers, Inc., 1987.
15. Humberstone N: Respiratory assessment and treatment. *In* Irwin S, Tecklin JS: *Cardiopulmonary Physical Therapy,* 2nd Ed. St. Louis, The C.V. Mosby Co., 1990.
16. Hurst JW, Schlant RC, Rackley CE, Sonnenblick EH, Wenger NK (eds.): *The Heart, Arteries and Veins,* 7th Ed. New York, McGraw-Hill Information Services Co., 1990.
17. Irwin S, Blessey RL: Patient evaluation. *In* Irwin S, Tecklin JS: *Cardiopulmonary Physical Therapy,* 2nd Ed. St. Louis, The C.V. Mosby Co., 1990.
18. Kloner RA (ed.): *The Guide to Cardiology,* 2nd Ed. New York, Le Jacq Communications, 1990.
19. Lee WR: *Essentials of Clinical Cardiology.* 1980.
20. Marriott HJL: *Practical Electrocardiography,* 5th Ed. Baltimore, Williams & Wilkins, 1972.
21. Phillips RE, Feeney MK: *The Cardiac Rhythms—A Systematic Approach to Interpretation,* 3rd Ed. Philadelphia, W.B. Saunders Co., 1990.
22. Sokolow M, McIlroy MB: *Clinical Cardiology,* 4th Ed. Los Altos, CA, Lange Medical Publications, 1986.

6

CARDIOPULMONARY PHYSICAL
THERAPY TREATMENT

Although many of the treatment techniques used in cardiopulmonary physical therapy require expertise beyond the realm of most practicing clinicians (as is true of all specialty areas), some of the techniques could and should be routinely incorporated in physical therapy treatment of patients with other pathologic conditions. This chapter uses a problem-oriented approach in presenting the problems commonly encountered in cardiopulmonary patients, as well as patients with many other medical and surgical diagnoses, and then describes the treatment techniques that are available to improve function. Specific recommendations and treatment modifications for particular patient diagnoses and therapeutic interventions are also provided in Chapters 1 through 3.

6.1 IMPAIRED EXERCISE TOLERANCE

The most common problem encountered in cardiac and pulmonary patients, as well as patients with any chronic disease, is progressively reduced activity/exercise tolerance or endurance. A vicious cycle develops of inactivity, reduced muscular inefficiency (i.e., deconditioning) causing increasing symptomatology, and further abatement of activity in order to avoid discomfort, as illustrated in Figure 6–1. The ultimate result is complete disability with inability to comfortably perform even the most basic activities of daily living; fortunately, most patients do not deteriorate fully to this level before death.

To increase exercise tolerance, a program of aerobic, or endurance, training is prescribed. Classically, this is described as exercise involving the large muscles of the body, which is sustained

continuously for at least 20 to 30 minutes at an intensity of 70% to 85% of maximal predicted heart rate (according to age) and performed at least 3 days per week. Needless to say, most deconditioned patients are incapable of performing exercise in this way, at least initially. However, even the most debilitated patient can gradually improve exercise tolerance with an appropriate individualized exercise prescription and attention to the basic principles of exercise training.

EXERCISE PRESCRIPTION

The four components of an exercise prescription include the mode of exercise, intensity, duration, and frequency; the key to how successfully any patient participates in an endurance training program lies in the therapist's ability to structure these components in accordance to the patient's interests, abilities, limitations, motivations, and lifestyle. If the patient is attending a formalized rehabilitation program, the novelty of the process and socialization with other participants may provide enough interest and motivation to keep the patient coming back. However, an entirely different situation exists when the patient is being seen just before discharge from the hospital, or as a home patient or outpatient, and will be performing the program independently with only occasional, if any, reinforcement.

- Asking questions regarding interests, abilities, limitations, motivations, and lifestyle and carefully listening to the patient, both what the patient says and does not say, are critical for success. Patience is required, for the individual may have little prior experience with regular exercise and may not know what will work best until after some trial and error.

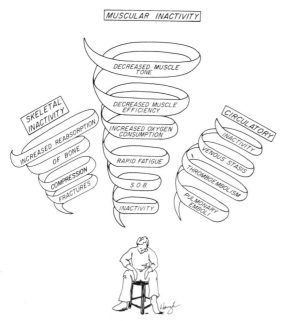

FIGURE 6–1. The effects of inactivity. SOB = shortness of breath. (From Frownfelter DL: *Chest Physical Therapy and Pulmonary Rehabilitation—An Interdisciplinary Approach*, 2nd Ed. Chicago, Year Book Medical Publishers, Inc., 1987. Used with permission.)

- The starting place for the endurance exercise prescription is the endurance evaluation described in the previous chapter, which is basically a submaximal exercise test designed to define a patient's physiologic responses to increasing exercise, including the patient's upper limit of comfortable tolerance. The results provide information about intensity, duration, and, indirectly, frequency.

Presented in this section are guidelines for duration, frequency, intensity, and mode that can be applied in prescribing an exercise training program designed to improve exercise tolerance. As will become apparent, there are relationships between intensity, frequency and duration so that a limitation in one of these may be compensated for by adjustments in the others. A summary of these guidelines is presented in Table 6–1.

MODE

Acceptable modes of exercise are any that use the large muscles of the body, are dynamic in nature, can be performed in a continuous manner, and, most importantly of all, are enjoyable for the individual. The most commonly used modes of exercise include walking and/or jogging (track or treadmill), bicycling (stationary or road/trail), swimming, aerobics, dancing, bench stepping, skating, cross-country skiing (snow or machine), stair stepping, and rowing machine.

- Participants in a cardiac or pulmonary rehabilitation program usually have the opportunity to work out using several different exercise modes in an interval fashion. Typically, these programs include walking and jogging, stationary cycling, and rowing machine. In addition, some offer arm ergometry (or set a stationary cycle up on a table) and four extremity modalities (e.g., Schwinn Airdyne, cross-country ski machine). Such variety enhances patient motivation and minimizes the potential for injury.
- Defining a practical yet enjoyable mode is a most challenging task when working with clients performing independent exercise at home. Walking or jogging is the simplest as far as equipment requirements are concerned but can pose problems in patients with joint disease or who live in areas that are not safe or where environmental factors, like extremes of weather or poor air quality, may have deleterious effects. It is advisable to investigate facilities in the community with controlled environments, such as shopping malls that open their doors a couple of hours early, which may be available as alternative walking sites. The more information and alternatives that can be given to patients, the easier it becomes for them to follow through and "just do it."
- For individuals who are interested in purchasing some type of home exercise equipment, one suggestion is to encourage them to try out various machines at, for example, fitness stores, friends' houses, and health clubs, in order to identify their favorite and then to peruse the want ads for exercise equipment for sale (which, more often than not, have been used only a handful of times, if at all, and cost only half as much as the standard price).

DURATION

The initial duration of the exercise program will be determined by the individual's fitness level and medical history and will be indicated by the endurance evaluation.

- Patients who are extremely deconditioned may not be able to walk even 5 minutes continuously without dyspnea or other symptoms of intolerance; these patients will benefit from multiple short intervals of activity with brief rest periods (1 to 2 minutes is usually adequate) interposed between them. Although these brief intervals are too short to be truly aerobic in nature, patients can often add 1 minute to one or more of the intervals each day and are thus able to walk up to 10 minutes continuously by the end of the first week.
- More typical, sedentary individuals can often perform 10 to 20 minutes of continuous exercise before the onset of peripheral fatigue or discomfort limits their ability to persist. If duration and especially intensity are initiated conservatively, patients are usually able to perform workouts 6 to 7 days per week without musculoskeletal distress, and thus progress fairly quickly.
- The goal should be to increase duration to at least 20 minutes of continuous exercise before any increase in intensity is instituted. Then, depending on patient goals and time constraints, the duration can be increased gradually to 45 to 60 minutes of continuous activity. If the individual's goal is to reduce body fat and weight or lower blood pressure, the exercise duration ideally should be increased to a minimum of 40 minutes of lower intensity exercise.[19]

TABLE 6-1. **Summary of Guidelines for Components of an Exercise Prescription**

COMPONENT	GUIDELINES
Mode	Any activity involving the large muscles of the body that is dynamic in nature and can be performed in a continuous manner (e.g., walking, jogging, bicycling, dancing, aerobics, swimming, cross-country skiing, rowing, stair climbing).
Duration	Depends on the individual's level of fitness initially, then the intensity: If very deconditioned individual, start with short intervals according to tolerance with brief (1–2 min) rests interposed between them, then increase the length of each interval (usually by about one min/day) and decrease the number of rest periods. If typical, sedentary-to-active individual, start with duration of tolerance (when onset of fatigue or discomfort appears), then increase by 1–2 min every day. Goal should be at least 20–30 min of continuous exercise if higher intensity or 40–60 min if low intensity. On days when sufficient time is not available, any amount of exercise is better than none; try to incorporate a number of 10-min periods throughout the day. Longer duration, lower intensity exercise is recommended for those trying to control weight, hypertension, or intermittent claudication.
Frequency	Depends on the duration and intensity: If continuous exercise duration is <15–20 min, frequency should be 2–3 times/day, every day if possible. If continuous exercise duration is >20 min, frequency can be once a day, 3–7 days/week, depending on intensity: If low-to-moderate intensity, program can be performed 5–7 days/week. If higher intensity program, frequency of 3–5 days/week is acceptable.
Intensity	Depends on fitness level, health status, and goals of program: For healthy, sedentary-to-active individual, intensity can be based on percentage of age-predicted or true maximal HR (e.g., 70–85% of HR_{max} or 60–75% of HR reserve + resting HR), with the percentage being determined by the individual's fitness level or tolerance. For patients with chronic disease and those on medications which affect HR, intensity is based on the results of an endurance evaluation (i.e., the defined upper limit of comfortable tolerance). If the patient goals are to reduce body fat, control hypertension, or relieve intermittent claudication, lower intensity, longer duration exercise is more beneficial than higher intensity exercise.

HR = heart rate, HR_{max} = maximal heart rate.

$$\boxed{\text{Target HR} = (\text{MHR} - \text{RHR}) \% + \text{RHR}}$$

FIGURE 6-2. Karvonen's formula for calculating training heart rate (HR) based on the HR reserve, or difference between maximal and resting HR (MHR and RHR, respectively).

- Of course, an individual's lifestyle and time schedule may impose additional constraints on the duration of exercise that an individual is able to perform. Some days (or weeks) just cannot accommodate 30 to 40 minutes of continuous exercise. In this case, any amount of exercise is better than none. Three exercise bouts of 10 minutes will probably not effect the same increase in aerobic fitness level as one 30 minute bout; however, it may offer advantages for increasing bone density and flexibility.[3]

FREQUENCY

The frequency, or number of days per week, of exercise participation is dependent on the duration, and to a lesser extent the intensity, the individual is able to exercise continuously.

- Until the patient is able to exercise for 15 to 20 minutes continuously, the patient should perform the program at least twice per day.

- When the patient can perform 15 to 20 minutes of continuous aerobic exercise, the frequency can be reduced to once a day, 5 to 6 days per week. As stated previously, if the intensity is conservatively established, patients can usually perform their program 6 to 7 days per week without any problems.
- Higher intensity exercise of 20 to 30 minutes can be scheduled for as few as three times per week while still continuing to improve aerobic fitness.
- Moderate intensity exercise of 20 to 30 minutes requires a frequency of 3 to 5 days per week to continue to show fitness gains.

INTENSITY

There are several different ways to prescribe exercise intensity.

- As mentioned earlier, the exercise intensity that has traditionally been recommended based on research documenting fitness increments is 70% to 85% of maximal heart rate (HR_{max}), which corresponds to 60% to 80% of maximal oxygen consumption. HR_{max} is determined either by performance of a maximal exercise stress test or by calculation based on age ($HR_{max} = 220 - \text{age}$).
- An alternative to using a percentage of HR_{max} as the training intensity is to use a percentage

FIGURE 6-3. Maximal heart rates and training zones, using a lower level of 70% and an upper level of 85% of maximal heart rate, according to age.

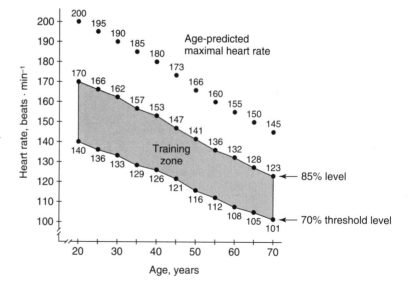

of the heart rate reserve, which takes into account the resting HR, and adds this to the resting HR. This calculation is called Karvonen's formula and is shown in Figure 6–2. Using this method, the training HR percentage range for the same oxygen consumptions mentioned above is 60% to 75%.

- Using either of these two methods, a training HR zone is defined within which the intensity of exercise is adequate to achieve a training effect. A chart showing training HR zones based on age is found in Figure 6–3. Using the lowest percentage classically associated with physiologic training (i.e., 70% of HR_{max} or 60% of HR reserve), the exercise intensity is moderate and can be sustained by most healthy individuals for a long time with little or no discomfort. Conversely, the top of the training zone results in exercise that is much more vigorous and difficult for most sedentary individuals to sustain for any period of time.

  - For healthy, sedentary individuals, the optimal training HR usually falls within this zone and is determined partly by the individual's genetics and partly by the individual's level of fitness. The lower the fitness level is, the lower will be the training HR.

  - For patients with chronic diseases and those on medications that affect HR, use of one of these formulas to determine training intensity is inappropriate, unless it is based on the results of a maximal symptom-limited exercise test performed with the patients taking their current medications. A training program based on an age-predicted maximal HR would be excessively intense for these individuals, and they would be unlikely to comply with it.

- A practical alternative is to define the intensity by using the rating of perceived exertion (RPE) scale, according to the procedures described for the endurance evaluation (see page 170). Because RPE is a valid and reliable indicator of the level of physical exertion during steady-state exercise, it is an effective means of monitoring exercise intensity during endurance training.[4] Using the 15-point scale (ranging from 6 to 20), a rating of 12 to 13 corresponds to approximately 60% of the HR range, whereas a rating of 16 corresponds to approximately 85%; thus, most individuals will exercise within the range of 12 to 16, or "somewhat hard" to "hard" (or 4 to 6 on the 10-point scale).

- Another method of prescribing exercise intensity is by using metabolic equivalents of energy expenditure, or METs. One MET is the amount of energy the body uses per kilogram of body weight per minute at rest, or approximately 3.5 mL O_2/kg/min. The energy cost of different activities can be compared by determining how many METs they consume. For example, walking 2.0 miles per hour (mph) uses about twice as much energy as sitting rest, or 2 METs, and walking 3.0 mph consumes about three times as much oxygen, or 3 METs.

  - To prescribe exercise using METs, the desired range of energy expenditure is determined (typically, 60% to 85% of maximal functional capacity) and stated in terms of METs, and activities that are known to require energy expenditures within the range are prescribed.

  - The energy cost of various recreational and household activities are listed in Table 6–2.

- Finally, the patient's goals for engaging in an endurance training program are taken into consideration when prescribing the intensity. For example, research has shown that lower intensity, longer duration exercise is more successful in promoting weight loss, control of hypertension, and relief of lower extremity claudication.[12,19,22,27] On the other hand, if the individual's goals include competition, exercise intensities in the higher range will be required.

PRINCIPLES OF TRAINING

Common to all the components of exercise training are some basic physiologic principles: the overload principle, specificity of training, individual variations in training responses, and the transient and reversible nature of training. Educating patients about these will promote better understanding of training and hopefully improve compliance.

OVERLOAD PRINCIPLE

This principle states that a physiologic overload must be applied to the body to attain a training

TABLE 6–2. **Energy Cost of Various Activities, Metabolic Equivalents of Energy Expenditure (METs)**

ACTIVITY	MEAN METS	RANGE	ACTIVITY	MEAN METS	RANGE
Back packing	–	5–11	Mountain climbing	–	5–10+
Badminton	5.8	4–9+	Music playing	–	2–3
Basketball			Paddleball, racquetball	9	8–12
Gameplay	8.3	7–12+	Running		
Nongame	–	3–9	12 min/mile	8.7	–
Bowling	–	2–4	10 min/mile	10.2	–
Canoeing, rowing, kayaking	–	3–8	8 min/mile	12.5	–
Calisthenic exercises	–	3–8+	6 min/mile	16.3	–
Climbing hills	7.2	5–10+	Sailing	–	2–5
Cycling			Self-care (washing, dressing, shaving, etc.)	–	2–4
Pleasure	–	3–8+			
10 mph	7.0	–	Shoveling snow	–	5–7
Dancing (social, square, tap)	–	3.7–7.4	Skating, ice and roller	–	5–8
Fishing			Skiing, snow		
From bank or boat	3.7	2–4	Downhill	–	5–8
Wading in stream	–	5–6	Cross-country	–	6–12+
Football (touch)	7.9	6–10	Skiing, water	–	5–7
Gardening (light to moderate)	–	4–6	Stairclimbing	–	4–8
Golf			Swimming	–	4–8+
Power cart	–	2–3	Table tennis	4.1	3–5
Walking (carrying bag or pulling cart)	5.1	4–7	Tennis	6.5	4–9+
			Volleyball	–	3–6
Handball	–	8–12+	Walking		
Hiking (cross-country)	–	3–7	2 mph	–	2
Housework			4 mph	–	4–6
Light to moderate	–	2–5			
Moderate to vigorous	–	4–8+			

effect. Overload can be achieved by manipulating the four components of the exercise prescription (frequency, duration, intensity, and mode) in such a way that the demands of the exercise are greater than normal.

SPECIFICITY OF TRAINING

Because different forms of exercise elicit different metabolic and physiologic adaptations within the systems of the body, this principle of exercise states that maximal aerobic fitness for any activity is accomplished only through overload involving the specific muscles engaged in the activity along with an exercise stress applied to the central cardiovascular system. For example, training for aerobic fitness in running is best achieved by performing running workouts, rather than bicycling or swimming workouts.

PRINCIPLE OF INDIVIDUAL DIFFERENCES

Because many factors influence how an individual responds to training, each person will accomplish the goal of exercise training in that person's own unique way, with individual differences in work rates and responses to specific training doses. Thus, this principle emphasizes the need to individualize each exercise prescription.

TRANSIENT AND REVERSIBLE NATURE OF TRAINING

Finally, when an individual stops exercising, detraining occurs very rapidly so that there are significant reductions in both metabolic and exercise capacity within 1 to 2 weeks. This principle acknowledges that even among highly trained athletes, the beneficial effects of exercise training are transient and reversible.

COMPLIANCE

One of the most difficult parts of an endurance training program is sticking with it. The typical dropout rate from supervised exercise programs is 50% at best and even lower for independent programs.[9] Strategies that increase the rate of compliance with exercise training include: identifying convenient times and locations, using cues and prompts to stimulate the desired behavior (e.g., exercise diary posted on the refrigerator), establishing short- and long-term goals, setting up behavioral contracts, maintaining a record of exercise performed, allowing rewards for reaching goals, and receiving positive reinforcement from others.[33] Another suggestion is to make exercising as social as possible; by involving friends or family members, it becomes more difficult to cancel planned workouts. Finally, one study has demonstrated higher compliance in obese and middle- to older-aged subjects who were given low-intensity exercise prescriptions rather than the standard intensity.[10]

6.2 ABNORMAL PHYSIOLOGIC RESPONSES TO EXERCISE

One difficulty that might be encountered in patients with cardiopulmonary dysfunction is abnormal physiologic responses to increasing activity. Common abnormalities include excessive increases in heart rate; hypertensive, blunted, or hypotensive blood pressure responses; increasing irregularity of the pulse or arrhythmias on electrocardiogram (ECG); excessive increases in respiratory rate; oxygenation desaturation; and other signs and symptoms of exercise intolerance, as discussed in Chapter 5 (see page 194).

- Whenever possible the cause of the abnormality should be identified and appropriate therapy instituted (e.g., drugs for arrhythmias, volume replacement for dehydration, supplemental oxygen for desaturation). Sometimes, the cause is simply deconditioning due to prolonged illness, with the usual tachycardia or orthostatic hypotension, and gradually increasing activity, including out of bed to chair and beginning ambulation, is indicated.

- For the physical therapist, the appropriate therapeutic intervention for this problem is continued clinical monitoring to allow as much activity as possible while still maintaining patient safety. The techniques for clinical monitoring are described in the previous chapter.

- It is also important to instruct the patient in self-monitoring of exercise intensity using pulse rate and rhythm, RPE, and/or symptoms. As both the therapist and the patient gain confidence in self-monitoring, the patient can progress to increasing levels of independence in the exercise program. Even patients who are in the high-risk group for morbidity and mortality following acute myocardial infarction and others who continue to exhibit abnormal responses to exercise should achieve independence in self-monitoring, since they are responsible for themselves during the remaining hours of the week when they are not in rehabilitation.

6.3 INABILITY TO MEET DEMANDS OF DAILY LIVING ACTIVITIES

Some patients with chronic diseases become so debilitated that they are unable to meet the physical demands of the various activities of daily living they are required to perform for independence. The options available to these patients consist of moving to an assisted living environment, such as a senior care facility or with a family member, receiving supplemental home care services within their current living situation, or learning techniques to reduce the demands of the activities they must perform, in addition to improving their ability to meet the demands of these activities through exercise training.

- Physical therapists play a key role in identifying this problem and the patient's level of need for assistance and initiating social service consultation for appropriate management.

- In addition, therapists are often involved in teaching patients energy conservation/work simplification techniques, which are summarized in Table 6–3.

TABLE 6–3. **Energy Conservation/Work Simplification Techniques**

1. Establish a Routine

Plan each day to include only what you can realistically accomplish.
Leave enough time for each task.
Allow a 30 to 60-min rest period after each meal and after any particularly strenuous activity (e.g., your exercise program, showering/bathing).
Do several different kinds of activity each day.
Include personal time for hobbies, going outside, reading, or other relaxing pursuits, as well as exercise time and time for daily tasks.

2. Pace Yourself

Allow ample time to complete each task.
Take your time with tasks and rest before you become really tired.
Alter your pace depending on the task, temperature, and time of day.
Work to music with a slower beat.

3. Sit Whenever Possible

Facing the task, sit in a chair or stool large enough to support your weight evenly, support your lower back, and allow placement of your feet flat on the floor.
Upper extremities should be supported.

4. Eliminate Unnecessary Tasks

Plan ahead and assemble all supplies for a task to minimize extra trips.
Use paper plates and cups when you want to save time and energy.
Straighten covers while still in bed to make bed making easier.
Let dishes air dry.
Cut hair short and get a permanent wave.
Delegate tasks to others when necessary.

5. Avoid Strenuous Arm Activities

Avoid straining or vigorous activities using arm motions: vacuuming, scrubbing, heavy carpentry, washing walls or windows, heavy gardening, painting walls, digging, etc.
Pace yourself during other arm activities, such as setting hair or strenuous clapping after a performance.
Seek consultation from an occupational therapist regarding adaptations to reduce the cost of favorite activites requiring arm work.

6. Keep Cool

Do more physically stressful activities during the cooler part of the day or evening.
Do your exercise program in a comfortable environment (e.g., an air conditioned mall or church hall).
Avoid excessively hot baths, showers, jacuzzis.
Make slow transitions with temperatures, such as moving from an air-conditioned building to the hot, humid outdoors, or diving into cool water on a hot day.

Data from Foderaro D: Energy Conservation and Work Simplification Techniques. Occupational Therapy Dept., Santa Clara Valley Medical Center, San Jose, Calif.

TABLE 6–3. Energy Conservation/Work Simplification Techniques *Continued*

7. Watch What You Eat

Avoid stimulants (e.g., caffeine, nicotine, over-the-counter drugs).
Watch the sodium content in foods, over-the-counter drugs, etc.

8. Increase Your Activity Level Gradually

Start easy, with low-level activities at first, taking frequent rest breaks as needed.
As you continue to feel better, add a little more each day.
Include one or two new activities per day.
Gradually increase the duration of your activity periods and shorten your rest periods.

9. Avoid Lifting

Avoid lifting chairs or other furniture, heavy grocery bags or laundry baskets, children, the corner of a mattress when making beds, etc.
Transport items on a wheeled cart if possible.
Divide groceries and laundry into small, easily handled parcels.

10. Organize Your Work Areas

Keep items that are used most often within easy reach.
Store items where they are used most. This does not mean cleaning out all of your drawers and closets; it usually means clearing out one or two easily accessible drawers or cabinets and moving a few frequently used items.

11. Avoid Isometric Contractions

Avoid pushing, pulling, or lifting heavy items.
Avoid breath holding during dressing or other activities requiring concentration.
Avoid the Valsalva maneuver.

12. Use Assistive Devices

Use a shower chair.
Use long-handled lower extremity bathing and dressing aids.
Use long-handled tools to avoid bending and reaching (e.g., reacher, long-handled dust pan, long-handled sponge).

13. Adjust Work Heights

The best work height for a table top is about two inches below your bent elbow

14. Avoid Sustained Positions

Change your posture, work height, and placement of objects used in an activity so you are not required to maintain any one position for a prolonged period of time.
Otherwise, take frequent short rest periods to ease the stress on your body.

When these individuals are hospitalized or otherwise referred for rehabilitation, their impaired activity tolerance may interfere with the physical therapy treatment plan. However, treatment modifications can usually permit effective participation (Table 6–4).

6.4 ELEVATED CORONARY RISK

Identifying the presence of coronary risk factors and providing guidance regarding their modification are appropriate roles for physical therapists, especially those who practice through direct access. Table 6–5 lists the major coronary risk factors and some physical therapy interventions designed to reduce them.

6.5 IMPAIRED VENTILATION AND OXYGENATION

Impaired ventilation, or hypoventilation, is manifested by elevated arterial carbon dioxide tension ($PaCO_2$ or PCO_2) with low arterial oxygen tension (PaO_2 or PO_2). The causes include respiratory muscle weakness, paralysis, or incoordination, reduced respiratory muscle endurance, restricted lung and/or thoracic compliance, retained secretions, and increased dead space ventilation. The physical therapy treatment of impaired ventilation and oxygenation varies with the cause, although there is quite a lot of overlap. Techniques to improve respiratory muscle strength and endurance, improve thoracic mobility, and reduce dead space ventilation are presented in this section. Refer to Section 6.6 for techniques to treat impaired secretion clearance.

AEROBIC EXERCISE

Any form of aerobic exercise of moderate to high intensity serves as a stimulus to increase respiratory muscle strength and endurance. Thus, the endurance training program prescribed to increase fitness level should also help improve respiratory muscle function.

VENTILATORY MUSCLE TRAINING

In addition, ventilatory muscle training using a resistive breathing device is specifically designed to improve respiratory muscle function. Several such devices, consisting of a mouthpiece and a chamber with adjustable resistance settings (progressively narrower airways), are commercially available (Fig. 6–4).

- Typically, patients begin using the device at a resistance of approximately 25% to 35% of the maximal negative inspiratory pressure measured at functional residual volume (or at an arbitrarily chosen low resistance that does not cause dyspnea, fatigue, or oxygen desaturation) for a duration of 15 to 30 minutes and a frequency of twice a day. When the patient can comfortably complete two 15- to 30-minute sessions a day at a particular setting, the resistance is increased to the next higher setting.
- Most of the research involving ventilatory muscle training has involved patients with chronic obstructive pulmonary disease (COPD) or quadriplegia. Improvements in ventilatory muscle function have been demonstrated; however, generalization to improved exercise tolerance, decreased dyspnea, and improved maximal

TABLE 6–4. Physical Therapy Treatment Modifications for Patients with Limited Tolerance

1. Avoid scheduling therapy sessions within an hour after meals so the demands of rehabilitation will not be superimposed on the extra work of digestion.
2. Schedule appointments so the patient has some rest time between the different rehabilitation services appointments.
3. Interject frequent brief rests while performing more strenuous rehabilitation activities, such as those involving the upper extremities, especially above shoulder level, and those performed in the quadruped position.
4. Monitor the patient's physiologic responses to activity to determine which activities cause problems and what modifications are effective in ameliorating them.
5. Use the rating of perceived exertion scale (see page 172) along with the patient's signs and symptoms to monitor exercise intensity and rate of progression.
6. Encourage coordination of breathing with activity to avoid the deleterious effects of breath holding and the Valsalva maneuver.

TABLE 6-5. **Physical Therapy Interventions for Modifying Major Coronary Risk Factors**

CORONARY RISK FACTOR	PHYSICAL THERAPY INTERVENTIONS
Hypertension	Encourage adherence to prescribed treatment.
	Inform physician if adequate blood pressure control is not maintained during rehabilitation activities (so medications can be adjusted).
	Educate patient regarding benefits of endurance training and provide appropriate exercise prescription.
	Monitor progress with exercise program and provide positive encouragement and feedback.
Cigarette smoking	Encourage smoking cessation and offer information regarding successful programs.
	Recommend exercise as a diversional activity for dealing with the urge to reach for a cigarette.
	Prescribe an endurance exercise program to counter weight gain.
↓HDL cholesterol	Prescribe appropriate endurance training program.
↑LDL cholesterol	Prescribe appropriate endurance training program.
	Encourage low-cholesterol, low-fat diet.
Diabetes mellitus or glucose intolerance	Encourage compliance with prescribed treatment.
	Educate regarding benefits of endurance training and provide appropriate exercise prescription.
Sedentary lifestyle	Prescribe appropriate endurance exercise program.
Stress	Instruct in relaxation exercises, offer biofeedback.
	Prescribe regular endurance exercise.
Obesity	Prescribe appropriate endurance exercise program.
	Encourage low-cholesterol, low-fat, high-fiber diet.

↓ = increased, ↑ = decreased, HDL = high-density lipoprotein, LDL = low-density lipoprotein.

work capacity has not been substantiated.[8,18,25] The role of ventilatory muscle training in the management of patients with other forms of restrictive lung dysfunction has not been defined and is an area worth further study.

Many patients also benefit from nocturnal ventilatory assistance, such as continuous positive airway pressure (CPAP), which allows the respiratory muscles to rest and avoid inefficient function due to fatigue.[1]

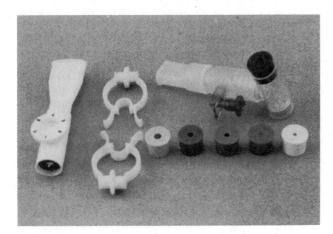

FIGURE 6-4. Two hand-held resistive breathing training devices: on the left, a P-flex, in which resistance is increased by changing to a higher number setting, and on the right, a DHD device, which uses stoppers with different size orifices inserted into its inspiratory port to change resistance. (From Frownfelter DL: *Chest Physical Therapy and Pulmonary Rehabilitation—An Interdisciplinary Approach,* 2nd Ed. Chicago, Year Book Medical Publishers, Inc., p. 228, 1987. Used with permission.)

Diaphragmatic Breathing Exercises

Diaphragmatic breathing exercises are traditionally performed to increase ventilation and improve oxygenation and thus alleviate dyspnea, reduce the work of breathing, and reduce the incidence of postoperative pulmonary complications. Yet, there is some controversy as to whether teaching diaphragmatic breathing exercises actually achieves any of these goals. However, as research continues, it seems prudent to continue with this treatment technique.

- The techniques for teaching diaphragmatic breathing exercises are as follows:
  - Have the patient assume a comfortable position, usually sitting supported, semifowler, or supine with the hips and knees flexed to relax the abdominal muscles.
  - Explain the purpose and goals of the exercise and then explain and demonstrate the desired result.
  - Place one hand on the patient's epigastric area while asking the patient to breathe slowly and comfortably; follow the patient's breathing with the hand.
  - After following several respiratory cycles, as the patient completes an exhalation, apply a firm counterpressure and ask the patient to "fill my hand with air" (the stretch caused by the counterpressure will facilitate the muscular response while the verbal command readies the patient for action) and notice the expansion under your hand; then instruct the patient to exhale normally.
  - Continue practicing the exercise until the patient can perform it correctly without manual stretch assistance.
  - Then, have the patient place his/her own hand on the epigastric area and repeat the same procedure while following the verbal cues from the therapist. Sometimes it helps to have the patient put the other hand on the sternum; instruct the patient to keep that motion to a minimum as the patient fills the first hand with air.
  - Continue practicing until the patient can perform the exercise without verbal cues.
- In breathing retraining, diaphragmatic breathing exercises can be progressed to higher levels of difficulty by having the patient perform the exercise while sitting unsupported, standing, and then walking, with cues initially and then sequentially removing the various cues.

Diaphragm Strengthening

For patients with less than normal diaphragmatic strength (determined by applying maximal manual resistance over the epigastric area during inspiration), diaphragmatic strengthening exercises may be indicated. As with all skeletal muscle, initial muscle strength determines the technique used for strengthening.

- Progressive resistive exercise can be used for greater than fair diaphragm strength. Resistance can be applied using weights, manual pressure, positioning, or incentive spirometry.
  - Weights are applied over the epigastric area with the patient in the supine position, thus providing resistance to diaphragmatic descent. The proper starting weight should permit full diaphragmatic excursion (i.e., full epigastric rise) using a coordinated, unaltered breathing pattern (no signs of accessory muscle contraction) for 15 minutes. As strength improves, additional weight can be added (exercising caution to avoid them toppling off the patient's abdomen at peak inspiration) until the patient demonstrates normal strength.
  - As an alternative, progressively increasing manual resistance can be applied in a similar manner.
  - Positioning uses the force of the abdominal contents to resist diaphragmatic contraction. This is accomplished by placing the patient in a gentle Trendelenburg position (a 15-degree head down tilt results in approximately 10 pounds of force against the diaphragm) and having the patient perform several series of three to five slow sustained deep diaphragmatic breaths with interposed rest periods.
- When diaphragm strength is fair or less (manifested as just normal or less than normal diaphragmatic excursion, or epigastric rise, in the supine position), care must be taken not to overstress the diaphragm so fatigue devel-

ops, since the diaphragm must continue to function throughout the day. Therefore, ventilatory muscle training devices (already described) or incentive spirometers are often used as described below.

- With the head of the bed raised 10 to 15 degrees to relieve the resistance applied by the abdominal contents, the patient is placed in the supine position and instructed to take four slow, easy breaths with normal exhalations in between.
- After the fourth inspiration, the patient exhales slowly but completely, places the mouthpiece in the mouth, forming a tight seal with the lips, and then performs a slow, deep diaphragmatic breath to elicit the visual cues of the apparatus (e.g., balls rising, lights flashing, etc.).
- The inspiration is sustained as long as possible (to allow collateral ventilation of the alveoli) before the mouthpiece is removed and the patient relaxes.
- This procedure is typically performed 10 times every hour while awake.
- For patients with "poor" diaphragm strength, breathing is usually most comfortable when the patient is in the resting supine position, since the diaphragm is unable to displace the abdominal contents but needs the mechanical advantage of the intestines holding it up in a more normal resting position. In addition, both the diaphragm and the accessory muscles are in a gravity-eliminated position in the supine position. In contrast, when the patient is in the upright position, as in sitting,

the abdominal contents shift inferiorly (and anteriorly if abdominal muscles are weak), pulling the diaphragm into a more horizontal position, where mechanical function is at an extreme disadvantage. In fact, in quadriplegics lower chest expansion can actually become negative (as demonstrated by a decreased circumference of $\frac{1}{2}$ to 1 inch measured at the xiphoid process) during inspiration.[37] Therefore, the use of an abdominal corset is recommended in patients with weak abdominal muscles to support the intestines and maintain the diaphragm in a better position, as illustrated in Figure 6–5. In patients with completely flaccid abdominal muscles, a body jacket, which provides rigid trunk support and has an anterior abdominal cutout for better diaphragmatic movement, often provides better postural and respiratory function.

THORACIC MOBILITY EXERCISES

Any exercise that affects the shoulders or trunk will help mobilize the chest. In addition, patients can be instructed in specific breathing exercises to increase chest expansion, segmentally and regionally. Finally, manual stretching and facilitation techniques can also be employed.

- A variety of *total body motions* can be used to increase chest mobility:
  - While sitting in a chair, the patient exhales while bending forward to touch the floor with the arms crossing at the feet. Then the patient extends up while taking a deep in-

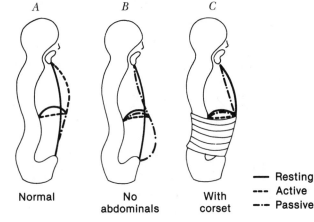

A   B   C

Normal   No abdominals   With corset

— Resting
--- Active
-·- Passive

FIGURE 6–5. The advantage of an abdominal corset in patients with poor abdominal strength. *(A),* Normal diaphragm position. *(B),* Weak abdominal muscles allow gravity to pull the diaphragm into a horizontal position. *(C),* Corset application supports optimal diaphragm positioning. (From Alvarez SE, et al.: Respiratory treatment of the adult patient with spinal cord injury. *Phys. Ther.* 61:1737–1745, 1980. Reprinted from *Physical Therapy* with the permission of the American Physical Therapy Association.)

spiration and lifts the arms up and out into a V above the head.

- While sitting in a chair with the right hand holding the left wrist, the patient exhales while bending and rotates to touch the floor lateral to the right ankle with the left hand. The patient then inspires while extending upward and rotates the left arm and hand up over the head and away from the left side. The procedure is then reversed to do the other side. As an alternative, this exercise can be performed with a cane or wand.

- With the patient lying in the supine position and the hips and knees flexed, the patient can perform modified sit-ups, or pelvic tilt with head lift, to strengthen the abdominal muscles. To add more thoracic mobility, the patient may stretch both arms overhead on inspiration and then reach past the knees on exhalation; or the patient may stretch the right hand up over the head and out to the right (160 degrees of abduction) during inspiration, then exhale while bringing the extended arm over and across the body, lifting the shoulders and head to reach past the left hip. If the patient needs more than one breath to complete the move, he can take an extra breath at the completion of each arc. He should rest for a few breaths before repeating the move with the opposite side.

- On hands and knees, the patient can rock forward during inspiration and then backward to heel-sitting with chin tucked during expiration. This move should be slow, relaxed, and rhythmic, pausing in the heel-sitting position for an additional breath or two. Repeat. As a variation, starting from the heel-sitting position, rock forward during inspiration, drop one elbow in to touch the floor on expiration, push back onto hands and knees on inspiration, and rock back to heel sitting on expiration.

- Standing with hands on a wall at shoulder height, the patient performs a modified pushup, exhales while bending the elbows, lowers the body to the wall, inhales while pushing away from the wall, returns to a standing position, and extends the arms. As strength improves, difficulty can be increased by having the patient use a high counter or sink instead of the wall. Careful

monitoring to ensure avoidance of the Valsalva maneuver is important.

- In addition, *exercises involving the shoulders and trunk* will mobilize the chest:
  - Sitting with arms extended at the sides, the patient inspires while flexing both arms up and over the head and expires while returning them to the sides (can also be done with a cane or wand).
  - Sitting with arms extended at the sides, the patient inhales while abducting both arms up and over the head and exhales while returning them to the sides.
  - Sitting with hands holding opposite forearms and resting on top of the head, the patient rotates the trunk to look past the right elbow, holds the position while taking two slow deep breaths, then repeats to the opposite side (can also be done with a cane or wand held overhead).
  - Sitting in a chair with arms at the sides, the patient abducts one arm out and over the head during inspiration, then continues the motion into a side bend towards the opposite side during expiration; the patient inhales while returning to an upright position and exhales while returning the arm to the side. Repeat on other side.
  - Sitting in a chair with hands behind the head, the patient inhales while extending up as tall as possible, then exhales while flexing forward, and brings the elbows toward each other in front.
  - Sitting in a chair, the patient inhales while lifting the hands up in front and toward the ceiling, exhales while reaching way behind the head leading with bent elbows, and lowers the hands behind the body.
  - In patients with neurologic deficits, proprioceptive neuromuscular facilitation (PNF) patterns involving the upper extremities and trunk coordinated with inspiration and expiration serve the same purpose.

- *Segmental, or localized, breathing exercises* use manual counterpressure as proprioceptive input to encourage expansion of specific parts of the chest. Hand placements (unilateral or bilateral) commonly used by therapists consist of the subclavicular areas for the upper lobes, anterior midchest for the right middle lobe and lingula, anterior lower ribs for the anterior basal segments of the lower lobes, lower lateral costal area for the lateral basal segments of the lower lobes, posterior lower chest for the posterior basal segments of the lower lobes, and posterior midchest (with scapulae abducted) for the superior segments of the lower lobes.

- After identifying the area of treatment, the therapist's hand(s) are placed on the appropriate part of the patient's chest, applying firm pressure at the end of expiration.
- The therapist then instructs the patient to take a slow, deep breath in through the nose right into the therapist's hand(s) while the therapist applies gradually diminishing resistance.
- Maximal inspiration is sustained for 2 to 3 seconds; then the patient exhales, which is sometimes assisted by the therapist's hand pressure.
- In addition, *PNF techniques* can be added:[28]
  - At the end of a deep inspiration, repeated stretches are applied as the patient is asked to breathe more, more, more (as in "ah-ah-ah-ah-choo!") in order to increase chest expansion.
  - Just before expansion, the patient is instructed to take a deep breath and a quick stretch is applied in order to increase the force of muscle contraction.
  - It is recommended that the therapist's hands be placed so the fingers are aligned with the contracting muscle fibers.
- In patients with poor intercostal strength, *manual chest stretching* can be used to maintain or increase chest wall mobility. It is applied segmentally to the lower, middle, and upper thoracic areas.[37]
  - With the patient in the supine position, the therapist places one hand under the patient's ribs with the fingers on the transverse processes of the spine and the other hand on the top of the patient's chest with the heel of the hand near the sternum.
  - The therapist then brings his/her hands together in a wringing motion, creating a motion at the costal articulation.
  - The therapist progresses up the chest, alternating hands, and then treats the opposite side of the chest in a similar manner.

PURSED-LIP BREATHING

Another technique that may be effective in improving ventilation and oxygenation is pursed-lip breathing.

- Pursed-lip breathing is often used spontaneously in patients with chronic obstructive lung disease (COPD) to relieve dyspnea, but the technique may also be taught by the physical therapist, as shown in Figure 6–6.
  - After having the patient assume a comfortable position, the therapist describes and demonstrates the technique for pursed-lip breathing and explains its expected benefits.
  - With a hand on the patient's midabdominal muscles, the therapist instructs the patient to inhale slowly through the nose.
  - The patient is then told to let the air escape gently through the pursed lips without any use of the abdominal muscles.

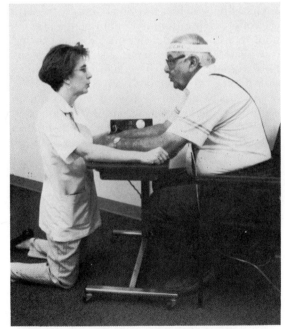

FIGURE 6–6. A physical therapist instructs a patient in the use of pursed-lip breathing and forward leaning posture in sitting to relieve dyspnea. (From Barr RN: Pulmonary rehabilitation. *In* Hillegass EA, Sadowsky HS: *Essentials of Cardiopulmonary Physical Therapy.* Philadelphia, W.B. Saunders Co., p. 684, 1994. Used with permission.)

- The patient is directed to stop exhaling when abdominal contraction is detected.
- When able to perform pursed-lip breathing without cues, the patient substitutes his/her own hand for the therapist's.
- Pursed-lip breathing has been shown to increase alveolar ventilation, increase oxygenation, and reduce the work of breathing and thus relieve dyspnea and increase exercise tolerance.[32] However, not all patients with airflow limitation show the same degree of benefit with this technique.
- In breathing retraining, pursed-lip breathing can be progressed in difficulty by eliminating the tactile feedback of the hand on the abdomen, advancing to standing, and finally proceeding to other activities.

POSITIONING

Changes in patient position can have a significant effect on arterial oxygenation in patients with lung disorders. Research involving both adults and neonates has documented the efficacy of prone positioning in improving oxygenation. In addition, sidelying on the side affected by unilateral lung disease is associated with significant decreases in oxygenation. In patients with disease affecting both lungs, left sidelying results in a greater drop in oxygen tension than right sidelying. Finally, patients who have undergone thoracotomy exhibit better oxygenation when lying on the unaffected side.

6.6 IMPAIRED SECRETION CLEARANCE

Secretion clearance can be a problem because of inadequate mucociliary function, impaired cough force, or excessive secretion production. Mucociliary transport can be impaired by cigarette smoking, anesthetics and analgesics, hypoxia or hypercapnia, dehydration, electrolyte imbalance, inhalation of dry gases, pollutants, and a cuffed endotracheal tube. Cough force can be affected by pain, weakness or incoordination of the ventilatory muscles, or structural abnormality. Excessive secretions are typically seen in chronic bronchitis, asthma, bronchiectasis, cystic fibrosis, and sometimes infection. A variety of physical therapy treatment techniques are available to improve secretion clearance.

BRONCHIAL DRAINAGE

Bronchial, or postural, drainage consists of positioning the patient according to bronchopulmonary anatomy so that a, or each, particular lung segment is placed with its bronchus perpendicular to gravity. The goal is to facilitate drainage of secretions into the segmental bronchus, from which they can be removed by coughing.

- The positions for bronchial drainage of the upper, middle, and lower lobes are illustrated in Figure 6–7 (for verbal description see page 214).
- There are some specific precautions and contraindications for bronchial drainage:
  - The Trendelenburg, or head-down, position is contraindicated in patients with pulmonary edema, increased intracranial pressure, unstable cardiovascular system, aortic aneurysm, recent esophageal anastamosis, untreated pneumothorax, poor diaphragmatic strength, hemoptysis, large pleural effusion, massive obesity, or ascites and in any patient who becomes agitated or anxious during treatment. Often, these patients can be placed in modified positions with the bed flat or near flat.
  - Caution is also indicated when positioning patients who are recovering from orthopedic surgery, such as total hip replacement or laminectomy, where certain movements or positions are to be avoided.
- The procedures involved in positioning patients for bronchial drainage include the following:
  - Explain the treatment to the patient and ask the patient to loosen any tight or binding clothing.
  - Observe any tubes or other equipment connected to the patient, making sure everything has enough slack to allow the position change without pulling taut or dislodging. Make any required adjustments.
  - Check the pulse, blood pressure, and oxygen saturation, if available, prior to positioning any patient who is critically ill or possibly unstable; monitor the patient during treatment.
  - For patients with large amounts of secretions, ask the patient to cough or perform suctioning prior to positioning.

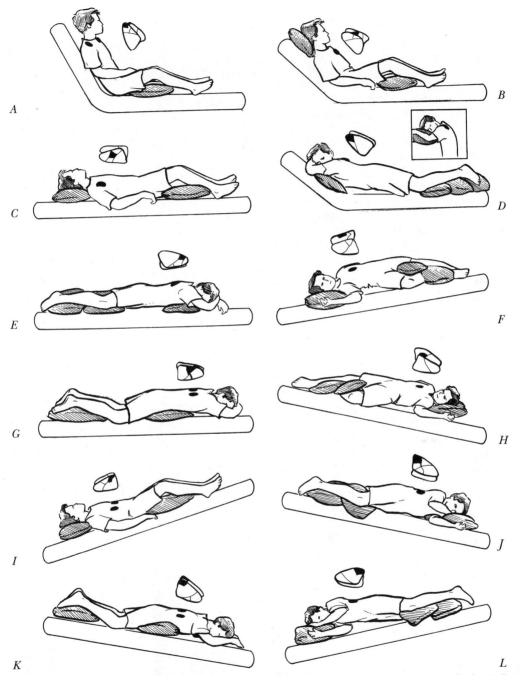

FIGURE 6–7. Bronchial drainage positions with treatment areas marked for percussion, if provided. *(A),* Both upper lobes, apical segments. *(B),* Left upper lobe, anterior segment. *(C),* Right upper lobe, anterior segment. *(D),* Left upper lobe, posterior segment, sitting or prone. *(E),* Right upper lobe, posterior segment. *(F),* Left upper lobe lingula. *(G),* Both lower lobes, superior segments (apical). *(H),* Right middle lobe. *(I),* Both lower lobes, anterior segments. *(J),* Right lower lobe, lateral segment. *(K),* Both lower lobes, posterior segments. *(L),* Left lower lobe, lateral segment (right lower lobe cardiac/medial).

- Place the patient in the proper, or modified, position, obtaining assistance from other staff, if necessary, and watch for any signs of intolerance.
- Maintain position for 5 to 20 minutes, depending on the quantity and tenacity of secretions and patient tolerance.
- Have the patient cough or perform suctioning before changing positions.
- If several positions are being used, it is best to limit total treatment time to 30 to 40 minutes because of the stress it places on the patient. Always treat the most critical areas first.
- Encourage the patient to cough periodically following treatment, as some secretions may take 30 to 60 minutes more to clear.
- Patients should never be left in head-down position unsupervised unless they are alert and able to reposition themselves.
- Manual techniques, such as percussion and vibration, are usually applied during bronchial drainage to augment the mobilization of secretions.

PERCUSSION

Percussion is a treatment technique which consists of rhythmically and alternately striking the chest wall over specific lung segments with cupped hands to mechanically jar and dislodge retained secretions (Fig. 6–8). The therapist molds her hand(s) to fit the contour of the area being treated and applies a force that is appropriate to the individual patient, depending on the patient's age and tolerance, condition of the chest, presence of pain, secretion density and amount, and anatomic site.

- Percussion is performed with the patient in the appropriate bronchial drainage position for each segment, although modified positions may be indicated, as stated under "Bronchial Drainage."
  - Upper lobes
    — Apical segments: the patient sits and leans back on pillows against a chair or the therapist at a 60-degree angle; percuss between the clavicle and the top of scapula on each side.
    — Posterior segment of left upper lobe: the patient leans forward over pillows or table at a 30-degree angle; percuss over the upper back on the left.
    — Anterior segment of left upper lobe: the patient lies on the back with the head elevated at a 30-degree angle; percuss between the clavicle and the nipple on the left side.
    — Anterior segment of right upper lobe: the patient lies flat on the back with the knees on a pillow; percuss between the clavicle and the nipple on the right side.
    — Posterior segment of right upper lobe: with the bed flat, the patient lies on the left side, then rolls the right shoulder 45 degrees forward with pillows placed for comfort; percuss over the upper back on the right side.
  - Right middle lobe and lingula
    — Right middle lobe: the patient lies on the left side with the head 15 degrees lower than the hips; then the patient rolls the right shoulder back 45 degrees onto a pillow; percuss over the right nipple area (or just above it on a female).

Figure 6–8. Chest percussion. Note cupped hands. (From Frownfelter DL: *Chest Physical Therapy and Pulmonary Rehabilitation—An Interdisciplinary Approach,* 2nd Ed. Chicago, Year Book Medical Publishers, Inc., p. 289, 1987. Used with permission.)

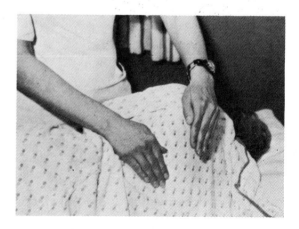

— Lingular segment of left upper lobe: the patient lies on the right side with the head 15 degrees lower than the hips; then the patient rolls the left shoulder back 45 degrees onto a pillow; percuss over the left nipple area (or just above it on a female).
- Lower lobes
  — Superior, or apical, segments: the patient lies in a prone flat position with pillow under the hips and ankles for comfort; percuss over midback just below scapula on each side.
  — Anterior segments: the patient lies in a supine position with the head 30 degrees lower than the hips; percuss over the lower ribs of each side.
  — Lateral segment of right lower lobe: the patient lies on the left side with a pillow between the knees for comfort and the head 30 degrees lower than the hips; percuss over the upper portion of lower ribs on the right side.
  — Posterior segments: the patient lies in a prone position with a pillow under the hips and ankles for comfort and the head 30 degrees lower than the hips; percuss over the lower ribs on each side.
  — Lateral segment of left lower lobe: the patient lies on the right side with a pillow between the knees for comfort and the head 30 degrees lower than the hips; percuss over the upper portion of the lower ribs on the left side.
- The force is adjusted according to patient tolerance and should not be uncomfortable, for it is not the force but the cupping that is effective.
- Percussion can be performed over a layer of thin cloth, such as a hospital gown.
- It should be continued for 2 to 5 minutes per lung segment, then followed with vibration and coughing or suctioning. When chest radiography or clinical assessment reveals a new atelectasis, treatment is continued with repeating cycles of percussion, vibration, and coughing/suction until resolution is clinically apparent and coughing/suction is no longer productive.
- Precautions and contraindications for percussion include:
  - Rib fractures or flail chest

- Low platelet count (20–40 K, varies according to physicians and facilities)
- Osteoporosis, prolonged steroid therapy, metastatic cancer to the ribs
- Unstable cardiovascular status
- Subcutaneous emphysema of the neck and thorax
- Recent spinal fusion
- Fresh burns, open wounds, skin infection in the thoracic area
- Untreated pneumothorax
- Resectable tumor
- Pulmonary embolism
- Anyone who does not tolerate the treatment
- Premedication for pain is important in postsurgical patients and others where ventilation and cough are limited by discomfort. Allow 20 to 30 minutes for analgesics to take effect before initiating treatment.
- For patients in whom percussion is contraindicated or who do not tolerate percussion, vibration can still be used effectively.

VIBRATION

Vibration consists of chest compression with manual vibration produced by tensing all muscles in the upper extremities in cocontraction. Performed during exhalation only, vibration aims at moving the mucous that was dislodged during percussion toward the larger airways.

- The therapist's hand placement for vibration can be on both sides of the patient's chest or one hand on top of the other, depending on therapist preference (Fig. 6–9).
- The patient is instructed to take a deep inspiration, and then chest compression with vibration are performed throughout exhalation for six to eight breaths. For patients with rapid respiratory rates, vibrations can be performed on every other breath, which may help reduce the breathing rate and allow better therapist coordination with exhalation.
- Patients unable to take a deep breath can be assisted with intermittent positive pressure breathing (IPPB) treatment or with a manual resuscitation bag.
- Caution is indicated in patients with a stiff, inelastic chest wall because of the risk of rib fracture with this technique.

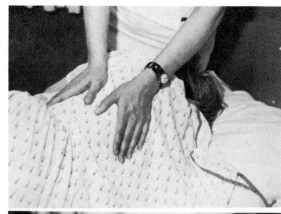

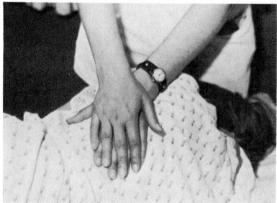

FIGURE 6–9. *(A),* Chest vibration with hands positioned on both sides of the chest. *(B),* Chest vibration with one hand placed on top of the other. (From Frownfelter DL: *Chest Physical Therapy and Pulmonary Rehabilitation—An Interdisciplinary Approach,* 2nd Ed. Chicago, Year Book Medical Publishers, Inc., p. 293, 1987. Used with permission.)

A

B

SHAKING AND RIB SPRINGING

Shaking is similar to vibration except that it consists of gentle thrusts in and out rather than vibrations with chest compression. Again, shaking is performed on exhalation only. A more vigorous form of shaking is termed rib springing, in which the ribs are "pumped" in a springing fashion three to four times during exhalation. Patients with rigid chest walls, osteoporosis or other bone abnormalities involving the chest, or pain should not be treated with rib springing. These techniques are claimed to achieve more rapid and efficient mobilization of secretions.

GLOSSOPHARYNGEAL BREATHING

Quadriplegics with high lesions are often instructed in glossopharyngeal breathing (GPB), a technique in which the patient swallows air into the lungs in order to increase vital ca-

pacity and thus can also be used to augment cough effectiveness.[28]

- The patient creates a pocket of negative pressure within the mouth by dropping the tongue to maximize the internal space while taking in a breath.
- The patient then closes off his lips and proceeds to force the air back and down his throat with a stroking maneuver of the tongue, pharynx, and larynx.

COUGHING

The cough serves as the primary means of clearing the first six to seven generations of airways of excess secretions and foreign material. Occurring either as a reflex or voluntarily, an effective cough consists of a deep inspiration, closure of the glottis with contraction of the abdominal muscles to increase intrathoracic and intraabdominal pressures, and opening of the glottis with expulsion of the trapped air by forceful abdominal contraction. Impairment of the cough mechanism can result from inadequate inspiratory volume, diminished expiratory force, or reduced maximal expiratory flow rates. Common causes of ineffective cough include weakness, paralysis, or incoordination of the ventilatory muscles, pain, COPD, and depression of the central nervous system. The result is retained secretions and bronchial obstruction.

- Different cough techniques are described in Table 6–6. Surgical patients should first be taught how to splint their incision prior to coughing.
- Most patients will cough better when sitting and possibly leaning forward slightly, although those with sternotomy incisions often do well with a high sidelying position because of the chest stabilization provided. Quadriplegics usually cough better with the head of the bed flat and often in a sidelying position.
- If secretions are extremely thick, extra hydration is indicated; if fluid intake is not restricted, the patient should be encouraged to drink more water during the day, or ultrasonic nebulizer or aerosol treatments can help thin the secretions.
- If inspiration is inadequate, the patient can be taught diaphragmatic or lateral costal breath-

ing. If pain is the limiting factor, regular doses of pain medication should be encouraged. If muscle strength is limited, patients can be assisted with IPPB treatment or with a manual resuscitation bag. Quadriplegics can use glossopharyngeal breathing (see page 216) to increase vital capacity and thus increase cough effectiveness.

ASSISTIVE COUGH TECHNIQUES

If expiratory muscles are weak, paralyzed, or subject to increased tone, the following assisted cough techniques can be used.[28]

Costophrenic Assist

- The costophrenic assist can be used in both the supine and sidelying positions.
- With the patient in the supine position, the therapist places the hands on the costophrenic angles of the patient's rib cage and at the end of expiration applies a quick stretch down and in on the patient's lower chest (to facilitate a stronger diaphragmatic and intercostal muscle contraction).
  - During the patient's inspiration, the therapist applies a series of three PNF repeated contractions, down and in (to encourage maximal inspiration), and the patient is asked to hold the deep inspiration.
  - While instructing the patient to cough, the

TABLE 6–6. **Various Cough Techniques**

COUGH TECHNIQUE	DESCRIPTION
Double cough	Following a deep inspiration, the patient performs two coughs in one breath; the second is usually more forceful than the first.
Controlled cough	The patient takes three deep breaths, exhaling normally after the first two and then coughing firmly on the third; the first two breaths are believed to decrease atelectasis and increase the volume of the cough.
Series of three coughs	The patient takes a small breath and gives a fair cough, then a bigger breath and gives a harder cough, and finally a really deep breath and gives a forceful cough; this technique allows patients to work their way up to a forceful cough.
Huffing	The patient takes a deep inspiration and then air is forcefully exhaled as in coughing except that the mouth is kept open (less stressful on the patient and more effective than constant forced coughing, especially in patients who tend to prolong the expiratory phase of a cough almost into a wheeze, such as asthmatics and others with COPD).
Pump coughing	The patient takes a deep breath and then gives three short easy coughs followed by three huffs (facilitates secretion clearance in patients with air trapping).

COPD = chronic obstructive pulmonary disease.

therapist applies strong pressure through the hands, up and in toward the central tendon of the patient's diaphragm.

- When the patient is in the sidelying position, the technique is performed as above except it is performed unilaterally on the upper side only, producing an asymmetric cough caused by the assistance primarily of the lung segments of the upper side.

Heimlich-Type Assist

The Heimlich-type assist can be used in both the supine and sidelying positions.

- With the patient in the supine position, the therapist places the heel of one hand just inferior to the patient's xiphoid process and below the patient's lower ribs.
  - The patient is instructed to take in a deep breath and hold it. Then just as the patient is instructed to cough, the therapist applies a quick push up and in under the diaphragm with the heel of the hand.
  - Patients with low neuromuscular tone or flaccid abdominal muscles tolerate this procedure the best.
- With the patient in the sidelying position, this technique is performed exactly as described above, with much fewer problems in patients with increased neuromuscular tone.

Combination of Heimlich-Type Assist and Costophrenic Assist

The technique can be used only when the patient is in the sidelying position.

- The therapist uses one hand to assist lateral compression of the chest (costophrenic assist), while the other hand performs a Heimlich-type assist, pushing up and in.
- Because it uses more planes of respiration, the combined technique is more effective at clearing secretions than either technique used alone.

Anterior Chest Compression Assist

This technique can be used only when the patient is in the supine position.

- The therapist puts one arm across the patient's pectoralis region to stabilize or compress the upper chest while the other arm is placed either parallel on the lower chest or,

like in the Heimlich-type technique, under the xiphoid process.
- Just as the patient is instructed to cough, the therapist applies a quick push up and in.

Massery Counterrotation Assist

The Massery counterrotation assist is performed in patients with spinal stability in the sidelying position with the patient's knees bent and arms out in front of the head or shoulders.

- The therapist works in a diagonal pattern (essential), placing the same hand as the side the patient is lying on on the patient's upper pectoralis region and the heel of the other hand firmly in the patient's upper gluteal fossa (compression/flexion position).
- After following the patient's breathing cycle and then applying an end-expiratory quick manual stretch on the diagonal (the hand over the pectoralis pulls the upper chest down and back diagonally while the other hand pushes the lower chest up and forward diagonally) to maximize a few inhalations, the therapist shifts hands to the expansion/extension position (upper hand over the scapula and lower hand over the iliac crest) to physically assist the patient in chest expansion (thus maximizing inspiration).
- This procedure is repeated three to five times to achieve good ventilation of all lung segments.
- Finally, the cough assist is performed by first giving an accentuated end-expiratory quick compression of the chest (hands in flexion position), then shifting hands quickly to perform the extension move as the patient takes a deep breath, which is held briefly at maximum, and finally shifting hands quickly back to the flexion position to perform a quick and forceful chest compression as the patient gives a strong cough.
- This technique is extremely effective even in patients who are incoherent or unresponsive.

Head Flexion Assist

Performed with the patient prone on elbows, this technique produces a weaker cough due to inhibition of the diaphragm, but it is one that quadriplegics who have good head and neck control and can roll independently can perform alone.

- The patient learns to take a deep inspiration while extending the head and neck up and back as far as possible and then coughs forcefully while throwing the head forward and down.
- The pattern can be assisted initially by the therapist to establish the desired moves and gradually progressed to a resisted pattern to strengthen the accessory muscles.

Quad-Long-Sitting Self-Assist

The patient performs a self-assisted cough while positioned in a long-sitting posture with arm support. The patient extends the head and body backward while taking a maximal inspiration and then coughs forcefully while throwing the head and upper body forward into a flexed position.

Para-Long-Sitting Self-Assist

The para-long-sitting self-assist is similar to above, except that the patient's hands may be placed on the back of the head in a butterfly position and the patient throws the body forward onto the legs during the cough/flexion phase, thereby using both the upper and lower chest.

Short-Sitting Self-Assist

The patient is placed in a short-sitting position (e.g., in a wheelchair or at the side of the bed), with one wrist over the other in the lap; the patient extends the head and trunk backward while taking a deep breath and then flexes forward and pulls the hands up and under the diaphragm while coughing forcefully.

Rocking

On hands and knees, the patient rocks all the way forward while looking up and taking a deep breath, then coughs with a flexed head while rocking backward to the heels.

SUCTIONING

If a patient is unable to clear secretions by coughing, suctioning is indicated. Because it is an invasive procedure with significant risk, suctioning must be performed using very careful technique:

- Preparation
  - Check that the suction apparatus is functioning properly and is connected, the suc-

tion is turned on, and the vacuum level is set between -80 and -120 cm H_2O.
  - Make sure the oxygen flow is turned on and attached to the self-inflating breathing bag.
  - Position the patient properly unless contraindicated: nasotracheal and pharyngeal suctioning are usually performed with the patient in the semi-Fowler position with the patient's neck hyperextended, whereas patients with a tracheostomy or endotracheal tube are suctioned in the supine flat position.
  - Have water soluble lubricant available if the patient is to be suctioned nasotracheally. Put on protective eyewear.
  - Lay out the sterile field containing gloves, catheter, and container for sterile water.
  - Using sterile technique, put on gloves, fill container with sterile water, and attach catheter to suction; squeeze out lubricant onto sterile field, if needed.
- Preoxygenation
  Using a self-inflating breathing bag and a mask or artificial airway connector, hyperventilate the patient with 100% oxygen.
- Lavage (optional)
  Instill 5 mL of sterile normal saline solution (NaCl) directly into the endotracheal or tracheostomy tube.
- Suction
  Using sterile technique throughout:
  - Wet the catheter in the sterile solution, or with the water soluble lubricant if nasotracheal suction is to be performed.
  - Insert the catheter (with no suction applied) into the airway until resistance is met or until a reflex cough is triggered.
  - Pull the catheter back slightly and then withdraw the catheter in a twirling motion while applying suction (should not take longer than 5 to 10 seconds).
  - Reoxygenate the patient with 100% oxygen.
  - Clean secretions from catheter by suctioning some of the sterile water.
  - Repeat process if necessary until there are no more secretions.
  - Suction the nasal and/or oral pharynges.
- Some of the complications that can develop include significant hypoxemia, arrhythmias, hypotension, and tissue trauma; however, proper technique minimizes the risk of morbidity.

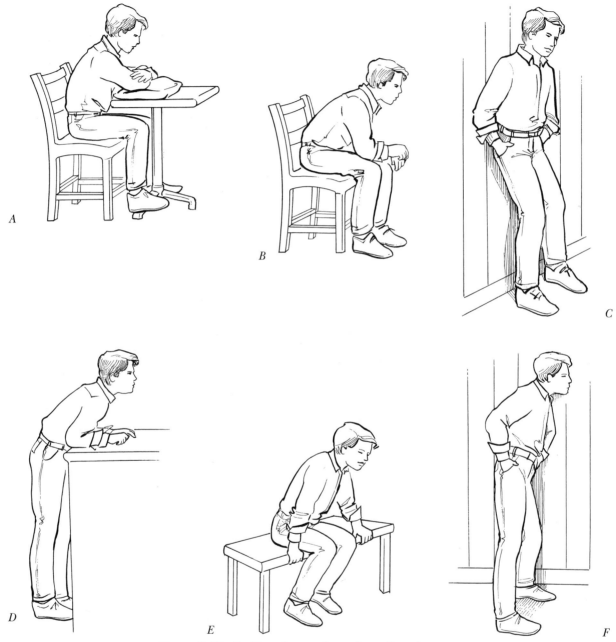

A

B

C

D

E

F

Figure 6-10. Positions frequently used to relieve dyspnea.

PROGRESSIVE ACTIVITY

One of the most effective means of improving secretion clearance is increasing activity. Frequent position changes in bed, sitting at the bedside, out of bed activities, and progressive ambulation serve to increase tidal volume and therefore assist in mobilizing secretions and improve cough force.

6.7 IMPAIRED ABILITY TO PROTECT AIRWAY

Patients with altered level of consciousness or bulbar muscle weakness or paralysis frequently develop pulmonary complications as a result of aspiration. In patients with a high risk of aspiration, bronchial hygiene techniques are often used prophylactically (see preceding section). In addition, patients can be placed on a swallowing program to teach them the proper swallowing mechanisms and thus improve cognition of the process and retrain the musculature. Patients with repeated episodes of aspiration pneumonia frequently require tracheostomy.

6.8 INCREASED WORK OF BREATHING

All the previously presented problems, as well as inefficient breathing patterns, serve to increase the work of breathing. The physical therapy techniques already described will succeed in reducing the work of breathing if they are effective in treating the causative problem(s). In addition, treatments to increase thoracic mobility will indirectly improve breathing mechanics. Other treatment options include instruction in controlling the breathing pattern (i.e., breathing retraining), dyspnea positioning, and relaxation techniques, as well as energy conservation/work simplification techniques (see Table 6-3).

BREATHING PATTERN CONTROL

During exertion or episodes of dyspnea, patients benefit from learning to maintain an uninterrupted breathing pattern through avoidance of breath holding, the Valsalva maneuver, or unnecessary talking.

Breathing retraining teaches patients specific breathing strategies (e.g., diaphragmatic breathing, pursed-lip breathing, see pages 208 and 211)

to reduce the work of breathing by slowing the respiratory rate or eliminating accessory muscle activity, especially during exertion, thus increasing the oxygen available to other tissues. However, this procedure is controversial, since it has been documented that patients with both obstructive and restrictive lung disease naturally assume a breathing pattern that requires the least energy and delays respiratory muscle fatigue.

POSITIONING TO RELIEVE DYSPNEA

Because patients with severe COPD often have flattened diaphragms and stiff, barrel-shaped chests and patients with severe restrictive lung dysfunction have reduced pulmonary compliance, use of the accessory muscles of inspiration (e.g., the sternocleidomastoid, levators, scalenes, pectoralis major) is a very important element in increasing thoracic dimension during inspiration. Therefore, when patients become dyspneic, positions that support the upper extremities are recommended to increase the mechanical efficiency of these muscles (by fixing their distal attachments) and thus reduce the cost of breathing (Fig. 6-10). In addition, leaning forward in the sitting position further assists the patient with COPD by increasing the intraabdominal pressure and pushing the diaphragm up into the thorax for a more optimal position for contraction. Positions that incorporate one or both of these strategies include:

- The professorial position in which the patient is sitting and leaning forward so that the elbows (or wrists) are supported by the knees
- Sitting and leaning forward with the elbows or upper body supported on a table
- Standing and leaning forward with the arms supported on a wall or other structure
- Leaning back against a wall or other structure with the spine straight and supported so that the neck and shoulders are relaxed and the hips are slightly flexed; in addition, hands can be placed in pockets or hooked into the waistband or belt loops to support the upper extremities

RELAXATION TECHNIQUES

Patients with severe lung disease tend to be anxious and tense, often worried about their next breath. Unfortunately, this tension compounds their respiratory problems by tightening the chest wall and spine. Several techniques are available that can help patients achieve a more relaxed state: Jacobsen's progressive relaxation, biofeedback, yoga, transcendental meditation, hypnosis, Benson's relaxation response, chest mobilization, and guided imagery or visualization. All include relaxed positioning in a quiet, comfortable atmosphere.

- Jacobsen's progressive relaxation exercises consist of sequentially tightening the various groups of muscles as strongly as possible and then completely relaxing them. In applying these techniques to pulmonary patients, attention is specifically focused on the upper chest, neck, shoulder, and abdominal muscles in order to improve ventilation.
- Autogenic training employs autosuggestion to achieve the relaxed state. The individual selects the preferred point of concentration for becoming relaxed:
  - Rhythm (e.g., breathing in ... out ... in ... out ...)
  - Sensation (e.g., relaxation, warmth, heaviness)
  - Imagery (e.g., imagining a favorite tranquil scene, such as the beach at sunset, and concentrating on being there; or imagining a peaceful descent, as on an escalator, from a place of high activity to one of quiet and rest)
- Biofeedback uses physiologic measurements to train voluntary control of autonomic responses, such as heart rate, blood pressure, and muscle tension. For pulmonary patients, the electrical activity of the muscles of the upper chest, neck, shoulders, and abdomen is selected in order to teach individuals to recognize their activity and gain control over them.
- Yoga is a form of exercise consisting of slow stretching and bending into different positions without strain or discomfort, and then holding that position for a period of time before releasing it as slowly as it was assumed. Breathing exercises are also included to increase the relaxation achieved.
- Transcendental meditation (TM) is an advanced form of autogenic relaxation, in which concentration on a specific word or phrase, called a mantra, is silently repeated to quiet

the body and still the mind. TM is usually performed for 15 to 20 minutes twice a day.
- Hypnosis involves the use of a somewhat altered level of consciousness to achieve a relaxed state. In addition, patients can be given suggestions that help them accomplish specific goals, such as smoking cessation.
- Benson's relaxation response is elicited using four important elements: a quiet environment, a mental device as a constant stimulus (e.g., a repeated word), a passive attitude, and decreased muscle tone related to a comfortable position that requires minimal work to maintain.
- Chest mobilization through rhythmic exercise involving the arms and trunk and the lower extremities can also serve to promote relaxation. Also, soft flowing music can be used to increase the sense of relaxation.
- Finally, guided imagery, or visualization, is a process that evokes mentally many senses to create detailed images, or daydreams, that assist an individual to relax. One of the more common images is walking to a beautiful, happy, and peaceful spot that becomes synonymous with a relaxing and rejuvenating escape, where all of an individual's worries and tensions are let go and the individual feels free.

6.9 SUMMARY

This chapter has presented the various techniques used to provide physical therapy treatment for patients with cardiopulmonary dysfunction. A problem-oriented approach was employed so that therapists can use at least some of the treatment techniques for any patient with one or more of the described problems, regardless of the referral diagnosis. Some are so simple that all the therapist needs is awareness of need (e.g., encouraging cough following changes of position and rehabilitation activities); others are routinely used by many therapists in all areas of practice (e.g., endurance exercise training). The most important points are reviewed below.

- Impaired exercise tolerance is a common problem of patients with a wide variety of chronic diseases. Therefore, endurance exer-

TABLE 6–7. Cardiovascular Effects of Endurance Training in Healthy Individuals and Cardiac Patients

VARIABLES	UNITS	CHANGES WITH ENDURANCE TRAINING	
		HEALTHY ADULTS	CARDIAC PATIENTS
Maximal values			
Oxygen uptake	mL · kg^{-1} · min^{-1}	Increase	Increase
Cardiac output	L/min	Increase	Unchanged*
Heart rate	Beats/min	Unchanged-decrease	Unchanged
Stroke volume	mL	Increase	Unchanged-increase*
Arteriovenous oxygen difference	m/100 mL blood	Increase	Increase
Systolic blood pressure	mm Hg	Unchanged	Unchanged?*
Rate-pressure product	Beats/min × mm Hg × 10^3	Unchanged	Unchanged?*
Endurance	sec	Increase†	Increase†
Ejection fraction	%	Increase‡	Unchanged-decrease*‡
Submaximal values§			
Oxygen uptake	mL · kg^{-1} · min^{-1}	Unchanged-decrease	Unchanged-decrease
Cardiac output	L/min	Unchanged-decrease	Unchanged
Heart rate	Beats/min	Decrease	Decrease
Stroke volume	mL	Increase	Increase
Systolic blood pressure	mm Hg	Decrease	Decrease
Rate-pressure product	Beats/min × mm Hg × 10^3	Decrease	Decrease
Resting values			
Oxygen uptake	mL · kg^{-1} · min^{-1}	Unchanged	Unchanged
Heart rate	Beats/min	Decrease	Decrease
Systolic blood pressure	mm Hg	Unchanged-decrease	Unchanged-decrease
Diastolic blood pressure	mm Hg	Unchanged-decrease	Unchanged-decrease
Rate-pressure product	Beats/min × mm Hg × 10^3	Decrease	Decrease

From Pollock ML, Wilmore JH: *Exercise in Health and Disease*, 2nd Ed. Philadelphia, W.B. Saunders Co., 1990. Used with permission.
*These values may increase in some patients with high-intensity training,
†The performance will improve, i.e., performance at a given distance will decrease, and performance time on a treadmill or cycle ergometer will increase.
‡Ejection fraction determined as a change from rest to exercise.
§Same absolute workload.

cise training becomes an important component of those patients' treatment programs because of its effectiveness in increasing exercise tolerance, improving respiratory muscle strength and endurance, and facilitating relaxation.

- In order to be effective, safe and enjoyable, careful attention must be directed toward creating an appropriate exercise prescription, including the proper mode(s), duration, frequency, and intensity.
- Initially, the individual's physiologic responses to exercise should be monitored, but the goal is for the individual to become independent in self-monitoring techniques. Rating of perceived exertion is a simple yet reliable means of monitoring exercise intensity and is effective for most individuals.
- The physiologic benefits of exercise training on healthy individuals and those with cardiac disease are listed in Table 6–7.
- Some individuals are so debilitated that it is difficult for them to perform the daily living activities required for independent living.
  - In addition to endurance exercise training, these individuals benefit from instruction in energy conservation and work simplification techniques, which may be provided by occupational or physical therapy.
  - For those who require rehabilitation, some physical therapy activities may be too demanding for their level of tolerance and therefore require modification. Recommended treatment modifications are listed in Table 6–4 (page 206).
- In addition, patients with pulmonary disease may require a number of other physical therapy treatment interventions to improve ventilation (e.g., breathing exercises, thoracic mobility exercises, ventilatory muscle training, bronchial hygiene techniques), oxygenation (e.g., those just listed plus pursed-lip breathing), secretion clearance (e.g., bronchial hygiene techniques: chest percussion, vibration, shaking, rib springing, coughing, suctioning), and reduce the work of breathing (e.g., breathing retraining, positioning, and relaxation techniques).

REFERENCES

1. Barr RN: Pulmonary rehabilitation. *In* Hillegass EA, Sadowsky HS: *Essentials of Cardiopulmonary Physical Therapy.* Philadelphia, W.B. Saunders Co., 1994.
2. Bellemare F, Grassino A: Force reserve of the diaphragm in patients with COPD. *J. Appl. Physiol.* 55:8–15, 1983.
3. Blair SN, Kohl HW, Paffenbarger RS, et al.: Physical fitness and all-cause mortality: A prospective study of healthy men and women. *JAMA* 262:2395–2401, 1989.
4. Borg GA: Psychophysical bases of perceived exertion. *Med. Sci. Sports Exer.* 14:377–387, 1982.
5. Bradley GW, Crawford R: Regulation of breathing during exercise in normal subjects and in chronic lung disease. *Clin. Sci. Mol. Med.* 51:575–582, 1976.
6. Cahalin LP: Cardiac muscle dysfunction. *In* Hillegass EA, Sadowsky HS (eds.): *Essentials of Cardiopulmonary Physical Therapy.* Philadelphia, W.B. Saunders Co., 1994.
7. Cahalin LP, Ice RG, Irwin S: Program planning and implementation. *In* Irwin S, Tecklin JS: *Cardiopulmonary Physical Therapy,* 2nd Ed. St. Louis, The C.V. Mosby Co., 1990.
8. Casciari RJ, Fairshter RD, Harrison A, et al.: Effects of breathing retraining in patients with chronic obstructive pulmonary disease. *Chest* 79:393–398, 1981.
9. Dishman RK (ed.): *Exercise Adherence: Its Impact on Public Health.* Champaign, Ill, Human Kinetics, 1988.
10. Dishman RK, Sallis JF, Orenstein D: The determinants of physical activity and exercise. *Public Health Rep.* 100:158–171, 1985.
11. Dodd DS, Brancatisano T, Engel LA: Chest wall mechanics in patients with severe chronic air flow obstruction. *Am. Rev. Respir. Dis.* 129:33–38, 1984.
12. Ersnt E, Matrai I: Intermittent claudication, exercise and blood rheology. *Circulation* 76:1110–1114, 1987.
13. Foderaro D: *Energy conservation and work simplification techniques.* Occupational Therapy Dept., Santa Clara Valley Medical Center, San Jose, Calif.
14. Frownfelter D: Breathing exercises and retraining, chest mobilization exercises. *In* Frownfelter DL: *Chest Physical Therapy and Pulmonary Rehabilitation—An Interdisciplinary Approach,* 2nd Ed. Chicago, Year Book Medical Publishers, Inc., 1987.
15. Frownfelter D: Cough. *In* Frownfelter DL: *Chest Physical Therapy and Pulmonary Rehabilitation—An Interdisciplinary Approach,* 2nd Ed. Chicago, Year Book Medical Publishers, Inc., 1987.

16. Frownfelter D: Postural drainage. *In* Frownfelter DL: *Chest Physical Therapy and Pulmonary Rehabilitation—An Interdisciplinary Approach,* 2nd Ed. Chicago, Year Book Medical Publishers, Inc., 1987.

17. Frownfelter D, Perlstein MF: Relaxation principles and techniques. *In* Frownfelter DL: *Chest Physical Therapy and Pulmonary Rehabilitation—An Interdisciplinary Approach,* 2nd Ed. Chicago, Year Book Medical Publishers, Inc., 1987.

18. Grassino A: A rationale for training respiratory muscles. *Int. Rehabil. Med.* 6:175–178, 1984.

19. Hagberg JM, Mountain SJ, Martin WH, Ehsani AA: Effects of exercise training on 60–69 year old essential hypertensives. *Am. J. Cardiol.* 64:348–353, 1989.

20. Hammon WE: Physical therapy for the acutely ill patient in the respiratory intensive care unit. *In* Irwin S, Tecklin JS: *Cardiopulmonary Physical Therapy,* 2nd Ed. St. Louis, The C.V. Mosby Co., 1990.

21. Hillegass E: The well individual. *In* Hillegass EA, Sadowsky HS: *Essentials of Cardiopulmonary Physical Therapy.* Philadelphia, W.B. Saunders Co., 1994.

22. Hollander W: Role of hypertension in atherosclerosis and cardiovascular disease. *Am. J. Cardiol.* 38:786–798, 1976.

23. Holtackers TR: Physical rehabilitation of the ventilator-dependent patient. *In* Irwin S, Tecklin JS: *Cardiopulmonary Physical Therapy,* 2nd Ed. St. Louis, The C.V. Mosby Co., 1990.

24. Humberstone N: Respiratory assessment and treatment. *In* Irwin S, Tecklin JS: *Cardiopulmonary Physical Therapy,* 2nd Ed. St. Louis, The C.V. Mosby Co., 1990.

25. Jones JL, Killian KJ, Summers E, et al.: Inspiratory muscle forces and endurance in maximum resistive loading. *J. Appl. Physiol.* 58:1608–1621, 1985.

26. Kuntz WT: The acute care setting. *In* Hillegass EA, Sadowsky HS: *Essentials of Cardiopulmonary Physical Therapy.* Philadelphia, W.B. Saunders Co., 1994.

27. Larsen OA, Lassen NA: Effect of daily muscular exercise in patients with intermittent claudication. *Lancet* ii:1093–1095, 1966.

28. Massery M: Respiratory rehabilitation secondary to neurological deficits: treatment techniques. *In* Frownfelter DL: *Chest Physical Therapy and Pulmonary Rehabilitation—An Interdisciplinary Approach,* 2nd Ed. Chicago, Year Book Medical Publishers, Inc., 1987.

29. Massery M: Respiratory rehabilitation secondary to neurological deficits: understanding the deficits. *In* Frownfelter DL: *Chest Physical Therapy and Pulmonary Rehabilitation—An Interdisciplinary Approach,* 2nd Ed. Chicago, Year Book Medical Publishers, Inc., 1987.

30. McArdle WD, Katch FI, Katch VL: *Exercise Physiology—Energy, Nutrition, and Human Performance,* 3rd Ed. Philadelphia, Lea & Febiger, 1991.

31. Meerhaeghe AV, Scano G, Sergysels R, et al.: Respiratory drive and ventilatory pattern during exercise in interstitial lung disease. *Bull. Eur. Physiopathol. Respir.* 17:15–26, 1981.

32. Mueller RE, Petty TL, Filley GF: Ventilation and arterial blood gas changes induced by pursed-lips breathing. *J. Appl. Physiol.* 28:784–789, 1970.

33. Oldridge NB, Donner A, Buck CW, et al: Predictive indices for drop-out: The Ontario Exercise Heart Collaborative Experience. *Am. J. Cardiol.* 51:70–74, 1983.

34. Pollock ML, Wilmore JH: *Exercise in Health and Disease,* 2nd Ed. Philadelphia, W.B. Saunders Co., 1990.

35. Regan K, Kleinfeld ME, Erik PC: Physical therapy for patients with abdominal or thoracic surgery. *In* Irwin S, Tecklin JS: *Cardiopulmonary Physical Therapy,* 2nd Ed. St. Louis, The C.V. Mosby Co., 1990.

36. Temes WC: Cardiac rehabilitation. *In* Hillegass EA, Sadowsky HS: *Essentials of Cardiopulmonary Physical Therapy.* Philadelphia, W.B. Saunders Co., 1994.

37. Wetzel JL, Lunsford BR, Peterson MJ, Alvarez SE: Respiratory rehabilitation of the patient with spinal cord injury. *In* Irwin S, Tecklin JS: *Cardiopulmonary Physical Therapy,* 2nd Ed. St. Louis, The C.V. Mosby Co., 1990.

38. Zadai CC: Rehabilitation of the patient with chronic obstructive pulmonary disease. *In* Irwin S, Tecklin JS: *Cardiopulmonary Physical Therapy,* 2nd Ed. St. Louis, The C.V. Mosby Co., 1990.

7
PEDIATRICS

In this chapter, some of the basic science of the most common cardiopulmonary problems encountered in neonates, infants, and children is presented. Attention is directed to the normal development of the cardiovascular and respiratory systems, problems that arise from developmental abnormalities, problems of prematurity, and commonly occurring diseases. Peculiarities of treatment specific to the pediatric population are also discussed.

7.1 PEDIATRIC CARDIOLOGY

Congenital heart disease represents the major portion of patients seen in pediatric cardiology practice. Most of these lesions probably result from disturbances in the complex embryologic development of the heart.

NORMAL EMBRYOLOGIC DEVELOPMENT OF THE HEART

The development of the heart can be broken down, for the sake of simplicity, into several grossly distinct phases, which are outlined in Table 7–1.

PRENATAL CIRCULATION

Because the developing fetus receives its oxygen and nutrition from the maternal circulation, there is no need to send large amounts of blood through the lungs or liver. Therefore, the fetus maintains a distinct prenatal circulatory pattern, shown in Figure 7–1, until the time of birth:

- Oxygenated blood returns from the placenta via the umbilical vein.
- Approximately half this blood flows through the ductus venosus to bypass the liver.

- Blood from the inferior vena cava flows primarily through the foramen ovale to the left atrium (LA), left ventricle (LV), aorta, and then to the coronary arteries, head and neck, and upper extremities.
- Blood from the superior vena cava and coronary sinus passes into the right ventricle (RV) and pulmonary trunk, where the majority of it flows through the ductus arteriosus into the aorta and out to the lower part of the body.

CIRCULATORY ADJUSTMENTS AT BIRTH

At birth, major circulatory adjustments occur as the lungs begin to function and the neonate moves to independent body functions:

- Occlusion of the placental circulation results in a reduction in blood pressure in the inferior vena cava and right atrium (RA) and an increase in blood pressure in the systemic arteries.
- At the onset of breathing, there is replacement of the fluid in the lungs by air causing pulmonary vascular resistance to fall dramatically.
- As blood flow to the lung increases, there is increased blood flow to the LA which elevates left atrial pressure so that it exceeds right atrial pressure, prompting closure of the foramen ovale.
- In addition, increased pulmonary blood flow along with rising arterial oxygen tensions results in constriction and closure of the ductus arteriosus.

CONGENITAL HEART DISEASE

Disturbances in the complex embryologic development of the heart often result in congenital

TABLE 7-1. **Gross Stages of Embryologic Development of the Heart**

TIME	EMBRYOLOGIC DEVELOPMENT
~Day 18	Cardiogenic cords are the first indications of cardiac development.
~Day 21–23	Fusion of the endocardial heart tubes, which formed from the canalized cardiogenic cords, into the pericardial cavity, plus elongation with development of the truncus arteriosus, bulbous cordis, ventricle, atrium, and sinus venosus.
~Day 24	The heart folds on itself and forms the bulboventricular loop.
~Day 25–35	Partioning of the major structures occurs:
	Development of the endocardial cushions divides the atrioventricular canal into right and left canals.
	Development of the septum primum and fusion with the endocardial cushions along with development of the septum secundum splits the atrium except at the foramen ovale.
	Growth of the interventricular septum toward the endocardial cushions divides the ventricle into two chambers, which communicate until complete closure via the interventricular foramen.
	Formation of the aortopulmonary septum divides the bulbus cordis and the trucus arterosus into the aorta and pulmonary trunk.
~Day 50	Complete development of the four-chambered heart.

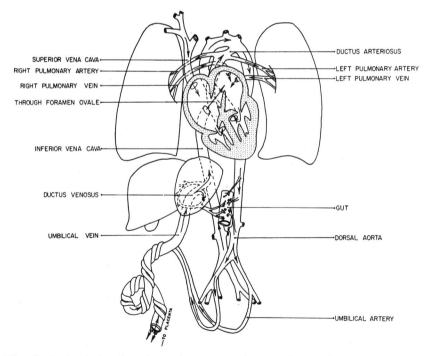

FIGURE 7-1. The fetal circulation has three shunts, one intracardiac and two extracardiac, which allow blood to bypass the lungs and the portal system. The ductus venosus shunts oxygenated blood from the placenta past the portal system directly to the inferior vena cava and right atrium, while the foramen ovale and the ductus arteriosus provide right-to-left shunting to minimize pulmonary blood flow. (From Avery ME: *The Lung and Its Disorders in the Newborn Infant,* 2nd Ed. Philadelphia, W.B. Saunders Co., p. 32, 1964. Used with permission.)

heart disease, which is the most common cause of pediatric cardiovascular disease. The incidence of congenital heart disease in the United States has been reported as approximately 1 per cent of live births.[14] The frequency of occurrence of the more common congenital cardiac defects is tabulated in Table 7–2. Congenital heart defects may occur in isolation, in combination, or may be a component of a number of congenital multisystem malformation syndromes, as listed in Table 7–3. The majority of defects are not life threatening, but one of every 500 newborns has severe heart disease requiring cardiac catheterization and/or surgery within the first year of life.[3]

CLINICAL MANIFESTATIONS OF HEART DISEASE IN INFANTS

- Tachycardia (or bradycardia if heart block)
- Signs and symptoms of respiratory distress
  - Tachypnea
  - Intercostal, suprasternal, subcostal, or substernal retractions
  - Nasal flaring
  - Expiratory grunting
  - Stridor
  - Head bobbing
  - Pallor, mottling, or webbing of skin versus cyanosis if severe

- Jugular venous distension
- Pulmonary rales
- Hepatomegaly
- Cyanosis
- Prominence of precordial chest wall
- Abnormal cardiac sounds, according to specific defect(s) (see pages 162 to 165)
- Failure to thrive

ACYANOTIC LESIONS

Acyanotic defects are usually associated with normal systemic arterial saturation. They can be divided into lesions with increased pulmonary blood flow due to left-to-right shunting through some communication between the two sides of the heart (e.g., atrial septal defect, patent ductus arteriosus, ventricular septal defect, arteriovenous malformation, endocardial cushion defect, and pulmonary hypertension due to any chronic left-to-right shunt) and lesions with normal blood pulmonary flow (e.g., coarctation of the aorta, mitral stenosis, pulmonary stenosis, aortic stenosis, endocardial fibroelastosis, and mitral regurgitation). The more common defects are described in this section; some of these defects occasionally result in shunt reversal (i.e., right-to-left shunting) when combined with other abnormalities, as noted under Pathophysiology.

TABLE 7–2. **Frequency of Occurrence of the More Common Congenital Cardiac Defects and Any Gender Preponderances for These Lesions[5,14,15]**

DEFECT	PERCENTAGE	GENDER PREPONDERANCE
Ventricular septal defect (VSD)	28–30	None
Atrial septal defect	9–10	Female
Patent ductus arteriosus	8.5–10	Female
Pulmonary stenosis (PS)	6.5–10	None
VSD with PS (includes tetralogy of Fallot)	6.5–7.5	Male
Aortic stenosis	6+*	Male (4:1)
Coarctation of the aorta	4–7	Male
Atrioventricular canal (partial and complete)	3.2–4.5	
Transposition of the great arteries	3.2–4.2	Male
Aortic atresia	2.2–2.8	Male (1.8:1)
Truncus arteriosus	1.4–2.0	None
Tricuspid atresia	1.0–1.5	None
Total anomalous pulmonary venous connection	1.0–1.5	
All others	15–18	—

*Incidence is probably greater since most patients with bicuspid aortic valve are not diagnosed until adulthood.

TABLE 7–3. Congenital Malformation Syndromes That May Have Associated Congenital Heart Defects[3,5]

SYNDROME	MAJOR CARDIOVASCULAR FEATURES	MAJOR NONCARDIAC FEATURES
Trisomy 21 (Down's syndrome)	Endocardial cushion defect, ASD, VSD, TOF	Hypotonia, hyperextensible joints, mongoloid facies, mental retardation
Trisomy 13	VSD, ASD, PDA	Single midline intracerebral ventricle with midfacial defects, polydactyly, nail changes, mental retardation
Trisomy 18	VSD, ASD, PDA, valvular defects	Clenched hand, short sternum, low-arch dermal ridge pattern on fingertips, mental retardation
XO (Turner's syndrome)	Coarctation of aorta, bicuspid aortic valve, aortic dilatation	Short female, broad chest, lymphedema, webbed neck
Congenital rubella	PDA, pulmonary valvular and/or artery stenosis, ASD	Cataracts, deafness, microcephaly
Marfan's syndrome	Aortic dilatation and dissection, aortic and mitral regurgitation	Gracile habitus, arachnodactyly with hyperextensibility, lens subluxation
Ehlers-Danlos syndrome	Arterial dilatation and rupture, mitral regurgitation	Hyperextensible joints, hyperelastic and friable skin
Osteogenesis imperfecta	Aortic incompetence	Fragile bones, blue sclerae
DiGeorge syndrome	Interrupted aortic arch, TOF, truncus arteriosus	Thymic hypoplasia or aplasia, parathyroid hypoplasia or aplasia, ear anomalies
Holt-Oram syndrome	ASD, VSD, others	Skeletal upper limb defect, hypoplasia of clavicles
CHARGE association (coloboma, heart, atresia choanae, retardation, genital and ear anomalies)	TOF, endocardial cushion defect, VSD, ASD	Colobomas, choanal atresia, mental and growth deficiencies, genital and ear anomalies
VATER association (vertebral, anal, tracheoesophageal, radial, and renal anomalies)	VSD	Vertebral anomalies, anal atresia, tracheoesophageal fistula, radial and renal anomalies
Williams syndrome	Supravalvular aortic stenosis, peripheral pulmonary stenosis	Mental retardation, elfin facies, loquacious personality, hoarse voice

ASD = atrial septal defect, PDA = patent ductus arteriosus, TOF = tetralogy of Fallot, VSD = ventricular septal defect.

Atrial Septal Defect

An atrial septal defect (ASD) is a through-and-through communication between the atria at the septal level, as shown in Figure 7–2. There are different anatomic types of ASD, but the classic ASD involves the region of the fossa ovalis.

PATHOPHYSIOLOGY

• An opening in the interatrial septum allows blood from the pulmonary veins in the LA to flow into the RA during both systole and diastole; (the magnitude of shunt depends on the size of ASD and the relative compliance of the ventricles, as well as the relative resistance in both the pulmonary and systemic circulations). This results in a large volume load on the RA and right ventricle (RV), while normal systemic flow is maintained so that there is enlargement of the RA and RV and dilation of the major pulmonary arteries (PAs) and pulmonary trunk.

• If there is coexisting pulmonary hypertension, RV hypertrophy (RVH) will develop along with atherosclerosis of the PAs, resulting in less left-to-right shunting and even possible shunt reversal with arterial desaturation and cyanosis.

NATURAL HISTORY

- The majority of children are asymptomatic, although probably most have some decreased exercise tolerance; a small number of infants develop congestive heart failure (CHF) in their first year.
- Symptoms become more common in the late teens and twenties, with the majority of individuals being symptomatic, some severely so, by age 40.
- Pulmonary vascular obstructive disease (Eisenmenger syndrome) affects ~15% of young adults.

TREATMENT

- If the child is asymptomatic: yearly follow-up with surgery recommended in preschool or preadolescent years.
- Earlier surgery if significant symptoms or CHF are present.

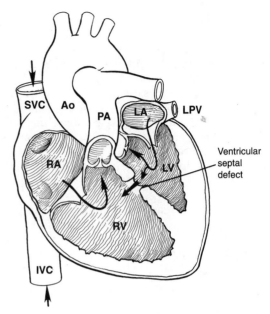

FIGURE 7–3. A ventricular septal defect usually allows blood to flow from the left ventricle into the right ventricle. Ao = aorta, IVC = inferior vena cava, LA = left atrium, LPV = left pulmonary vein, LV = left ventricle, PA = main pulmonary artery, RA = right atrium, RV = right ventricle, SVC = superior vena cava.

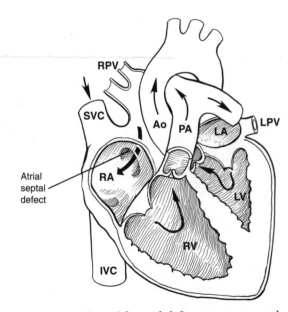

FIGURE 7–2. An atrial septal defect most commonly results in shunting of blood from the left atrium to the right. Ao = aorta, IVC = inferior vena cava, LA = left atrium, PA = pulmonary artery, LPV = left pulmonary vein, LV = left ventricle, PA = main pulmonary artery, RA = right atrium, RPV = right pulmonary vein, RV = right ventricle, SVC = superior vena cava.

Ventricular Septal Defect

A ventricular septal defect (VSD) is an opening between the ventricles at the septal level (Fig. 7–3); most are paramembranous.

PATHOPHYSIOLOGY

- In general, the functional effects of VSD depend on the size of the defect and the reaction of the pulmonary vascular bed:
  - If there is a VSD with no other lesions (usually small and quite restrictive) and pulmonary vascular resistance is normal, there will be a left-to-right shunt, which will be proportional to the size of the lesion.
    - If the VSD is small and/or PA pressure is elevated, the left-to-right shunt will be small.
    - If the VSD is large, there will be a large left-to-right shunt (which is inversely proportional to the level of resistance to pulmonary flow) and markedly elevated RV

and PA systolic pressures so that they become equal to LV and aortic pressure. Thus, there is an increased volume load on the RV, PA, LA, and LV, which results in higher LV end-diastolic volume and pressure.

— At birth, there is greater resistance to flow in the pulmonary vasculature so the left-to-right shunt is small; but over the first few weeks of life, pulmonary vascular resistance decreases and there is a progressive rise in shunting; in some infants, CHF develops (usually between 3 and 12 weeks of age).

• If there is increased resistance to LV emptying (e.g., aortic stenosis or coarctation), LV pressures will rise and the left-to-right shunting will increase.

NATURAL HISTORY

• Extremely variable, ranging from spontaneous closure (~24%), persistent small, asymptomatic VSD (most common), to CHF and possible death in early infancy.

• Possible complications may develop:
  • RV outflow tract obstruction in 5% to 10% of patients leads to right-to-left shunt (with cyanosis, etc.).
  • Aortic regurgitation in ~5% of patients.
  • Pulmonary vascular obstruction results in progressive irreversible pulmonary hypertension (HTN) (Eisenmenger syndrome).

TREATMENT

• If isolated asymptomatic VSD: semiannual or annual follow-up with elective catheterization between ages 3 and 6.
  • If small shunt (pulmonary/systemic flow <1.5 to 2:1): no surgery, but subacute bacterial endocarditis (SBE) prophylaxis.
  • If larger shunt: elective surgery to close VSD prior to elementary school.
• If symptomatic: early surgery to close VSD.

Patent Ductus Arteriosus

Persistent patency of the ductus arteriosus, which normally allows blood to be shunted from the pulmonary artery to the aorta in the fetus, past the first few weeks of life when it should constrict and close is termed *patent ductus arteriosus* (PDA) and is illustrated in Figure 7–4. PDAs can be narrow, allowing little blood flow from

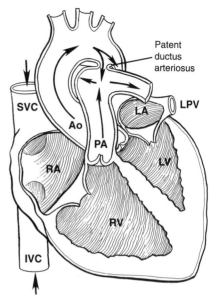

FIGURE 7–4. A patent ductus arteriosus (PDA) usually results in blood flow from the aorta back to the pulmonary arteries and lungs. Ao = aorta, IVC = inferior vena cava, LA = left atrium, LPV = left pulmonary vein, LV = left ventricle, PA = main pulmonary artery, RA = right atrium, RV = right ventricle, SVC = superior vena cava.

the aorta through the PDA so the RV remains unaffected, or wide, in which case there is a large aortopulmonary shunt and the RV hypertrophies.

PATHOPHYSIOLOGY

• PDA may result in CHF in some infants, whereas in other infants with certain coexisting cardiac malformations it may provide the only life-sustaining conduit to preserve systemic or pulmonary arterial blood flow.

• In premature infants, immaturity interferes with the normal mechanisms for postnatal ductal closure. In the vast majority of preterm infants under 1500 g birthweight, patency of the ductus arteriosus is prolonged; in approximately one third of these, a large aortopulmonary shunt results in significant cardiopulmonary deterioration.

• In full-term infants and children with PDA, flow across the defect is determined by the pressure relation between the aorta and the PA and the cross-sectional area and length of the PDA.

- Most commonly, PA pressures are normal so there is a persistent gradient and shunt from the aorta to the PA throughout the cardiac cycle, which results in increased pulmonary flow, enlargement of the LA and LV, and possible flow murmurs across the mitral and aortic valves.
- If there is heart failure or pulmonary HTN, the pressure gradient across the PDA will be less and there will be less flow through the PDA to the pulmonary arterial system.
- If there is severe pulmonary vascular obstructive disease and pulmonary HTN, flow through the PDA will reverse and there will be preferential shunting of unoxygenated blood to the descending aorta, producing cyanosis and clubbing of the toes but not the fingers.

NATURAL HISTORY

- Full-term infants usually do well for years.
- However, possible complications include: increased risk of infective endocarditis with age, possible pulmonary HTN with aneurysm formation and the potential of compressing recurrent laryngeal nerve, embolization of septic material to the lungs, or pulmonary aneurysm rupture.
- If there is a PDA with a large shunt, there is a higher risk of CHF and sudden death.
- Also, over the years, progressive damage of the pulmonary vascular bed results in irreversible pulmonary vascular obstructive disease and premature death in late adolescence or young adulthood.

TREATMENT

- Primary prevention of premature birth is important.
- In asymptomatic premature infants with small left-to-right shunts, no intervention is required because of probable spontaneous closure with maturation.
- If there is a significant PDA along with respiratory distress syndrome, indomethacin is given to stimulate constriction and closure of the ductus, and control of CHF is attempted

using medical management; if this is unsuccessful, surgical closure of PDA is required.
- Because infective endocarditis and heart failure are major causes of morbidity in older children, surgical ligation or division is recommended at age 1 to 2 years.

Coarctation of the Aorta

A coarctation of the aorta is a discreet narrowing of the distal segment of the aortic arch, most commonly in the vicinity of the former ductus, as depicted in Figure 7–5.

PATHOPHYSIOLOGY

- Narrowing of the aorta results in elevated systolic LV and aortic pressures proximal to the coarctation (i.e., to the brain and the upper extremities) and reduced systolic blood pressure distal to the defect (i.e., to the kidneys, etc., and lower extremities), which leads to LV hypertrophy (LVH), decreased capacity and distensibility of the proximal aorta, and the development of collateral blood vessels along the aorta.

NATURAL HISTORY

- Most infants with uncomplicated coarctations do well with medical management.

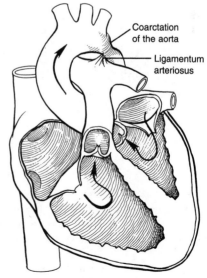

FIGURE 7-5. Coarctation of the aorta with narrowing of the aorta in the juxtaductal location.

- Some infants with simple coarctation, as well as those with coarctation complicated by association with other defects (e.g., VSD, PDA) develop CHF by the second week of life; those who do not respond well to medical management and those with complicated coarctations, require prompt surgical correction for survival.
- Following surgical repair, a few patients develop rapidly recurrent coarctation or moderate-to-severe mitral stenosis or regurgitation.
- In addition, restenosis of a surgically corrected defect may develop if the area of repair does not grow with the child.
- If surgical correction is not performed, persistent HTN by adolescence or early adulthood results in aortic rupture or intracranial hemorrhage, CHF often complicated by mitral or aortic valve disease, and atherosclerosis by age 40; the average age of death is 34 years.
- There is an increased risk of infective endocarditis.

TREATMENT
- Medical management until age 4, then surgical repair using a dacron aortic graft.
- Earlier repair if systolic blood pressure >155 to 160 mm Hg.
- If coarctation is complicated by other lesions:
  - If PDA plus coarctation: surgical correction of both defects.
  - If VSD plus coarctation: surgical correction of coarctation, ? banding of PA, ? VSD closure.
- Balloon valvuloplasty for restenosis.
- Antibiotics for endocarditis prophylaxis.

Pulmonary Stenosis
Narrowing of the pulmonary valve orifice is most commonly due to fusion of the valve cusps during mid to late fetal development. It is often accompanied by hypertrophy of the septal and parietal bands narrowing the RV infundibulum.

- The pathophysiologic and clinical manifestations of pulmonary stenosis (PS) can be found on page 79; typical pediatric variations include the following:
  - The clinical manifestations of PS depend on the severity of obstruction and the degree of development of the RV and its outflow tract,

the tricuspid valve, and the pulmonary arterial tree.
  - Most infants and children are asymptomatic; the small percentage with severe PS will have symptoms related to heart failure and diminished pulmonary blood flow and may have cyanosis if there is a patent foramen ovale or atrial septal defect.
  - The severity of stenosis may increase over time.

Aortic Stenosis
A congenitally narrowed aortic valve orifice, aortic stenosis (AS) usually results from thickening of the valve tissue with varying degrees of commissural fusion. In infants and small children with severe AS, the aortic valve ring may be relatively underdeveloped.

- The pathophysiologic and clinical manifestations of AS have been described on page 78; however, some variations that occur in the pediatric population are mentioned here:
  - AS in infants is occasionally responsible for profound and intractable heart failure; it is considered a medical emergency in the seriously ill newborn.
  - Myocardial ischemia is often a significant problem in infants and children with AS despite normal coronary arteries; in infants with severe AS, rupture of the LV papillary muscles may occur with resultant acute mitral regurgitation and precipitate or intensify heart failure.
  - The symptomatic child usually has critical stenosis (a peak systolic gradient of >75 mm Hg or a calculated effective orifice <0.5 cm^2/m^2 body surface area) and is at risk for sudden death.

CYANOTIC CONGENITAL HEART DISEASE
Cyanotic conditions are characterized by reduced systemic arterial saturation usually due to shunting of systemic venous blood into the arterial circulation. They can be divided according to lesions that have decreased pulmonary blood flow (e.g., severe pulmonary stenosis, pulmonary atresia ± VSD, tetralogy of Fallot, tricuspid atresia, transposition of the great arteries with pulmonary stenosis, truncus arteriosus with hypoplastic pulmonary arteries, and Ebstein's anomaly) versus those with increased pulmonary

blood flow (e.g., hypoplastic left heart syndrome, total anomalous pulmonary venous connection, transposition of the great arteries ± VSD, single ventricle, tricuspid atresia with transposition, and truncus arteriosus). Because of persistent cyanosis or right-to-left shunts, these patients often have characteristic extracardiac complications, including polycythemia, relative anemia, central nervous system abscess, thromboembolic stroke, gum disease, gout, digital clubbing and hypoxic arthropathies, infectious diseases, and failure to thrive. Surgical procedures performed for the palliation of congenital heart disease are listed in Table 7–4 and those performed for correction are recorded in Table 7–5.

Tetralogy of Fallot

Tetralogy of Fallot (TOF) is a syndrome consisting of four defects: a large nonrestrictive VSD, severe RV outflow tract obstruction, overriding of the aortic root over the ventricular septum,

and RVH (Fig. 7–6). If there is an ASD in addition, it is called "pentalogy/pentad of Fallot." A right aortic arch occurs in 25% to 30% of patients.

PATHOPHYSIOLOGY

- A large VSD and severe RV outflow tract obstruction result in right-to-left shunting with equal pressure in both ventricles and the aorta, arterial unsaturation, and polycythemia.
  - The degree of shunting is a function of the relative pulmonary and systemic resistances, as well as the amount of systemic venous return.
- The circulation to abnormal lungs is via bronchial and other collateral arteries.
- Hypoxic or hypercyanotic ("tet") spells occur in some infants leading to increased cyanosis.

NATURAL HISTORY

- The prognosis is poorest in very young infants with cyanosis because of the severity of ob-

TABLE 7–4. Palliative Procedures for Congenital Heart Disease

PROCEDURES	LESION	COMMENTS
Blalock-Taussig Teflon tube graft or shunt (subclavian artery to ipsilateral pulmonary artery, usually right sided)	TOF, pulmonary valve atresia	Improves pulmonary blood flow; most common shunting procedure
Waterston shunt (aorta to right pulmonary artery)	TOF, pulmonary valve atresia, tricuspid atresia	Improves pulmonary blood flow
Balloon atrial septostomy (Rashkind procedure)	TGA, tricuspid atresia	Improves oxygenation with increased atrial mixing
Operative atrial septostomy (Blalock-Hanlon operation)	TGA	
Catheter balloon dilating valvotomy (balloon angioplasty)	Pulmonary valve stenosis. Aortic valve stenosis	Increases valve patency
Operative valvotomy	As above for balloon plus pulmonary atresia	Increases valve patency; resultant pulmonary valve insufficiency enhances RV growth
Prostaglandin (PGE₁) infusion	Pulmonary atresia, tricuspid atresia, TOF, coarctation of aorta, interrupted aortic arch	Maintains pulmonary blood flow via PDA
Pulmonary artery banding	VSD, endocardial cushion defects. Single ventricle	Decreases pulmonary blood flow, prevents heart failure
Device occlusion (embolization, umbrella, foams); correction/closure	PDA, VSD, ASD, arteriovenous malformations	New and experimental

From Liebman J, Freed MD: Cardiovascular system. *In* Behrman RE, Kliegman R: *Nelson Essentials of Pediatrics.* Philadelphia, W.B. Saunders Co., p. 465, 1990. Used with permission.
TOF = tetralogy of Fallot, TGA = transposition of the great arteries, VSD = ventricular septal defect, ASD = atrial septal defect, PDA = patent ductus arteriosus, RV = right ventricle.

TABLE 7–5. **Corrective Procedures for Congenital Heart Disease**

PROCEDURE	LESION	EFFECT
Repair of septal defects (patching)	ASD, VSD, endocardial cushion defects	Complete repair
Valve replacement	Aortic, mitral, pulmonic stenosis, Ebstein's anomaly	Repair but prosthetic valve complications
Aortic graft, or subclavian flap angioplasty	Interrupted arch, coarctation of aorta	Repair but possible late recoarctation
Total correction possible	TOF, anomalous venous return, PDA	Complete repair
Mustard procedure (atrial switch by an intraatrial baffle)	TGA	RV remains systemic ventricle
Jatene procedure (arterial switch)	TGA	Anatomic correction
Fontan procedure (right atrium to pulmonary artery anastomosis)	Tricuspid atresia, single ventricle, pulmonary atresia	Alleviates shunting, enhances pulmonary blood flow. Atrium functions as right ventricle
Norwood procedure	Hypoplastic left heart	Two-staged procedure with variable success
Heart transplant	Hypoplastic left heart	Normal heart with risk of immune-mediated rejection
Heart-lung transplant	Eisenmenger syndrome; cor pulmonale?	Normal organs with risk of rejection

From Liebman J, Freed MD: Cardiovascular system. *In* Behrman RE, Kliegman R: *Nelson Essentials of Pediatrics.* Philadelphia, W.B. Saunders Co., p. 466, 1990.
LV = left ventricle, TOF = tetralogy of Fallot, TGA = transposition of the great arteries, VSD = ventricular septal defect, ASD = atrial septal defect, PDA = patent ductus arteriosus, RV = right ventricle.

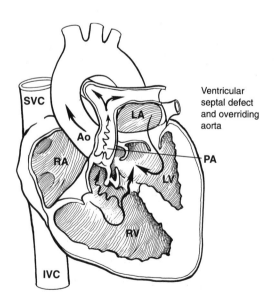

Ventricular septal defect and overriding aorta

FIGURE 7–6. Classic tetralogy of Fallot: biventricular origin of the aorta, large ventricular septal defect, right ventricular hypertrophy, and obstruction to pulmonary flow. Ao = aorta, IVC = inferior vena cava, LA = left atrium, LV = left ventricle, PA = main pulmonary artery, RA = right atrium, RV = right ventricle, SVC = superior vena cava.

struction, small size of the pulmonary arteries, and frequent hypoxic spells.

- Increasing cyanosis and polycythemia result in progressive obstruction to pulmonary blood flow, even to the point of atresia.
- Polycythemia increases the risk of cerebrovascular accidents (CVAs) and brain abscesses.
- Polycythemia combined with reduced pulmonary blood flow leads to multiple thrombi in small pulmonary vessels.
- The risk of infective endocarditis is markedly increased.
- Without surgery, one third of patients die by age 1, one half by age 3, three fourths by age 10, and 95% by age 30.[4]

TREATMENT

- Medical management to prevent and treat complications
- High-concentration oxygen and morphine sulfate for hypoxic ("tet") spells
- Antibiotics for endocarditis prophylaxis
- Elective surgical correction in early childhood versus two-stage repair in symptomatic infants (see Tables 7–4 and 7–5)

Transposition of the Great Arteries

Transposition of the great arteries (TGA) is an anomaly where the origin of the aorta arises from the morphologic RV while the PAs arise from the morphologic LV so that there are two separate and parallel circulations; although almost all patients have an ASD, two thirds have a PDA, and one third have a VSD (see Fig. 7–7).

PATHOPHYSIOLOGY

- Bidirectional shunts must exist since unidirectional shunting would result in progressive depletion of circulating volume in either the pulmonary or systemic vascular bed.
- The major determinant of systemic arterial oxygen saturation is the amount of blood exchanged between the two circulations by the intercirculatory shunts.
- There is an increased risk of pulmonary vascular obstructive disease leading to progressive irreversible pulmonary HTN (Eisenmenger syndrome).
- Often there is preferential blood flow to the right lung, which produces greater pulmonary

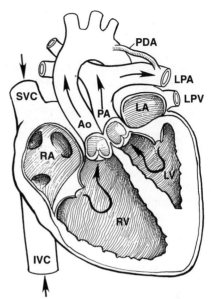

FIGURE 7-7. Complete transposition of the great arteries. When the interventricular septum is intact, there is usually a patent foramen ovale and enlarged bronchial arteries (Br. Art.). Otherwise, the ventricular septal defect allows connection of the systemic and pulmonary circulations. Ao = aorta, IVC = inferior vena cava, LA = left atrium, LPA = left pulmonary artery, LPV = left pulmonary vein, LV = left ventricle, PA = main pulmonary artery, PDA = patent ductus arteriosus, RA = right atrium, RV = right ventricle, SVC = superior vena cava.

vascular obstructive disease on the right and more pulmonary thrombosis on the left.

NATURAL HISTORY

- Without treatment, ~30% of infants die in the first week of life, 50% within the first month, 70% in the first 6 months, and 90% in the first year.[3]
- The clinical course is determined by the degree of tissue hypoxia, the ability of each ventricle to sustain the increased workload in the presence of reduced coronary arterial oxygenation, the nature of associated cardiovascular anomalies, and the anatomic and functional status of the pulmonary vascular bed.

TREATMENT

- Medical management if possible (oxygen, digitalis, diuretics, iron, sodium bicarbonate)

- Prostaglandin E_1 to dilate the ductus arteriosus in early neonatal period to increase pulmonary blood flow and enhance intercirculatory mixing
- Balloon catheter inflation to create or enlarge an ASD and thus improve intercirculatory mixing
- Surgical intervention (see Tables 7–4 and 7–5)

OTHER CARDIAC DISORDERS SEEN IN CHILDHOOD

Cardiovascular disease in children sometimes results from infection or inflammation involving the cardiac structures, trauma, drug toxicity, cardiomyopathy, or involvement of the heart by systemic diseases.

MYOCARDITIS

Inflammation of the myocardium can occur at any age. In children, myocarditis most frequently results from viral infection, such as coxsackie B virus, and presents as acute heart failure, or sometimes shock, with a dilated heart and marked ST abnormalities on electrocardiography. Following intensive therapy in a critical care unit, most children recover completely; however, some children die and some develop chronic dilated cardiomyopathy, which can be severe (see pages 80 to 81).

CARDIOMYOPATHIES

In addition to myocarditis, myocardial disease can develop in children as a result of a number of abnormalities, such as familial/hereditary diseases (e.g, muscular dystrophy, Friedreich's ataxia, hemachromatosis, and endocardial fibroelastosis), drug toxicity (e.g., adriamycin, ipecac), anomalous left coronary artery, sickle cell disease, hypertrophic cardiomyopathy, and metabolic, nutritional, and endocrine disorders (e.g., thiamine deficiency, selenium deficiency, and hypo- and hyperthyroidism). Cardiomyopathy not due to myocarditis carries a poorer prognosis; although some children stabilize, others rapidly deteriorate and heart transplantation becomes the only hope for survival. Refer to pages 80 to 81 for more information on cardiomyopathies.

ENDOCARDIAL FIBROELASTOSIS

Usually a secondary rather than a primary disorder seen in infants and children, endocardial fibroelastosis (EFE) is characterized by a proliferation of elastic and collagenous fibers within the endocardium, most commonly of the LV, which becomes abnormally thickened. EFE is typically associated with left-sided congenital heart disease, such as aortic stenosis, coarctation of the aorta, and anomalous origin of the coronary artery from the pulmonary trunk, or it may occur as a nonspecific response to some cardiomyopathies. It presents clinically as a dilated cardiomyopathy with severe heart failure and frequently severe mitral regurgitation and is treated accordingly (see pages 74 and 81).

RHEUMATIC FEVER

Acute rheumatic fever (ARF) most commonly affects children 5 to 15 years of age and is related to an immune reaction to untreated group A, β-streptococcus infection.

- Because of the wide variety of clinical manifestations and the similarity to many other diseases, ARF can be difficult to diagnose. It typically presents 2 to 6 weeks after a sore throat or other presumed streptococcal infection with any of the following manifestations: polyarthritis, carditis, chorea, erythema marginatum, and/or subcutaneous nodules. The usual duration is less than 3 months, although it may continue for 6 months or more in cases with severe carditis.
- Treatment for ARF depends on the manifestations and severity of the attack but generally consists of bed rest, antibiotic therapy, and aspirin or corticosteroids once the diagnosis is established. In addition, permanent antibiotic prophylaxis is essential to avoid repeated episodes of ARF, for the healing rate of rheumatic carditis is remarkably high if recurrences are prevented. However, some patients do develop chronic rheumatic heart disease (RHD) with valvular dysfunction.
- Chronic RHD usually results in mitral and/or aortic valvular disease, most commonly regurgitation or stenosis plus regurgitation, which is treated according to the specific defect(s), as described on pages 78 to 80.

PERICARDITIS

In children, inflammation of the pericardium most commonly results from viral or bacterial infections and immune-mediated disease (e.g., postinfectious immune complexes, connective tissue diseases, and the presence of autoantibody), but it may also be due to uremia, hypothyroidism, trauma, postpericardiotomy, and malignancy. It is discussed in more detail on page 83.

ARRHYTHMIAS

Intrinsic abnormalities of the myocardium or the conduction system and extrinsic factors that alter the excitability of the heart can cause arrhythmias in children. These include infections/postinfections (e.g., endocarditis, Lyme disease, diptheria, myocarditis, Guillain-Barré, and rheumatic fever), drugs (e.g., antiarrhythmic agents, caffeine, bronchodilators, ephedrine, tricyclic antidepressants), structural lesions of the heart (e.g., congenital defects, mitral valve prolapse, ventricular tumor), metabolic-endocrine disorders (e.g., electrolyte disturbances, uremia, thyrotoxicosis, cardiomyopathy, pheochromocytoma, prophyria), and others. Arrhythmias commonly seen in children and their treatment are presented in Table 7–6.

CLINICAL IMPLICATIONS FOR PHYSICAL THERAPY

- During the postoperative period following heart surgery, children, especially those with Down's syndrome or preexisting lung disease, have an elevated risk of developing pulmonary complications, including atelectasis, infection, and airway obstruction; therefore, children should be instructed in splinted coughing techniques and encouraged to participate in activities that increase ventilation and progress mobility. Bronchial hygiene treatments are usually required only for patients who are unable to clear their secretions or those with chronic lung disease.
- To counter the tendency to splint their incision, children should be encouraged to perform arm, shoulder, and trunk movements, using songs and games for the younger ones (e.g, "The Itsy Bitsy Spider").
- Pediatric cardiac rehabilitation has been shown to be safe and effective in children with acquired or congenital heart disease and children at risk for developing atherosclerotic heart disease; supervised programs using moderate intensity (70% to 80% of maximal heart rate) are effective in achieving the following beneficial effects:
  - Lowering resting blood pressure
  - Increasing peak oxygen consumption
  - Improving exercise tolerance
- The size of the child may limit the types of exercise the child can perform, especially for ex-

TABLE 7–6. **Arrhythmias in Children and Their Treatment**

TYPE	TREATMENT
Sinus tachycardia	Treat fever, remove sympathomimetic agents (e.g., caffeine, bronchodilators, ephedrine)
Atrial flutter	Digoxin, cardioversion
Supraventricular tachycardia (SVT)	Vagal stimulation (e.g., ice water to face, Valsalva maneuver), digoxin, verapamil in older children, cardioversion if acutely ill
First-degree AV block	Observe, obtain digoxin level if on therapy
Mobitz type I (Wenckebach) second-degree AV block	Observe, correct underlying electrolyte or other abnormalities
Mobitz type II second-degree AV block	Observe, consider pacemaker
Complete third-degree AV block	Permanent pacemaker, especially if rate <50 or hemodynamic instability
Premature ventricular complex (PVC)	None if asymptomatic, otherwise lidocaine, procainamide, quinidine
Ventricular tachycardia	Lidocaine, cardioversion, procainamide, propranolol, bretylium, phenytoin
Ventricular fibrillation	Nonsynchronized cardioversion/defibrillation, automatic implantable cardioverter defibrillator (AICD) if chronic

AV = atrioventricular.

ercise testing. Keeping the workouts fun and interesting is a major challenge!

- Exercise training following heart transplantation is very important:
  - Initially, it helps with airway clearance.
  - Gradually, it allows the child to attain a higher functional level than the child's previous deconditioned state.
  - The ultimate goal is to maintain a healthy lifestyle and possibly to slow the development of premature atherosclerosis observed in some patients.
  - Prolonged warm-up and cool-down are essential in these patients because of denervation of the heart.

7.2 PEDIATRIC PULMONOLOGY

Disorders of the respiratory system are fairly common in children and may result from infection, immaturity (e.g., respiratory distress syndrome), genetics (e.g., cystic fibrosis), congenital anomalies (both pulmonary and cardiac), immunologic abnormalities, iatrogenic causes (e.g., oxygen toxicity), and accidents. The more common disorders are presented in this section.

NORMAL EMBRYOLOGIC DEVELOPMENT OF THE LUNGS

The respiratory system begins its development around 24 days' gestation and continues into postnatal life. The different phases of embryo-logic development are described briefly in Table 7–7; however, the lung continues to develop during early postnatal life, especially proliferation of the alveoli and terminal sacs, which continues until the age of 8 years or so.

PHYSIOLOGIC TRANSITIONS AT BIRTH

At the time of birth, major physiologic alterations occur in the respiratory system. The emergence of the fetus from the birth canal produces a number of strong respiratory stimuli, the fluid within the airways is rapidly cleared, and the infant usually takes his first breath soon after birth. Almost immediately, there is a tremendous increase in pulmonary blood flow allowing a shift of gas exchange from the placenta to the lungs. In addition, the pulmonary vascular resistance initially falls very rapidly (then more slowly for the first 6 to 8 weeks of life) and the ductus arteriosus closes, which results in the abrupt reduction of pulmonary artery pressure and facilitates increased pulmonary blood flow.

NORMAL DIFFERENCES BETWEEN INFANT AND ADULT RESPIRATORY SYSTEMS

There are a number of anatomic and physiologic differences between the respiratory systems of full-term infants and older children and

TABLE 7–7. **Phases of Development of the Respiratory System**

PHASE	GESTATIONAL AGE	EMBRYOLOGIC DEVELOPMENT
Pseudoglandular	~24–28 days	Development of primordial lungs and major bronchi
	~4–12 weeks	Separation of the trachea from the esophagus, formation of the larynx, and rapid growth and repeated preacinar branching of the bronchi
	~12–16 weeks	Distinction of lung lobes with complete airway branching pattern, formation of bronchial arteries
Canalicular	~16–24 weeks	Development of airway epithelium and submucosal glands; formation of preacinar pattern of blood supply; initial appearance of alveoli at end of phase
Saccular/alveolar	~24–44+ weeks	Rapid proliferation of the alveoli; increasing airway diameter and length, vessel size and number, cartilage mass, and gland growth

TABLE 7–8. Anatomic Differences Affecting Pulmonary Function in Infants and Sometimes Small Children Compared with Adults

ANATOMIC DIFFERENCE	EFFECT(S)
High larynx	Allows infant to breathe and swallow simultaneously, but also creates the possibility of obligatory nose breathing, in which case any narrowing of the nasal passageways will result in ↑ work of breathing
Enlarged lymphatic tissue	Possibility of upper airway obstruction
Alveolar surface area of only 5% of adult's	Because alveoli continue to develop rapidly during the first year of life, then more slowly until age 8, this protective difference allows any early disease-related lung damage to become less significant over time
↓ Airway diameter and structural support	↑ Risk of airway obstruction and collapse
↓ Number of collateral ventilation channels	↑ Incidence of right middle and upper lobe atelectasis in neonates
Horizontal configuration of cartilagenous rib cage	↓ Efficiency of ventilation + ↑ distortion of rib cage

↑ = increased, ↓ = decreased.

adults, which increase the infant's susceptibility to respiratory dysfunction.

- The anatomic differences that affect pulmonary function in infants are described in Table 7–8.
- The physiologic differences affecting pulmonary function in infants are described in Table 7–9.
- Some of these differences tend to be even more pronounced in premature infants, which combined with the lack of maturity

of a number of pulmonary structures significantly increases the risk of pulmonary dysfunction.

Neonatal Respiratory Disorders

Because of the differences in their respiratory systems, discussed above, and relative immaturity, neonates are particularly vulnerable to pulmonary dysfunction. Prematurity adds an additional burden.

TABLE 7–9. Physiologic Differences Affecting Pulmonary Function in Infants and Sometimes Small Children Compared with Adults

PHYSIOLOGIC DIFFERENCE	EFFECT(S)
↓ Lung compliance in neonate	Need for ↑ inflation pressures → ↑ work of breathing
↑ Irregularity of respiratory pattern	↑ Risk of apnea
Respiratory compensation via ↑ rate rather than ↑ depth	↓ Efficiency of ventilation → ↑ work of breathing
↓ Pulmonary reserve	↑ Risk of serious pulmonary dysfunction with any abnormality
↑ Time spent in rapid eye movement (REM) sleep	↑↑ Work of breathing
↓ Percentage of type I, high-oxidative fibers in diaphragm	↑ Vulnerability to respiratory muscle fatigue

↑ = increased, ↑↑ = much increased, ↓ = decreased, → = leads to.

INFANT RESPIRATORY DISTRESS SYNDROME

Infant respiratory distress syndrome (IRDS), also called hyaline membrane disease (HMD), is a disorder of prematurity or lack of complete lung maturation in neonates born before 36 weeks of gestation, resulting in inadequate amounts of surfactant in the alveoli.

- The severity of the signs and symptoms is inversely related to the gestational age.
- Fortunately, new treatments may avert the development of IRDS in many premature infants.

Pathophysiology

- Inadequate surfactant increases the retractive forces in the lungs, resulting in diminished lung compliance, additional work of breathing, and progressive diffuse microatelectasis, which leads to alveolar collapse, greater ventilation-perfusion mismatching, and impaired gas exchange (due to increased dead space ventilation and decreased alveolar ventilation, see page 90), as shown in Figure 7–8.
- Abnormal alveolar epithelial and endothelial permeability in the immature lung causes disruption of the bronchiolar epithelium during mechanical ventilation along with pulmonary edema and the generation of hyaline membranes.
- Increased compliance of the proximal and distal airways (as opposed to decreased compliance of alveoli) in infants results in disruption, dilation, and deformation of the airways during mechanical ventilation with the high pressures required to adequately ventilate the infant's lungs.
- If there is a persistent PDA, intracardiac left-to-right shunt increases pulmonary blood flow and pressures leading to possible pulmonary edema and further interference with surfactant production.

Common Complications

- Intracranial hemorrhage
- Sepsis
- Pneumonia
- Pneumothorax
- Pulmonary hemorrhage
- Pulmonary interstitial emphysema
- Bronchopulmonary dysplasia

Clinical Manifestations

- Signs and symptoms of respiratory distress
  - Rapid, labored breathing with expiratory grunt on auscultation
  - Significant intercostal and substernal retractions
  - Nasal flaring, grunting
  - Cyanosis
- Weak cry
- Decreased lung volumes, especially functional reserve capacity and vital capacity
- Decreased PO_2, increased PCO_2, and decreased pH on examination of arterial blood gas
- Bradycardia

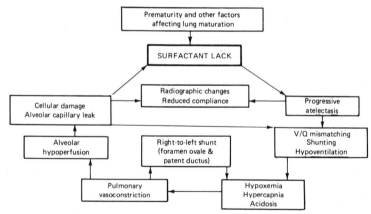

FIGURE 7–8. Pathogenesis and pathophysiology of infant respiratory distress syndrome. The central abnormality is the lack of surfactant. Note several vicious cycles in the scheme. (From Farzan S: *A Concise Handbook of Respiratory Diseases,* 3rd Ed. Norwalk, CT, Appleton & Lange, p. 375, 1992. Used with permission.)

- Fine reticulogranular pattern on chest x-ray examination, possibly air bronchograms

Treatment
- Corticosteroids for mother prior to delivery
- Supportive care
  - Neutral thermal environment
  - Nutritional support, hyperalimentation
  - Fluid and electrolyte replacement
  - Supplemental oxygen
  - Continuous positive airway pressure (CPAP)
- Bronchial drainage techniques
- Exogenous or semisynthetic surfactant

AIR LEAKS

Neonates with pulmonary dysfunction requiring positive pressure ventilation often develop air leaks with accumulation of air in the pleural space (i.e., pneumothorax), the pericardial sac (i.e., pneumopericardium), the mediastinum (i.e., pneumomediastinum), and/or between the layers of lung tissue (i.e., pulmonary interstitial emphysema). Of these, pneumothorax creates the greatest threat to the neonate (see page 95).

BRONCHOPULMONARY DYSPLASIA

Bronchopulmonary dysplasia (BPD) is a form of chronic obstructive lung disease (see page 84) that develops in some survivors of IRDS who have received mechanical ventilation with high concentrations of oxygen over a prolonged period of time. It is sometimes called *pulmonary fibroplasia* or *ventilator lung*.

Pathophysiology
- Prolonged oxygen exposure along with barotrauma results in interstitial edema, atelectasis, mucosal metaplasia, interstitial fibrosis, necrotizing obliterative bronchiolitis, and overextended alveoli, which leads to a further need for prolonged oxygen therapy with a slow weaning process and greater risk of recurrent pulmonary infections.
- Infants with BPD have an increased risk of pulmonary HTN, right heart failure, poor growth, elevated oxygen consumption, and emotional and behavioral problems.

Clinical Manifestations
- Severe chest retractions
- Oxygen dependence
- Hypercapnia

- Compensatory metabolic alkalosis
- Pulmonary HTN, RVH on chest radiograph
- Signs and symptoms of cor pulmonale
- Reactive airway bronchoconstriction

Treatment
- Supportive care
  - Supplemental nutrition
  - Diuretics
  - Oxygen
  - Mechanical ventilation
  - Possible tracheostomy
- Steroid therapy?

MECONIUM ASPIRATION SYNDROME

Airway obstruction and chemical pneumonitis develops in 10% to 30% of infants who are meconium-stained at birth (meconium aspiration syndrome, MAS). Release of meconium, the dark, sticky, fecal material that accumulates in utero, occurs in 10% to 20% of births, especially those that are full- or postterm.

Pathophysiology
- Aspiration of meconium causes a "ball-valve" type of obstruction with air-trapping and air leaks, hypoxemia, hypercapnia, and persistent fetal circulation, which results in pulmonary HTN.
- In addition, aspiration of meconium produces severe necrotizing chemical pneumonitis with inflammation of the airways, which increases airway resistance, ventilation-perfusion abnormalities, and work of breathing. Some infants develop respiratory muscle fatigue and respiratory failure.

Clinical Manifestations
- Suction fluid positive for meconium
- Possible wheezes, decreased expiration over area(s) of obstruction
- Signs and symptoms of respiratory distress (see page 229)

Treatment
- Intrapartum oropharyngeal suctioning and immediate postpartum intubation for direct tracheal suctioning
- Supportive care
  - Supplemental nutrition
  - Diuretics
  - Oxygen
  - Mechanical ventilation

- Extracorporeal membrane oxygenation (ECMO)

CLINICAL IMPLICATIONS FOR PHYSICAL THERAPY

- Although overwhelming, an intensive care unit is the safest place to evaluate and treat any patient because of the constant monitoring provided and ready availability of additional trained personnel.
  - Always check with the infant's nurse before giving any treatment for the most current information on the infant's condition, recent events, and interventions.
  - Some situations that would indicate the need to delay physical therapy intervention include very recent extubation, untreated pneumothorax, immediately status post placement of a chest tube (before chest radiograph results), unstable blood gases, recent feeding (unless stomach is bypassed), and intolerance to handling (e.g., increased apnea, bradycardia, skin color changes)
  - Ask questions or for help whenever appropriate.
- Physiologic monitoring is extremely important in these infants due to their lack of tolerance for increased activity, which further stresses their cardiorespiratory systems, and includes:
  - Heart rate
  - Blood pressure (if arterial line in place; otherwise very difficult)
  - ECG
  - Transcutaneous or pulse oximetry
  - Skin color changes
  - Respiratory rate and pattern
- Sometimes a neonate may tolerate physical therapy intervention better if the amount of oxygen is increased; however, this requires a physician's orders. Also, the oxygen must always be turned back down when treatment is completed.
- Positioning can affect ventilation-perfusion balances and airway clearance, as well as neuromusculoskeletal patterns.
  - Prone positioning is the optimal position for ventilation in a normal tone infant but could cause problems in a patient with an enlarged abdomen or one with decreased tone.
  - Careful monitoring of the infant is essential when attempting new position changes.
- The more severe the infant's medical problems and the longer the stay in intensive care, the more prone the infant is to developmental delay and consequently the need for neuromusculoskeletal physical therapy interventions.

PEDIATRIC PULMONARY DISORDERS

Some pulmonary disorders affecting infants and children result from genetic disorders (e.g., cystic fibrosis and immotile cilia syndrome); most of the others are due to infection, asthma, or accidents.

CYSTIC FIBROSIS

Cystic fibrosis (CF) is an autosomal recessive disorder due to a defect of chromosome 7, which results in dysfunction of the exocrine glands of the body, with abnormal secretions in the respiratory tract, sweat glands, and mucosal glands of the small intestine, the pancreas, and bile ducts of the liver. However, 90% of morbidity and mortality is due to involvement of the pulmonary system, which occurs in >98% of patients, although the degree is extremely variable.

Pulmonary Pathophysiology

- Hypertrophy and hyperplasia of bronchial mucous glands with thick, tenacious mucus causes obstruction of small bronchi and bronchioles and impairment of mucociliary clearance. Atelectasis and frequent pulmonary infections are common, which lead to even more mucus production and impaired secretion clearance.
- If chronic suppurative bronchitis develops, there is destruction of normal ciliated epithelium and squamous metaplasia, resulting in bronchiectasis, peribronchial fibrosis, pneumonitis, and/or multiple abscesses. Profound ventilation-perfusion mismatching produces marked hypoxemia, hypercapnia, and pulmonary HTN, which leads to RVH and eventual cor pulmonale (see page 99).
- In addition, the markedly elevated work of breathing (especially during acute infections) increases the possibility of respiratory muscle fatigue and respiratory failure (see page 98).

Pulmonary Clinical Manifestations

- Tachypnea
- Irritability
- Cyanosis during crying spells or on exertion, and later possibly at rest
- Chronic bronchial infections and often upper respiratory infections, bronchiectasis
- Blood-streaked mucous, hemoptysis
- Easily fatigued, decreased exercise tolerance
- Increased use of accessory muscles of respiration
- Increased anteroposterior diameter of chest, possible costal flaring and intercostal retractions
- Digital clubbing, possible hypertrophic pulmonary osteoarthropathy
- Decreased breath sounds with prolonged expiration, wheezes, localized or generalized crackles
- Hypoxemia, possible hypercapnia and respiratory acidosis
- Possible signs and symptoms of pulmonary HTN, RVH, cor pulmonale, and/or respiratory failure (see pages 98 to 99)

Treatment

- Usually coordinated by a tertiary referral center
- Physical measures
  - Bronchial hygiene techniques
  - Exercise
- Pharmacologic therapy
  - Bronchodilators
  - Mucolytic agents
  - Corticosteroids, inhaled or oral
  - Antibiotics
  - Oxygen, diuretics for cor pulmonale
- Possible heart-lung or single lung transplantation for end-stage disease
- Nutrition
  - Pancreatic enzymes
  - Supplemental nutrition

Clinical Implications for Physical Therapy

- Since bronchial hygiene is a critical part of the successful management of CF, the physical therapy treatment plan usually includes instruction for the family.
- Another important component of treatment is aerobic exercise, which is generally recommended to increase cardiopulmonary fitness, increase muscle strength and endurance, improve posture, increase chest mobility, and assist with airway clearance.[17]
  - However, exercise is *not* a substitute for bronchial drainage.[19]
  - As the patient grows, exercise has beneficial effects on self-confidence, self-image, socialization, and quality of life.
  - In adolescents, strengthening exercises can help with self-image, and postural exercises are beneficial in countering the tendency towards kyphosis.
- The role of supplemental oxygen in the management of CF is controversial: although it can help reduce periods of desaturation, it may not improve an individual's ability to do work.

ASTHMA

Between 5% to 10% of all children are affected by asthma, which is described in detail on page 87. The majority of children experience bronchoconstriction with both extrinsic and intrinsic stimuli, and up to 95% of children with asthma experience exercise-induced bronchoconstriction, especially in cold air. However, regular aerobic exercise, following bronchodilator administration, is an important component of the treatment of children with asthma since improved cardiorespiratory fitness increases the threshold at which provocation of symptoms occurs and seems to improve the child's tolerance of bronchospasm. In addition, children who are more fit tend to require less medication, have higher self-esteem and self-confidence, and have fewer absences from school. Other areas of physical therapy involvement in asthma cases include patient and family education in breathing control, relaxation, effective coughing, and occasionally bronchial hygiene techniques. Fortunately, most children who develop asthma before age 5 years "outgrow" it.

BRONCHIOLITIS

Usually caused by respiratory syncytial virus, acute bronchiolitis is the most common severe lower respiratory tract infection in infants under 2 years of age. Its peak incidence coincides with the coldest months of the year, typically November through March. Bronchiolitis results in bronchiolar edema, necrosis and shedding of the epithelial cells, and increased mucous secretion, which leads to airway obstruction. The result is gross hyperinflation of the lungs along with localized areas of atelectasis. The predominant diagnostic feature on auscultation consists of widespread fine crackles, usually accompanied by diffuse high-pitched wheezes. Treatment consists of close monitoring, supplemental oxygen, and on rare instances mechanical ventilation, fluids, and often bronchial drainage with percussion and vibration, although the use of bronchial hygiene techniques is considered controversial by some. Although complete recovery usually occurs within 7 to 21 days, up to 80% of infants will have recurrent attacks of coughing and wheezing over the subsequent 2 to 3 years, and respiratory sequelae may continue into adulthood as asthma, increased airway resistance, and abnormal arterial oxygen levels.[21]

IMMOTILE CILIA SYNDROME

Immotile cilia syndrome (ICS) is an inherited disorder in which ultrastructural abnormalities in the cilia result in absent or disordered movement; there are a number of variants of this syndrome. Lack of or ineffective cilia motion results in the accumulation of secretions in the airways so that frequent bacterial infections occur in both the upper and the lower airways. Bronchiectasis is common by early adulthood. Daily prophylactic bronchial hygiene treatments are a major component of the management of children with ICS. In addition, regular aerobic exercise is recommended to assist with airway clearance and improve cardiorespiratory fitness.

α-1-ANTITRYPSIN DEFICIENCY

α-1-Antitrypsin deficiency is a rare inherited condition in which the level of antiproteases is only about 10% to 20% of normal; also called a-1-protease inhibitor deficiency. Because the proteases released by the normal phagocytic cells in the lungs are not inhibited, there is progressive damage to the pulmonary connective tissue and destruction of the alveolar walls. Emphysema often develops as early as age 30, especially in smokers and those with recurrent pulmonary infections (see page 85). However, dyspnea may occur as the initial manifestation during adolescence.

ASPIRATION SYNDROMES

Aspiration of material into the lungs is common in children and can range from asymptomatic to fatal. The most common causes of aspiration are foreign body aspiration, aspiration due to gastroesophageal reflux, and drowning.

- Aspiration may result in obstruction and/or inflammation of one or more airways, causing pneumonia, bronchiectasis, severe ventilation-perfusion abnormalities, and possible pulmonary edema and/or loss of surfactant. Because the right main stem bronchus is a more direct continuation of the trachea, aspiration tends to involve the right lung more frequently than the left lung. Severe gastroesophageal reflux with recurrent aspiration can result in chronic pulmonary disease and ultimately bronchiectasis.
- Clinical manifestations include unilateral absence of breath sounds and/or localized wheezing, stridor, bloody sputum, and possible respiratory distress.
- The best approach to treatment is prevention through parental education. Foreign objects must be removed by rigid bronchoscopy, whereas other causes of aspiration may require supportive care and antibiotics.

7.3 CARDIOPULMONARY DYSFUNCTION ASSOCIATED WITH NEUROLOGIC AND NEUROMUSCULAR DISORDERS

Neurologic dysfunction often affects respiratory function as a result of altered control of breathing, loss of protective reflexes, or abnormal control of the respiratory muscles. Neuromuscular disorders directly affect the function of the respiratory muscles, resulting in hypoventilation, impaired cough force, chronic aspiration, and ultimately respiratory failure; they may also affect the heart directly (see page 106). The most common disorders seen in infants and children are presented here: cerebral palsy, Down's syndrome, and Duchenne's dystrophy. Neurologic impairment can also develop during childhood due to infection, intracranial mass, cerebrovascular accident (usually secondary to congenital anomalies), or trauma. Other neuromuscular disorders that can affect children include Guillain-Barré syndrome, spinal cord injury, Werdnig-Hoffman's syndrome, Kugel-Welander disease, and familia disautonomia (Riley-Day syndrome).

CEREBRAL PALSY

Cerebral palsy (CP) includes a variety of nondegenerating neurologic disabilities caused by injuries in the prenatal and perinatal period that result in abnormalities of motor function.

- Depending on the extent of injury, there may be mental retardation, seizures, learning disabilities, language problems, sensory deficits, hearing impairment, and orthopedic problems; the motor difficulties may involve the lower extremities more than the upper extremities (i.e., spastic diplegia), all four extremities (i.e, spastic quadriplegia), or only one side of the body (i.e., spastic hemiplegia), or they may be characterized by hypotonia, choreoathetosis, and dystonic movements occurring later in life (i.e., extrapyramidal CP), or by marked hypotonia but brisk reflexes (i.e., atonic CP). Alternatively, there may be mixed forms of CP due to combinations of insults to multiple cerebral areas.
- Consequently, the effects on the respiratory system are extremely variable. However, children with CP often develop problems with poor chest expansion, abnormal breathing patterns, reduced cough effectiveness, abnormal chest wall configurations, and impaired phonation. In addition, general mobility is usually reduced.

DOWN'S SYNDROME

Also called trisomy 21 syndrome, Down's syndrome is the most common autosomal chromosomal abnormality in humans. The clinical manifestations include development delays, lower-than-average intelligence (although the range is wide), typical craniofacial features, and smaller stature than same-aged peers.

- Congenital heart disease occurs in almost 40% of Down's children and most commonly consists of endocardial cushion defect, atrial septal defect, ventricular septal defect, or tetralogy of Fallot (see pages 230 to 238).
- In addition, about 80% of infants with trisomy 21 syndrome are hypotonic at birth, which usually improves with age. These children often have poor airway clearance of both the upper and lower airways and are therefore more susceptible to pulmonary infections. In addition, postural abnormalities can also lead to restrictive lung dysfunction in older children.

MUSCULAR DYSTROPHIES

A group of hereditary conditions characterized by progressive degeneration of the striated muscles, the muscular dystrophies (MD) result in increasingly severe weakness. The most common type is Duchenne's dystrophy, which affects the proximal muscles of young children so that they are usually unable to walk by adolescence.

- Respiratory muscle weakness becomes a major problem by the teens, and most patients die of respiratory failure, usually related to pulmonary infection, by age 20.
- Cardiac involvement is also extremely common, with scarring of the posterobasal LV evidenced by typical ECG changes, multifocal dystrophic involvement of the conduction system manifested as arrhythmias and conduction disturbances, possible mitral valve prolapse or mitral regurgitation due to dystrophic involvement of the posteromedial papillary muscle, and cardiomyopathy.

CLINICAL IMPLICATIONS FOR PHYSICAL THERAPY

- Bronchial hygiene techniques may be indicated to assist with the removal of secretions, especially in more severely involved patients.
- Games and activities involving coordination of breathing patterns and increased ventilation are recommended to improve the efficiency of ventilation.
- Manual stretching and mobilization of the rib cage are beneficial for patients with reduced thoracic compliance resulting from muscle weakness, paralysis, or spasticity.

- Diaphragmatic strengthening exercises using abdominal weights, inspiratory resistive devices, or incentive spirometry (see page 208) are important for patients with neuromuscular disorders and can generally be performed by school-age children (or sometimes younger if they are part of a game).
- Coughing techniques should be taught and reinforced, especially following any activity.
- Activity level and ability to exercise varies a great deal according to the specific disorder and each child's degree of involvement.
  - Neurodevelopmental interventions are generally safe, but children at risk should be monitored (see below).
  - Generally speaking, the physical therapy program should include activities designed to increase or maintain chest wall mobility, improve posture, increase cardiorespiratory fitness, promote airway clearance, and improve level of function.
- Physiologic monitoring of exercise responses is indicated in high-risk children and usually consists of:
  - Heart rate
  - Blood pressure if arterial line in place (accurate cuff blood pressures are very difficult to obtain in these children)
  - Respiratory rate and pattern
  - Oxygen saturation, pulse oximetry
  - Skin color changes

7.4 PEDIATRIC PATIENT ASSESSMENT

The cardiopulmonary physical therapy assessment of infants and children is similar to that performed on adults, except for modifications required because of age and size.

MEDICAL CHART REVIEW

As with adults, a careful review of the physician and nursing admission and progress notes is extremely important. In the case of neonates and infants, special attention is directed to the following items:

- Complete history of labor and delivery
- Apgar scores (Table 7–10)
- Dubowitz gestational age scores
- Clinical course from birth to the present
- Any history of respiratory distress, oxygen use, and ventilatory assistance
- Arterial blood gas history and chest x-ray reports
- Mode and frequency of feedings
- Medical orders

DISCUSSION WITH THE NURSE OR PHYSICIAN

When dealing with infants and small children who are not able to express themselves clearly, it is critical to check in with the primary caretakers before any intervention is attempted. Important information to obtain includes:

- Current status of the infant or child
- Any evaluation or treatment procedures performed during the past few hours
- Time and mode of the last feeding
- Infant's response to handling (e.g., changes in heart rate, respiratory rate, and transcutaneous oxygen values)

TABLE 7–10. **Apgar Score for Newborn Infants**

	POINTS		
SIGNS	0	1	2
Heart rate	Absent	<100/min	>100/min
Respiration	Absent	Weak cry	Vigorous cry
Muscle tone	Limp	Some flexion of extremities	Arms, legs well flexed
Reflex irritability	None	Some motion	Cry, withdrawal
Color of body	Blue, pale	Pink body, blue extremities	Pink all over

The score is first taken 60 seconds after birth and may be repeated at 1- to 5-minute intervals until the total score reaches at least 8.

TABLE 7–11. **Important Observations When Assessing Infants and Children with Cardiopulmonary Dysfunction**

OBSERVATION	COMMENTS
Signs of respiratory distress	
Retractions	Can be suprasternal, substernal, intercostal, and subcostal in location; mild retractions are normal in infants.
Nasal flaring	A reflex that reduces airway resistance in the nasal passages.
Expiratory grunting	Increases functional residual capacity and improves the distribution of ventilation and the ventilation-perfusion relationship.
Stridor	Occurs on inspiration because of obstruction or collapse of the upper airway.
Head bobbing	Results from accessory muscle use to assist ventilation in infants with heavy heads.
Bulging of intercostal muscles	Occurs when obstruction to expiration creates high pleural pressures during expiration.
Chest configuration	A barrel-shaped chest indicates hyperinflation or air trapping within the lungs.
	Pectus excavatum (funnel chest) can result from prolonged periods of sternal retractions during the first month of life.
Skin color	
Cyanosis	When present (usually in the mucous membranes and around the lips and mouth), significant hypoxemia exists.
Plethora	Redness may be noted in infants with polycythemia.
Pallor, mottling, webbing	Commonly seen in distressed infants; may be associated with hypoxemia, sepsis, intraventricular hemorrhage, and other problems.
Breathing pattern	
Tachypnea	Respiratory rate >50/min; indicates respiratory distress.
Irregularity of respiration	Respiration is normally irregular in neonates; premature infants often display "periodic breathing" with 5 to 10-second apneic pauses not associated with cyanosis or bradycardia.
Apnea	Pauses in breathing of 20 or more seconds; indicates respiratory distress, sepsis, intraventricular hemorrhage, and other stresses in premature infants.
Coughing and sneezing	Normal protective mechanisms for the infant's airways; sneezing occurs more frequently in neonates; important to document if either occurs spontaneously or if coughing can be stimulated.
Other	
Vital signs	Vary with age (see Table 7–12).
Transcutaneous oxygen ($TcPO_2$)	Values obtained generally run 5–10 mm Hg below arterial values as a result of some absorption by skin.
Oxygen saturation (SaO_2)	Values must be interpreted within the context of infant's respiratory and metabolic status, since shifts of the oxygen-hemoglobin curve will change the affinity of oxygen and hemoglobin; motion artifact can be a problem.
Peripheral circulation	Pallor, cyanosis, weblike markings of extremities, cool extremities, and poor correlation of $TcPO_2$ and PaO_2 values indicate poor circulation.
Skeletal system	↓ Calcium, ↓ phosphate, and other vitamin deficiencies can result in rickets or osteoporosis; scoliosis can cause thoracic deformity and restrictive lung dysfunction.
Neuromuscular system	Often affected by prematurity, hypoxia, and various pre- and perinatal problems; evaluation should include assessment of primitive reflexes, muscle tone, limb movements and patterns, sucking and swallowing, deep tendon reflexes, behaviors, state of quiet alertness, and range of motion.
Nutritional support	Mode of feeding may affect treatment (e.g., infants fed orally or orogastrally are often kept on their right sides for 20–30 min to assist in gastric emptying); also, abdominal distension may interfere with ventilation, especially in the head-down position.

PHYSICAL ASSESSMENT

As with adults, the physical assessment of infants and children consists of inspection/observations, auscultation, palpation, and percussion. However, in neonates and small infants, the techniques are modified because of the small body size.

- Important observations that provide information specific to the cardiopulmonary status of infants and small children are presented in Table 7–11. Otherwise the items of observation are similar to those of adults, except for the normal values for vital signs, which vary with age and are presented in Table 7–12.
- Because of their thin chest walls, proximity of major airways, and enhanced transmission of sound, auscultation of the breath sounds is a gross assessment, at best, in infants and children, especially if mechanical ventilation is being used. Auscultation of the heart may reveal the murmurs of persistent fetal circulation (e.g., PDA or atrial septal defect, which can develop as a result of hypoxic vasoconstriction and pulmonary HTN due to neonatal lung disease) or congenital heart disease.
  - To improve the accuracy of findings, any water within the ventilator tubing should be emptied and auscultation of the mechanically assisted breaths should be performed.
  - Whenever possible, the infant's head should be in the midline position, since breath sounds will be decreased on the opposite side of a turned head.
  - In infants, the location of abnormal breath sounds does not necessarily correspond with the underlying lung segment; therefore, findings should be correlated with chest x-ray findings prior to treatment.
- Palpation is mainly performed in order to assess tracheal, and thus mediastinal, deviation and to document subcutaneous emphysema, edema, or rib fracture.
  - Because the chest walls of tiny infants move very little, the symmetry of their expansion is usually not palpated.
  - However, symmetry of motion can be assessed in older infants and children, and paradoxical chest motion can be palpated in the neonate.
- The technique for performing percussion varies according to the size of the infant, as do the indications.
  - Direct, or immediate, percussion is used in small infants mainly for determining the presence of pneumothoraces, diaphragmatic hernia, enlarged liver, and masses.

TABLE 7-12. **Changes in Vital Signs as a Function of Age**

AGE	MEAN HEART RATE ±2 S.D.	MEAN BLOOD PRESSURE (MM HG)	MEAN RESPIRATORY RATE (BPM)
Premature neonate	125 ± 50	35–56 systolic (birth to 7 days)	40–60
Full-term neonate	140 ± 50	75/50	30–40
Infant			
1–6 months	130 ± 45	80/46	30–40
6–12 months	115 ± 40	96/65	30
Preschool			
1–2 years	110 ± 40	99/65	25–30
2–6 years	105 ± 35	100/60	25
School			
6–8 years	95 ± 30	105/60	20–25
8–12 years	95 ± 30	110/60	20
Adolescence			
12–14 years	82 ± 25	118/60	16–20
14–18 years	82 ± 25	120/65	14–18
Adult	72 ± 25	127/76	12–15

- Mediate, or indirect, percussion is used in the usual manner in larger infants and children, as described in Chapter 5 (see page 169).

7.5 CARDIOPULMONARY PHYSICAL THERAPY TREATMENT

The principles of physical therapy treatment for infants and children with cardiopulmonary dysfunction are the same as for adults; however, treatment modifications are necessary because of size, physiologic differences, and psychosocial immaturity. Specific modifications are presented in this section.

BRONCHIAL HYGIENE TECHNIQUES

The techniques used with infants and small children include bronchial drainage positioning, chest percussion and vibration, cough stimulation, and airway suctioning. For older children, all the treatment techniques used with adults can be used, although more creativity is required in order to obtain cooperation of most children. As with adults, treatment modifications may be required because of the specifics of each patient's condition. In the sick neonate, especially a premature infant, careful assessment of the risks and benefits of treatment and each specific procedure is required because of the infant's intolerance of stimulation, including routine care. The most appropriate and safe treatment program must be individually designed to meet the needs of each infant.

- Bronchial drainage employs the same 12 positions used in adults since the neonate's bronchial tree is completely developed (see description on page 212).
  - Infants and small children can be positioned on the therapist's lap or on pillows, as shown in Figure 7–9, which is often soothing to the child.
  - Essential points for performing bronchial drainage in infants are listed in Table 7–13.
  - Precautions and contraindications for bronchial drainage in the neonate are presented in Table 7–14.
  - Positioning, especially prone, can also be used to increase ventilation and improve ventilation-perfusion matching.

- The manual techniques of chest percussion and vibration, which are used in conjunction with bronchial drainage to assist in the removal of secretions, are often modified to conform to the size of the infant or child.
  - There are many precautions and contraindications for the use of these techniques, especially chest percussion and vibration, in the neonate, which are listed in Tables 7–15 and 7–16.
  - When chest percussion is employed to treat small infants, a commercially available or adapted percussion device can be utilized (Fig. 7–10) or the hand position can be modified (Fig. 7–11 and 7–12).
  - Vibration is performed with only one hand on premature and small infants, as demonstrated in Figure 7–13.
  - Essential points for performing chest percussion and vibration in small infants are listed in Table 7–17.
- Following bronchial drainage with or without chest percussion and vibration, infants usually need assistance in clearing the loosened secretions.
  - Suctioning is required, but is always potentially dangerous for the infant.
  - Otherwise, the nasal and oral pharynges can be suctioned and an attempt at cough stimulation can be made. If the infant has an adequate cough, suctioning should be deferred.
  - The suggested procedure for performing suctioning is described in Table 7–18.
  - Hypoxemia and hyperoxemia can be minimized during suctioning if transcutaneous oxygen levels are monitored.
- Older children should be encouraged to cough or huff to clear secretions. Use of games and stories to elicit coughing is usually the most successful (e.g., stickers as rewards, *The Three Little Pigs*).
- Other treatment techniques (described in Chapter 6) that can be used with older children include:
  - Instruction in positions for breathlessness
  - Deep breathing exercises and breathing retraining
  - Shaking
  - Coughing
  - Physical exercises and conditioning
  - Postural exercises

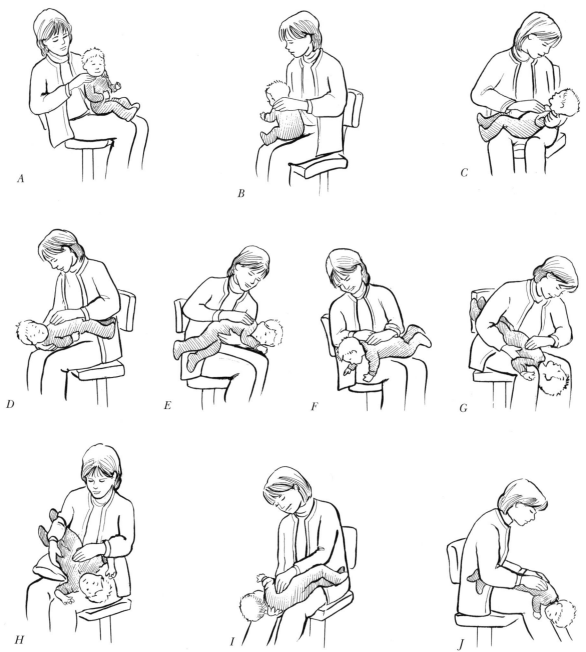

FIGURE 7–9. The 12 positions for bronchial drainage in infants performed on the lap or using pillows. *(A),* Apical segments of both upper lobes (BUL). *(B),* Posterior segment of left upper lobe (LUL). *(C),* Anterior segment of LUL. *(D),* Anterior segment of right upper lobe (RUL). *(E),* Posterior segment of RUL. *(F),* Superior, or apical, segments of both lower lobes (BLL). *(G),* Anterior segments of BLL. *(H),* Right middle lobe (also done on other side for lingular segment of LUL). *(I),* Lateral segment of right lower lobe (RLL) (also done on other side for lateral segment of left lower lobe (LLL). *(J),* Posterior segments of BLL.

TABLE 7-13. **Essential Points in Performing Bronchial Drainage in Infants**

1. Care should be taken to coordinate any change in the infant's position with other nursing procedures to avoid unnecessary stimulation.
2. Infants should never be left unattended when in a head-down position.
3. Vital signs should be monitored closely by respiration and heart rate monitors. The alarms should be turned on!
4. The infant's chest should be auscultated for bilateral breath sounds after positioning.
5. While the infant is in a drainage position, secretions will be more easily mobilized. The infant's trachea or endotracheal tube should be suctioned as needed.
6. Avoid placing the infant in a head-down position for approximately 1 hour after eating to avoid aspiration of regurgitated food.
7. Any change in the infant's position should be done slowly to minimize stress on the cardiovascular system.
8. Infants with umbilical arterial lines *may* be placed on their abdomens. However, one should always check that the line has not been kinked.
9. Some infants might require modified drainage positions. Infants with severe cardiovascular instability or suspected intracranial bleeding should not be placed in a head-down position.

From Crane L: The neonate and child. *In* Frownfelter DL: *Chest Physical Therapy and Pulmonary Rehabilitation,* 2nd Ed. Chicago, Year Book Medical Publishers, Inc., p. 679, 1987. Used with permission.

TABLE 7-14. **Precautions and Contraindications for Bronchial Drainage in Neonates**

POSITION	PRECAUTION	CONTRAINDICATION
Prone	Umbilical arterial catheter Continuous positive airway pressure in nose Excessive abdominal distention Abdominal incision Anterior chest tube	Untreated tension pneumothorax
Trendelenburg position (head-down)	Distended abdomen SEH/IVH (grades I and II) Chronic congestive heart failure or cor pulmonale Persistent fetal circulation Cardiac dysrhythmias Apnea and bradycardia Infant exhibiting signs of acute respiratory distress Hydrocephalus Less than 28 weeks' gestational age	Untreated tension pneumothorax Recent tracheoesophageal fistula repair Recent eye or intracranial surgery Intraventricular hemorrhage (grades III and IV) Acute congestive heart failure or cor pulmonale

From Crane LD: Physical therapy for the neonate with respiratory disease. *In* Irwin S, Tecklin JS: *Cardiopulmonary Physical Therapy,* 2nd Ed. St. Louis, The C.V. Mosby Co., p. 406, 1990. Used with permission.
SEH/IVH = subependymal hemorrhage/intraventricular hemorrhage.

TABLE 7-15. **Precautions and Contra-indications for Chest Percussion in Neonates**

PRECAUTIONS	CONTRAINDICATIONS
Poor condition of skin	Intolerance to treatment as indicated by low TcPO$_2$ values
Coagulopathy	
Presence of a chest tube	
Healing thoracic incision	Rib fracture
Osteoporosis and rickets	Hemoptysis
Persistent fetal circulation	
Cardiac dysrhythmias	
Apnea and bradycardia	
Signs of acute respiratory distress	
Increased irritability during treatment	
Subcutaneous emphysema	
Bronchospasm, wheezing, rhonchi	
Subependymal hemorrhage/intraventricular hemorrhage (SEH/IVH)	
Prematurity (less than 28 weeks gestational age)	

From Crane LD: Physical therapy for the neonate with respiratory disease. *In* Irwin S, Tecklin JS: *Cardiopulmonary Physical Therapy,* 2nd Ed. St. Louis, The C.V. Mosby Co., p. 408, 1990. Used with permission.

TABLE 7-16. **Precautions and Contra-indications for Vibration in Neonates**

PRECAUTIONS	CONTRAINDICATIONS
Increased irritability/crying during treatment	Untreated tension pneumothorax
Persistent fetal circulation	Intolerance to treatment as indicated by low TcPO$_2$ values
Apnea and bradycardia	Hemoptysis

From Crane LD: Physical therapy for the neonate with respiratory distress. *In* Irwin S, Tecklin JS: *Cardiopulmonary Physical Therapy,* 2nd Ed. St. Louis, The C.V. Mosby Co., p. 408, 1990. Used with permission.

ENDURANCE EXERCISE TRAINING

Children with chronic lung and heart disease usually have reduced exercise tolerance compared with their healthy peers. However, most can safety participate in monitored exercise programs and achieve the same benefits of training as other children. Careful monitoring initially helps to avoid overexertion and deleterious responses, but the monitoring can be reduced and eliminated as the child progresses through the program. The principles of exercise training for children are the same as those for adults (see Chapter 6), although aerobic activities need to

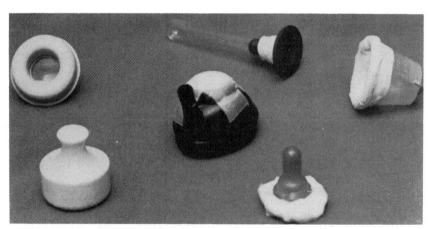

FIGURE 7-10. Commercially available and adapted devices for chest percussion on small infants (From Crane LD: Physical therapy for the neonate with respiratory disease. *In* Irwin S, Tecklin JS: *Cardiopulmonary Physical Therapy,* 2nd Ed. St. Louis, The C.V. Mosby Co., p. 409, 1990. Used with permission.)

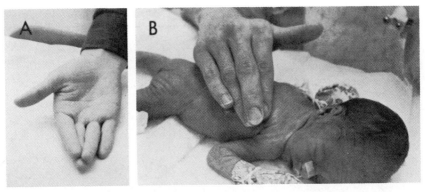

FIGURE 7-11. Tenting of the fingers for performing manual chest percussion on premature or small infants. (From Crane L: The neonate and child. *In* Frownfelter DL: *Chest Physical Therapy and Pulmonary Rehabilitation,* 2nd Ed. Chicago, Year Book Medical Publishers, Inc., 1987. Used with permission.)

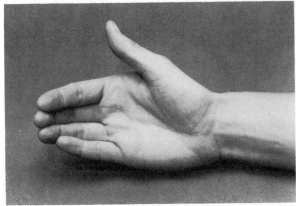 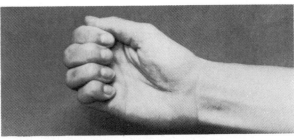

A   *B*

FIGURE 7-12. Hand modifications that can be used for performing manual chest percussion on infants and small toddlers. *(A),* Four fingers cupped for percussion. *(B),* Thenar and hypothenar surfaces for percussion. (From Crane LD: Physical therapy for the neonate with respiratory disease. *In* Irwin S, Tecklin JS: *Cardiopulmonary Physical Therapy,* 2nd Ed. St. Louis, The C.V. Mosby Co., p. 409, 1990. Used with permission.)

FIGURE 7-13. Manual chest wall vibration of a premature infant. (From Crane L: The neonate and child. *In* Frownfelter DL: *Chest Physical Therapy and Pulmonary Rehabilitation,* 2nd Ed. Chicago, Year Book Medical Publishers, Inc., p. 690, 1987. Used with permission.)

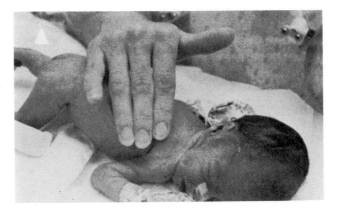

TABLE 7–17. **Essential Points for Performing Chest Percussion and Vibration in Small Infants**

1. Chest percussion can be administered manually or with one of a variety of percussion devices; the choice is personal and depends on the size of the therapist's hand, the infant, and the shape of the area to be treated. Regardless of the method used, a cupping effect should be maintained.
2. Although most percussion techniques cover a larger area than the specific lung segment being treated, it is important to avoid percussing over the liver, spleen, and kidneys by paying close attention to the borders of the lungs and surface anatomy.
3. In most cases a thin sheet or article of clothing can be used to cover the area being treated. The exception is when careful observation of anatomic landmarks and signs of respiratory distress is important.
4. The infant's chest should be supported firmly during percussion.
5. Vibration can be applied manually or using a mechanical vibrator or an electric toothbrush with foam padding of the bristle portion.
6. The time necessary for effective drainage is considered to be a minimum of 3–5 min per position, but sometimes has to be shortened if a position is not tolerated well.
7. Since bronchial drainage is often fatiguing, the areas of greatest involvement should be treated first, followed by the less involved areas.
8. Careful attention to the infant's responses to treatment is important, particularly in sick neonates; heart rate, respiratory rate, and transcutaneous oxygen values should be monitored, if available.

TABLE 7–18. **Procedure for Suctioning Infants**

STEP	PROCEDURES
1. Preparation	Place the infant in the supine position, preferably with the head in the midline position.
	Check that the suction apparatus is functioning properly and is connected, the suction is turned on, and the vacuum level is set between −60 and −80 cm H_2O.
	Make sure the oxygen flow is turned on and attached to the self-inflating breathing bag and the pressure manometer is connected.
	Check to see what pressures the ventilator is delivering or what pressure is required to properly ventilate the infant.
2. Hyperventilation	Using a self-inflating bag, an artificial airway connector, and the pressure noted in Step 1, hyperventilate the infant at approximately 20 bpm above the rate set on the ventilator (maximum of 60 bpm).
	Hyperoxygenate the infant using an oxygen concentration 10–20% higher than the level set on the ventilator; if the FIO_2 is 0.5 or higher, use 100% oxygen.
	Hyperventilation and hyperoxygenation should precede and follow each pass with the suction catheter.
3. Lavage (optional)	Instill 0.5–1.0 mL, or 2–3 drops, of sterile normal saline solution (NaCl) directly into the endotracheal or tracheostomy tube.
4. Suction	Using sterile technique:
	Wet the catheter in the sterile solution.
	Insert the catheter (with no suction applied) into the airway until resistance is met.
	Pull the catheter back slightly and then withdraw the catheter while applying intermittent suction and turning the catheter (should not last longer than 10 seconds).
	Repeat if necessary until there are no more secretions.
	Suction the nasal and oral pharynges.

bpm = breaths per minute, FIO_2 = fraction of inspired oxygen.

be fun and varied for the children to maintain interest. Noncompetitive games are usually the most successful.

REFERENCES

1. Aloan CA: *Respiratory Care of the Newborn: A Clinical Manual.* Philadelphia, J.B. Lippincott Co., 1987.
2. Bates DW: *Respiratory Function in Disease,* 3rd Ed. Philadelphia, W.B. Saunders Co, 1989.
3. Behrman RE, Kliegman R: *Nelson Essentials of Pediatrics.* Philadelphia, W.B. Saunders Co, 1990.
4. Bertranaou EG, Blackstone EH, Hazelrig JB, et al.: Life expectancy without surgery in tetralogy of Fallot. *Am. J. Cardiol.* 42:458, 1978.
5. Braunwald E (ed.): *Heart Disease— A Textbook of Cardiovascular Medicine,* 4th Ed. Philadelphia, W.B. Saunders Co, 1992.
6. Brewis RAL, Gibson GJ, Geddes DM (eds.): *Respiratory Medicine.* London, Bailliére Tindall, 1990.
7. Burton GG, Hodgkin JE, Ward JJ (eds.): *Respiratory Care. A Guide to Clinical Practice,* 3rd Ed. Philadelphia, J.B. Lippincott Co., 1992.
8. Cherniack RM, Cherniack L: *Respiration in Health and Disease,* 3rd Ed. Philadelphia, W.B. Saunders Co, 1983.
9. Crane L: Physical therapy for neonates with respiratory dysfunction. *Phys. Ther.* 61:1764, 1981.
10. Crane L: The neonate and child. *In* Frownfelter DL: *Chest Physical Therapy and Pulmonary Rehabilitation,* 2nd Ed. Chicago, Year Book Medical Publishers, Inc., 1987.
11. Crane LD: Physical therapy for the neonate with respiratory disease. *In* Irwin S, Tecklin JS: *Cardiopulmonary Physical Therapy,* 2nd Ed. St. Louis, The C.V. Mosby Co., 1990.
12. Farzan S: *A Concise Handbook of Respiratory Diseases,* 3rd Ed. Norwalk, CT, Appleton & Lange, 1992.
13. Flenley DC: *Respiratory Medicine,* 2nd Ed. London, Bailliére Tindall, 1990.
14. Hoffman JI: Congenital heart disease. *Ped. Clin. North Am.* 37:25–43, 1990.
15. Hurst JW (ed.): *The Heart, Arteries and Veins,* 7th Ed. New York, McGraw-Hill Information Services Co., 1990.
16. Johnson TR, Moore WM, Jeffries JE (eds.): *Children Are Different: Developmental Physiology,* 2nd Ed. Columbus, OH, Ross Laboratories, 1978.
17. Kaplan TA, ZeBranek JD, McKey RM: Use of exercise in the management of cystic fibrosis. *Pediatr. Pulmonol.* 10:205–207, 1991.
18. Kloner RA (ed.): *The Guide to Cardiology,* 2nd Ed. New York, Le Jacq Communications, 1990.
19. Lannefors L, Wollmer P: Mucus clearance with three chest physiotherapy regimes in cystic fibrosis. A comparison between postural drainage, PEP, and physical exercise. *Eur. Resp. J.* 5:748–753, 1992.
20. McFadden R: Decreasing respiratory compromise during infant suctioning. *Am. J. Nurs.* 81:2158, 1981.
21. Sly PD, Hibbert ME: Childhood asthma following hospitalization with acute viral bronchiolitis in infancy. *Pediatr. Pulmonol.* 7:153–158, 1989.
22. Sokolow M, McIlroy MB: *Clinical Cardiology,* 4th Ed. Los Altos, CA, Lange Medical Publications, 1986.
23. Wyngaarden JB, Smith LH Jr., Bennett JC (eds.): *Cecil Textbook of Medicine,* 19th Ed. Philadelphia, W.B. Saunders Co., 1992.

8

LABORATORY MEDICINE

This chapter contains normal reference values for many common laboratory tests, as well as a few diagnostic profiles. Because each clinical laboratory has its own set of reference values, depending on its specific assaying techniques, the listed values should be used only as a general guide. The reader should compare a patient's test results to the reference values produced by the laboratory that ran the tests. The main purpose of this chapter is to provide the most common causes of abnormally high or low values for each analyte.

8.1 SHORTHAND FOR LABORATORY VALUES

To simplify recording of patients' laboratory values, some shorthand notations have been developed, which are commonly found in medical charts. They are illustrated in Figure 8–1.

8.2 SERUM CHEMISTRY

Analysis of blood chemistry is commonly performed as an adjunct to physical examination to determine the presence of medical problems, clarify a diagnosis, and monitor the progression of disease. Many laboratories offer "panel" tests, whereby multiple determinations are performed on a single blood sample. For example, the SMA-6 includes sodium, potassium, chloride, carbon dioxide, blood urea nitrogen, and glucose; the ASTRA-7 consists of the SMA-6 plus creatinine; and the SMA-12 is composed of the SMA-6 plus creatinine, lactate dehydrogenase, serum

glutamic-oxaloacetic transaminase, serum glutamic-pyruvic transaminase, protein, and albumin.

- Normal reference values for serum chemistry analytes according to the Massachusetts General Hospital[4] are listed in Table 8–1, along with some causes of abnormally high or low values.[1–3,5–9]

8.3 HEMATOLOGY

Analysis of the blood cells themselves is achieved through the complete blood cell count, which indicates the number of red and white blood cells in a cubic millimeter of blood, the erythrocyte indices, hematocrit, and differential percentages of the various types of white blood cells.

- Table 8–2 lists normal reference values for the complete blood cell count[4] and some common causes of abnormally high and low values.[1,2,5,9]
- Other hematologic analytes, including erythrocyte sedimentation rate, ferritin, folate, and reticulocyte count, are presented with some more common causes of excessively high and low values in Table 8–3.[1,2,5,9]
- Common terminology for various hematologic abnormalities and their clinical definitions are depicted in Table 8–4.

8.4 COAGULATION STUDIES

Another important function that can be monitored via blood tests is the control of blood coagulation so that there is neither excessive bleeding nor clot formation.

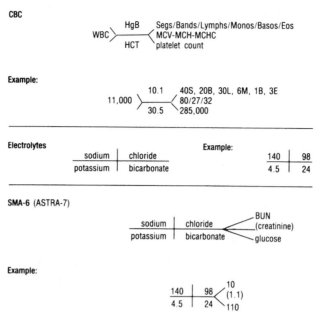

FIGURE 8–1. Shorthand notation for recording laboratory values. The ASTR-7 is identical to the SMA-6 except that the creatinine is also noted. (From Gomella LG (ed.): *Clinician's Pocket Reference,* 7th Ed. Norwalk, CT, Appleton & Lange, 1993. Used with permission.)

- Normal reference values for coagulation studies[4] and some common causes of abnormalities are listed in Table 8–5.[1,2,5,9]

8.5 SELECTED IMMUNOLOGIC STUDIES

Immunologic studies allow medical personnel to monitor the immune system, the presence of antigen-antibody reactions, and related changes within the blood.

- Table 8–6 enumerates selected immunologic analytes, their normal reference values,[4] and common causes of abnormalities.[1,2,5,9]

8.6 ARTERIAL BLOOD GASES

Arterial blood gases (ABGs) are used to assess the adequacy of ventilation, oxygenation, and acid-base status.

- Normal values for ABGs are listed in Table 8–7.
- Information related to the interpretation of ABGs can be found on pages 189 to 191.

HYPOXIA

- Low concentrations of oxygen in the arterial blood can result from several disorders, as described in Chapter 3. In summary, hypoxia may result from:
  - Ventilation-perfusion abnormalities (e.g., chronic obstructive pulmonary disease (COPD), restrictive lung dysfunction)
  - Alveolar hypoventilation (e.g., skeletal abnormalities, neuromuscular disorders)
  - Decreased pulmonary diffusion capacity (e.g., pulmonary edema, pulmonary fibrosis)
  - Right-to-left shunt (e.g., congenital heart defects)

Text continued on page 269

TABLE 8-1. **Normal Reference Values for Serum Analytes***

ANALYTE	REFERENCE VALUES	SOME CAUSES OF ABNORMAL RESULTS
Alanine aminotransferase (ALT, SGPT)	F: 7–30 U/L M: 10–55 U/L	Increased: liver disease (hepatitis, cirrhosis, Reye's syndrome; alcoholism), muscle trauma, rhabdomyolysis, acute pancreatitis, myositis, drugs (heparin, salicylates), obesity, severe preeclampsia, acute MI.
Albumin	3.1–4.3 g/dL	Increased: dehydration, IV albumin infusions. Decreased: malnutrition, malabsorption, ↑ need (hyperthyroidism, pregnancy), impaired synthesis (liver disease, chronic infection, hereditary analbuminemia), ↑ breakdown (neoplasms, infection, trauma), ↑ loss (edema, ascites, burns, hemorrhage, nephrotic syndrome, protein-losing enteropathies), dilutional (IV fluids, SIADH, water intoxication).
Aldolase	0–7 U/L	Increased: cell destruction (acute MI, burns, hemolytic anemia, acute hepatitis, acute pancreatitis, muscular dystrophies, myopathies, polymyositis, prostate cancer; gangrene, rhabdomyolysis). Decreased: ↓ muscle mass, late stages of muscular dystrophy.
Alkaline phosphatase	F: 30–100 U/L M: 45–115 U/L	Increased: ↑ deposition of calcium in bone (hyperparathyroidism, Paget's disease, osteoblastic bone tumors, osteogenesis imperfecta, osteomalacia, rickets, late pregnancy, childhood), liver disease with obstruction of the biliary system (stone, carcinoma, metastatic tumor, abscess, cyst, TB, amyloid, sarcoid, leukemia), drugs (phenobarbital, phenytoin). Decreased: excess vitamin D, milk-alkali syndrome, scurvy, hypothyroidism, celiac disease, malnutrition.
Ammonia (plasma)	12–55 μmol/L	Increased: severe liver disease, GU tract infection with distention and stasis, transient ↑ in newborn, moribund children, drugs (methicillin, ammonia cycle resins, chlorthalidone, spironolactone). Decreased: renal failure, drugs (neomycin, tetracycline, lactulose, MAO inhibitors).
Amylase	53–123 U/L	Increased: acute pancreatitis, pancreatic duct obstruction (stones, stricture, tumor, sphincter spasm due to drugs), mumps, renal disease, peptic ulcers, cholecystitis, diabetic ketoacidosis, parotiditis, intestinal obstruction. Decreased: advanced chronic pancreatitis, cystic fibrosis, hepatic necrosis.

*All reference values are those used at the Massachusetts General Hospital[a] unless otherwise footnoted.
↓ = decreased, ↑ = increased, ACTH = adrenocorticotropic hormone, ADH = antidiuretic hormone, ANS = autonomic nervous system, CHF = congestive heart failure, CML = chronic myelogenous leukemia, CNS = central nervous system, DM = diabetes mellitus, F = female, GI = gastrointestinal, GU = genitourinary, IM = intramuscular, IV = intravenous, M = male, MAO = monoamine oxidase, MI = myocardial infarction, NG = nasogastric, PTCA = percutaneous transluminal coronary angioplasty, RA = rheumatoid arthritis, SIADH = syndrome of inappropriate secretion of antidiuretic hormone, SVT = supraventricular tachycardia, TB = tuberculosis.

Continued on following page

Continued on following page

TABLE 8–1. Normal Reference Values for Serum Analytes *Continued*

ANALYTE	REFERENCE VALUES	SOME CAUSES OF ABNORMAL RESULTS
Angiotensin converting enzyme (ACE level)	10–50 U/L	Increased: sarcoidosis, primary biliary cirrhosis, alcoholism, hyperthyroidism, hyperparathyroidism, DM, amyloidosis, multiple myeloma, lung disease (asbestosis, berylliosis, silicosis, allergic alveolitis, coccidioidomycosis), Gaucher's disease, leprosy. Decreased: azotemia, chronic renal dialysis; factitiously in diabetic ketoacidosis, beriberi, severe liver disease.
Arterial blood gases	See page 274.	
Antistreptolysin O titer (ASO Titer)[2]	≤160 Todd units/mL	Increased: acute or recent streptococcal infections (pharyngitis, scarlet fever, rheumatic fever, glomerulonephritis), RA and other collagen vascular diseases.
Aspartrate aminotransferase (AST, SGOT)	F: 9–25 U/L M: 10–40 U/L	Increased: acute MI, liver disease, musculoskeletal diseases (including trauma, surgery, IM injections), acute pancreatitis, other organ infections, local radiation therapy, burns, heat exhaustion.
Bicarbonate (HCO$_3^-$)	22–26 mEq/L (varies according to age)	Increased: respiratory acidosis (emphysema, respiratory failure), compensated metabolic alkalosis (severe vomiting, NG suction), primary aldosteronism, Barter's syndrome. Decreased: respiratory alkalosis (hyperventilation, severe CNS damage), compensated metabolic acidosis (ketoacidosis, lactic acidosis), renal failure, toxins, adrenal insufficiency, drugs (salicylates, acetazolamide).
Bilirubin	Total: 0–1.0 mg/dL Direct: <0.5 mg/dL	Increased: hepatic cellular damage, biliary obstruction, hemolytic diseases, prolonged fasting. Decreased: drugs (barbiturates).
Blood urea nitrogen (BUN)	8–25 mg/dL	Increased: renal failure, prerenal azotemia (CHF, salt and water depletion, shock), postrenal azotemia, GI bleed, acute MI, stress, drugs (aminoglycosides). Decreased: severe liver disease (drugs, poisoning, hepatitis), ↑ use of protein for synthesis (late pregnancy, infancy, acromegaly, malnutrition, anabolic steroids), diet (low protein and high carbohydrate, IV feedings only, impaired absorption [celiac disease], malnutrition), nephrotic syndrome, SIADH.
Calcium (Ca^{++})	Total: 8.5–10.5 mg/dL Ionized (plasma): 1.14–1.3 mmol/L	Increased: hyperparathyroidism, malignant tumors, vitamin D intoxication, milk-alkali syndrome, acute osteoporosis (immobilization of young patients, Paget's disease), granulomatous diseases, (sarcoidosis, TB, mycoses, berylliosis), some patients with hyperthyroidism or hypothyroidism, following renal transplantation, polyuric phase of renal failure, drugs (diuretics, thyroid hormone, estrogens, androgens, progestins, tamoxifen, lithium). Decreased: hypoparathyroidism, malabsorption of Ca^{++} and vitamin D, obstructive jaundice, hypoalbuminemia, acute pancreatitis, chronic renal disease, osteomalacia, rickets, starvation, late pregnancy, drugs (citrated banked blood, mithramycin, fluoride intoxication, gentamycin, phenobarbital, phenytoin, cisplatinum, loop diuretics, calcitonin), respiratory distress, asphyxia, cerebral injuries, neonates with high bilirubinemia.

Test	Reference Value	Interpretation
Carcinoembryonic antigen (CEA)	0–3.0 ng/mL	Increased: carcinoma (colon, pancreas, lung, stomach), smokers, nonneoplastic liver disease, Crohn's disease, ulcerative colitis.
Chloride (Cl⁻)	100–108 mmol/L	Increased: metabolic acidosis due to prolonged diarrhea or renal disease, respiratory alkalosis (hyperventilation, severe CNS damage), diabetes insipidus, intestinal fistulas, dehydration, ureterosigmoidostomy, certain drug excesses (ammonium chloride, IV saline, steroids, salicylates, acetazolamide). Decreased: prolonged vomiting or NG suction, metabolic acidosis with accumulation of organic anions, chronic respiratory acidosis, salt-losing renal diseases, water intoxication, adrenocortical insufficiency, SIADH, primary aldosteronism, hyponatremia, CHF, burns.
Cholesterol	Desirable: <200 mg/dL Borderline: 200–239 mg/dL High risk: ≥240 mg/dL	Increased: hyperlipoproteinemia, idiopathic hypercholesterolemia, biliary obstruction, nephrosis, hypothyroidism, DM, pregnancy, MI, drugs (steroids, phenothiazines, oral contraceptives). Decreased: starvation, malabsorption, sideroblastic anemia, thalassemia, hyperthyroidism, hypolipoproteinemias, liver failure, Cushing's syndrome, multiple myeloma, CML, myeloid metaplasia, myelofibrosis.
Creatine kinase (CK, CPK)	F: 40–150 U/L M: 60–400 U/L	Increased: muscle damage (acute MI, myocarditis, muscular dystrophy, trauma, IM injections, after surgery, status epilepticus, thermal and electrical burns), brain infarction, rhabdomyolysis, myositis, hypothyroidism, acromegaly, malignant hyperthermia, late pregnancy and parturition, vigorous exercise.
CK (MB fraction)	0–7.5 ng/mL (≤5%) Relative index: 0–3%	Increased: necrosis of myocardial cells (acute MI, contusion, PTCA, cardioversion, surgery, pericarditis, prolonged SVT), skeletal muscle disease or trauma, alcoholism, Reye's syndrome, acute cholecystitis, carcinomas, hypothyroidism, drugs (aspirin, tranquilizers).
Creatinine	0.6–1.5 mg/dL	Increased: ingestion of raw meat, acromegaly, gigantism, azotemia, impaired renal function. Decreased: not clinically significant.
Erythrocyte sedimentation rate	See page 270.	
Gamma-glutamyl transpeptidase (GGT) (plasma)	1.0–60.0 U/L	Increased: liver disease, pancreatitis, acute MI, alcoholism, drugs (barbiturates, phenytoin), neoplasms, CHF.
Glucose (fasting) (plasma)	70–110 mg/dL	Increased: DM, hemochromatosis, Cushing's syndrome, acromegaly, gigantism, ↑ circulating epinephrine (adrenaline injection, pheochromocytoma, stress [emotional], burns, shock, acute MI, anesthesia), ↓ vitamin B, pancreatitis, some CNS lesions, drugs (estrogens, corticosteroids, alcohol, phenytoin, thiazides, propranolol, chronic ↑ vitamin A). Decreased: pancreatic disorders, neoplasms (adrenal gland, stomach, fibrosarcoma, others), hepatic disease [diffuse or severe], endocrine disorders (Addison's disease, hypopituitarism, hypothyroidism, early DM), functional disturbances (following gastrectomy or gastroenterostomy, ANS disorders), malnutrition, alcoholism, some pediatric anomalies and enzyme diseases.

Continued on following page

TABLE 8-1. Normal Reference Values for Serum Analytes *Continued*

ANALYTE	REFERENCE VALUES	SOME CAUSES OF ABNORMAL RESULTS
High-density lipoprotein (HDL) cholesterol[2]	F: ≥43 mg/dL M: ≥33 mg/dL	Decreased: uremia, diabetes, liver disease, ↓ apoproteins, Tangier's disease.
Lactate dehydrogenase (LDH)	110–210 U/L	Increased: acute MI, cardiac surgery, prosthetic heart valve, hepatitis, malignant tumors, pulmonary embolus and infarction, myelogenous leukemia, diseases of muscle, burns, trauma, renal diseases (nephrotic syndrome, nephritis), hemolytic anemia, pernicious anemia, various infections and parasitic diseases, hypothyroidism, collagen vascular diseases, acute pancreatitis, intestinal obstruction, sarcoidosis. Decreased: x-ray irradiation.
LDH isoenzymes:	LDH_1 17–27% LDH_2 28–38% LDH_3 18–28% LDH_4 5–15% LDH_5 5–15%	If $LDH_1/LDH_2 > 1.0$: recent MI (level starts to rise at 12–48 hours). If $LDH_5 > LDH_4$: liver disease.
Lactic acid (plasma)	0.5–2.2 mmol/L	Increased lactic acidosis due to hypoxia, hemorrhage, shock, sepsis, cirrhosis, exercise.
Lipase	4–24 U/dL	Increased: acute pancreatitis, pancreatic duct obstruction, fat embolus syndrome, perforated peptic ulcer, mumps.
Low-density lipoprotein (LDL) cholesterol	Desirable: ≤ 129 mg/dL Borderline: 130–159 mg/dL High risk: ≥ 160 mg/dL	Increased: excess dietary saturated fats, acute MI, DM, primary hyperlipoproteinemia, primary biliary cirrhosis, nephrosis, hypothyroidism.
Magnesium (Mg^+)	1.5–2.0 mEq/L	Increased: renal failure, hypothyroidism, Mg^+-containing antacids, Addison's disease, diabetic coma, severe dehydration, lithium intoxication.
Osmolality	280–296 mOs/kg H_2O	Increased: hyperglycemia, alcohol ingestion, ↑ sodium with dehydration (diarrhea, vomiting, fever, ↓ water intake, hyperventilation, diabetes insipidus, osmotic diuresis), ↑ sodium with normal hydration (hypothalamic disorders), ↑ sodium with overhydration ($NaHCO_3$ for respiratory distress or cardiac arrest, infants given feedings with high Na^+ content). Decreased: hyponatremia with hypovolemia (adrenal insufficiency, renal losses, GI tract loss [diarrhea, vomiting], burns, peritonitis, pancreatitis), hyponatremia with normal or ↑ hydration (CHF, cirrhosis, nephrotic syndrome, SIADH).
pH (arterial)	7.35–7.45	See page 269.
Phosphorus (inorganic)	2.6–4.5 mg/dL	Increased: ↑ phosphate load (↑ vitamin D intake, massive transfusions, phosphate enemas, laxatives or infusion), excess tissue turnover (neoplasms, trauma, rhabdomyolysis, chemotherapy), acromegaly, hypoparathyroidism with ↓ Ca^{++}, high intestinal obstruction, ↓ Mg^+, sarcoidosis.

Phosphorus (inorganic)—cont'd		Decreased: renal or intestinal loss (diuretics, renal tubular defects, hyperthyroidism, hyperparathyroidism, $\downarrow K^+$, $\downarrow Mg^+$, others), $\downarrow$ intestinal absorption (malabsorption, malnutrition, $\downarrow$ vitamin D, osteomalacia, diarrhea, vomiting, phosphate-binding antacids), alcoholism, DM, hyperalimentation, nutritional recovery syndrome, alkalosis, drugs (salicylate poisoning, anabolic steroids, epinephrine, glucagon, insulin, IV glucose).
Potassium (K^+)	3.5–5.0 mmol/L	Increased: impaired excretion (renal failure, oliguria, severe dehydration, $\downarrow$ blood volume, $\downarrow$ mineralocorticoids, Addison's disease), K^+ redistribution (acute acidosis, insulin, intravascular hemolysis, drugs [succinylcholine, digitalis toxicity, β-adrenergic blockade, arginine infusion]), release of extracellular K^+ (burns, crush injury, severe infections, rhabdomyolysis), $\uparrow$ supply of K^+ (factitiously if thrombocytosis or leukocytosis, hemolysis of sample, incomplete separation of serum and clot, prolonged use of tourniquet or hand exercise when drawing blood).
		Decreased: hyperglycemia, nephropathies, mineralocorticoid excess, drugs (diuretics, insulin, adrenergics, antibiotics [amphotericin B, gentamicin, carbenicillin, ticarcillin]), GI loss (vomiting, diarrhea, NG suction, bowel obstruction, small bowel or biliary fistula, laxative abuse, neoplasms), skin loss (excess sweating, cystic fibrosis, severe burns, draining wounds), alkalosis, severe eating disorders, dietary deficiency, licorice abuse.
Protein, total	6.0–8.0 g/dL	Increased: hypergammaglobulinemias, hypovolemic states, dehydration, multiple myeloma, Waldenstrom's macroglobulinemia, sarcoidosis, collagen vascular diseases.
		Decreased: nutritional deficiency, $\downarrow$ or ineffective protein synthesis (severe liver disease, agammaglobulinemia), $\uparrow$ loss (renal [nephrotic syndrome], GI [protein-losing enteropathies or surgical resection], severe skin disease, burns), $\uparrow$ catabolism (fever, inflammation, hyperthyroidism, malignancy, chronic diseases), dilutional (IV fluids, SIADH, water intoxication).
Serum gamma-glutamyl transpeptidase	See GGT, page 263.	
Serum glutamic-oxalacetic Transaminase	See AST, page 262.	
Serum glutamic-pyruvic transaminase	See ALT, page 261.	
Sodium (Na^+)	135–145 mmol/L	Increased: osmotic diuresis (glycosuria, mannitol, urea), excess sweating, diabetes insipidus, respiratory loss (hyperpnea), administration of hypertonic $NaHCO_3$ or dialysis, salt tablets.
		Decreased: nephrotic syndrome, CHF, cirrhosis, renal failure, SIADH, hypothyroidism, adrenal insufficiency, urea, $\downarrow$ mineralocorticoids, GI or skin loss (vomiting, diarrhea, burns, pancreatitis, peritonitis), renal loss (diuresis, ketonuria, metabolic alkalosis, salt-losing nephritis, renal tubular acidosis), drugs that stimulate ADH release (chlorpropamide, tolbutamide, clofibrate, morphine, barbiturates, carbamazepine, acetaminophen, isoproterenol, indomethacin).

Continued on following page

TABLE 8-1: **Normal Reference Values for Serum Analytes** *Continued*

ANALYTE	REFERENCE VALUES	SOME CAUSES OF ABNORMAL RESULTS
Sweat chloride[3]	<60 mEq/L	Increased: Cystic fibrosis (not valid in infants <3 weeks)
Triglycerides	40–150 mg/dL	Increased: hyperlipoproteinemias (see page 274), hypothyroidism, liver diseases, alcoholism, pancreatitis, acute MI, nephrotic syndrome, DM, pregnancy, estrogens, glycogen storage disease.
		Decreased: malnutrition, congenital abetalipoproteinemia, drugs (clofibrate).
Uric acid	F: 2.3–6.6 mg/dL M: 3.6–8.5 mg/dL	Increased: gout, renal failure, asymptomatic hyperuricemia, ↑ destruction of nucleoproteins (leukemia, multiple myeloma, polycythemia, lymphoma [especially following radiation therapy], other disseminated neoplasms, cancer chemotherapy, hemolytic anemia, sickle cell anemia, resolving pneumonia, toxemia of pregnancy), diet (high-protein weight loss, excess nucleoproteins [sweetbreads, liver]), lead poisoning, polycystic kidneys, sarcoidosis, hypoparathyroidism, hypothyroidism, metabolic acidosis, drugs (diuretics, small doses of salicylates).
		Decreased: ACTH therapy, drugs (probenecid, cortisone, allopurinol, coumarins, high doses of salicylates, glycerol guaiacolate), x-ray contrast agents, Wilson's disease, Fanconi's syndrome.

TABLE 8–2. Normal Reference Values for a Complete Blood Cell Count and Some Common Causes of Abnormalities*

ANALYTE	REFERENCE VALUES	SOME CAUSES OF ABNORMAL RESULTS
White blood cell count (WBC, leukocytes)	$4.3–10.8 \times 10^3/mm^3$	Increased: most commonly related to ↑ numbers of neutrophils, lymphocytes, eosinophils, or monocytes (see Differential, next page). Decreased: viral infections, hypersplenism, bone marrow suppression due to drugs (antimetabolites, barbiturates, antibiotics, antihistamines, anticonvulsants, antithyroid meds, arsenicals, cancer chemotherapy, cardiovascular drugs/analgesics, antiinflammatory drugs), primary bone marrow disorders (leukemia, myeloma, aplastic anemia, congenital disorders, myelodysplastic syndromes), immune-associated neutropenia, marrow-occupying diseases (fungal infection, metastatic tumor).
Red blood cell count (RBC, erythrocytes)	$4.15–4.9 \times 10^6/mm^3$	Increased: polycythemia vera, smokers, high altitude, cardiovascular disease, congenital heart disease, chronic lung disease, renal cell carcinoma, other erythropoetin-producing neoplasms, stress, hemoconcentration/dehydration. Decreased: anemias, hemolysis, chronic renal failure, hemorrhage, marrow failure, Hodgkin's disease, lymphoma, multiple myeloma, leukemia, SLE, Addison's disease, rheumatic fever, SBE.
Hemoglobin (Hb)	F: 12–16 g/dL M: 13–18 g/dL	Increased: hemoconcentration, dehydration, COPD, CHF, high altitude. Decreased: hemorrhage, anemia, hyperthyroidism, cirrhosis, hemolysis.
Hematocrit (Hct)	F: 37–48% M: 42–52%	Increased: polycythemia vera, erythrocytosis, smoking, COPD, high altitude, severe dehydration, hypovolemia, shock. Decreased: hemorrhage, anemia, pregnancy, leukemia, hyperthyroidism, cirrhosis, hemolysis.
Mean corpuscular hemoglobin (MCH)	28–33 pg/cell	Increased: macrocytic anemias. Decreased: microcytic anemias.
Mean corpuscular hemoglobin concentration (MCHC)	32–36 g/dL	Increased: spherocytosis, intravascular hemolysis, high-titer cold agglutins, severe plasma lipemia. Decreased: hypochromatic anemia, iron deficiency, macrocytic anemias, anemia of chronic disease.
Mean corpuscular volume (MCV)	86–98 μm^3	Increased: ↓ vitamin B, ↓ folic acid, chronic liver disease, alcoholism, reticulocytosis, myelodysplastic syndromes, myelofibrosis, hypothyroidism, cytotoxic chemotherapy. Decreased: chronic ↓ iron, thalessemia, other hemoglobinopathies, anemia of chronic disease, CRF.

*Normal values used at Massachusetts General Hospital.[4]
↓ = decreased, ↑ = increased, ACTH = adrenocorticotrophic hormone, AIDS = acquired immunodeficiency syndrome, AML = acute myelogenous leukemia, ARC = AIDS-related complex, CHF = congestive heart failure, CLL = chronic lymphocytic leukemia, CML = chronic myelogenous leukemia, CMV = cytomegalovirus, COPD = chronic obstructive pulmonary disease, CRF = chronic renal failure, HIV = human immunodeficiency virus, ITP = idiopathic thrombocytopenic purpura, MI = myocardial infarction, MS = multiple sclerosis, PMNs = polymorphonuclear leukocytes, RA = rheumatoid arthritis, SBE = subacute bacterial endocarditis, SLE = systemic lupus erythematosus, TB = tuberculosis, URI = upper respiratory infection.

Continued on following page

TABLE 8-2. **Normal Reference Values for a Complete Blood Cell Count and Some Common Causes of Abnormalities** *Continued*

ANALYTE	REFERENCE VALUES	SOME CAUSES OF ABNORMAL RESULTS
Red cell distribution width (RDW)	11.5–14.5%	Related to MCV level: *If normal RDW and* ↑ *MCV:* aplastic anemia, preleukemia. *If normal RDW and normal MCF:* normal, anemia of chronic disease, acute blood loss or hemolysis, CLL, CML, others. *If normal RDW and* ↓ *MCV:* anemia of chronic disease, heterozygous thalassemia. *If* ↑ *RDW and* ↑ *MCV:* ↓ vitamin B, ↓ folate, autoimmune hemolytic anemia, cold agglutins, CLL with high count, neonates. *If* ↑ *RDW and normal MCV:* early iron deficiency, early ↓ vitamin B, early ↓ folate, sickle cell diseases, myelofibrosis, sideroblastic anemia. *If* ↑ *RDW and* ↓ *MCV:* iron deficiency, RBC fragmentation, thalassemia intermedia.
Platelets	150–350 × 10³/mm³	Increased: malignancy (especially disseminated or advanced), myeloproliferative diseases, following splenectomy, collagen disorders, iron deficiency anemia, pseudothrombocytosis, acute infections, chronic pancreatitis, cirrhosis, cardiac disease. Decreased: thrombocytopenia (acquired and hereditary).
Differential count (leukocytes)		
Segmented neutrophils (segs, mature neutrophils, PMNs)	45–74%	Increased: acute bacterial infections, tissue breakdown (trauma, burns, tumors, gangrene, acute MI, stress), myelogenous leukemia, hemolysis, uremia, diabetic acidosis, acute gout, seizures, severe exercise, late pregnancy and labor, many drugs.
Bands (stabs, early mature neutrophils)	0–4%	Decreased: viral infections, aplastic anemia, agranulocytosis, immunosuppressive drugs, radiation therapy to bone marrow, drugs (antibiotics, antithyroid drugs), lymphocytic and monocytic leukemias.
Eosinophils (eos)	0–7%	Increased: allergies, eczema, contact dermatitis, reactions to certain drugs (iodides, sulfa drugs, chlorpromazine), chronic granulomatous diseases (sarcoidosis), parasitic infections, lymphomas, lung cancer, pulmonary infiltrates with eosinophilia (PIE), hypereosinophilic syndrome, polycythemia, subacute infections, polyarteritis nodosa, inflammatory bowel diseases. Decreased: adrenal steroid production due to bodily stress (burns, post surgery, SLE), acute infections, infectious mononucleosis, CHF, Cushing's syndrome, drugs (ACTH, epinephrine, throxine, prostaglandins), infections with neutrophilia, neutropenia.

TABLE 8–2. **Normal Reference Values for a Complete Blood Cell Count and Some Common Causes of Abnormalities** *Continued*

ANALYTE	REFERENCE VALUES	SOME CAUSES OF ABNORMAL RESULTS
Differential count (leukocytes)—cont'd		
Basophils (basos)	0–2%	Increased: leukemia, inflammatory processes, polycythemia vera, Hodgkin's disease, hemolytic anemia, following splenectomy or radiation therapy, myeloid metaplasia. Decreased: stress reactions (acute MI, bleeding ulcer), hypersensitivity reactions, steroids, pregnancy, hyperthyroidism.
Lymphocytes (lymphs)	16–45%	Increased: chronic infections, infectious mononucleosis and other viral infections (CMV, URIs, etc.), lymphocytic leukemias, ulcerative colitis, hypoadrenalism, ITP. Decreased: AIDS, ARC, bone marrow suppression from chemotherapy, aplastic anemia, neoplasms, steroids, adrenocortical hyperfunction, neurological disorders (MS, myasthenia gravis Guillain-Barré syndrome), SLE, burns, trauma, chronic uremia, TB, Cushing's syndrome.
Monocytes (monos)	4–10%	Increased: viral diseases, recovery phase of various acute infections, neoplasms, disseminated TB, inflammatory bowel disease, SBE, collagen diseases, hematologic disorders (AML, CML, polycythemia vera, lymphoma, multiple myeloma). Decreased: aplastic anemia, lymphocytic leukemias, hairy cell leukemia, prednisone, RA, HIV.

- Oxygen saturation at any given P_{O_2} is influenced by body temperature, pH, and the level of 2,3-diphosphoglycerate (DPG) inside the red blood cells.

ACID-BASE DISORDERS

Acid-base disturbances are very common clinical problems and are of two basic types: acidosis and alkalosis. The primary causes of acid-base disorders are dysfunction of the respiratory system and/or the metabolic/renal system.

RESPIRATORY ACIDOSIS

Alveolar hypoventilation leads to increased arterial P_{CO_2} levels and reduced pH.

- Acute causes
  - Inadequate ventilation during general anesthesia, mechanical ventilation, or resuscitation
  - Respiratory suppression due to drugs or central nervous system (CNS) disease/trauma
  - Respiratory muscle weakness or paralysis
  - Impaired ventilation (e.g., bronchospasm, laryngospasm, foreign body aspiration, pneumothorax, chest trauma, pneumonia)
  - Impaired diffusion (pulmonary edema, interstitial pneumonitis)
  - Impaired perfusion (e.g., pulmonary embolus (PE), right ventricular failure; decreased cardiac output—congestive heart failure (CHF), arrhythmias, myocardial infarction)

TABLE 8–3. Other Hematologic Analytes*

ANALYTE	REFERENCE VALUES	SOME CAUSES OF ABNORMAL RESULTS
Erythrocyte sedimentation rate (ESR, sed rate)	F: 0–30 mm/hr M: 1–13 mm/hr (Westergren scale)	Increased: severe anemia, macrocytosis, collagen diseases, hypercholesterolemia, infections, acute rheumatic fever, carcinoma, acute MI, nephrosis, pregnancy, chronic inflammatory diseases, ↑ fibrinogen, gamma or beta globulins, toxemia. Decreased: polycythemia, abnormal RBCs (especially sickle cell disease), microcytosis, ↓ fibrinogen, cachexia, ↑ WBC, over-anticoagulation, CHF.
Ferritin	>20 ng/ml	Increased: hyperthyroidism, inflammatory diseases, liver disease, neoplasms, iron replacement therapy, heochromatosis, chronic renal disease. Decreased: iron deficiency anemia.
Folate (folic acid)	Normal >3.2 ng/ml Borderline: 13–30 ng/ml	Decreased: folic acid deficiency (inadequate intake, malabsorption, alcoholism), drugs (methotrexate, trimethoprim, phenytoin, oral contraceptives, aminopterin, azulfadine), vitamin B_{12} deficiency, hemolytic anemia.
Reticulocyte count	0.5–2.5% red cells	Increased: hemolytic anemias, hemorrhage, sickle cell crisis, thalassemia, autoimmune hemolysis, postanemia therapy (folic acid, ferrous sulfate, vitamin B_{12}).

*Normal reference values according to Massachusetts General Hospital.[4]
CHF = congestive heart failure, F = female, M = male, RBC = red blood cell, WBC = white blood cell.

- Chronic causes
  - Lung disease (e.g., chronic bronchitis, emphysema, pulmonary fibrosis)
  - Chest wall disorders (e.g., cervical spine injury, neuromuscular diseases, chest trauma or surgery, kyphoscoliosis)
  - Abdominal interference (e.g., ascites, massive obesity, upper abdominal incision)

METABOLIC ACIDOSIS

A low pH can also result from many metabolic disturbances:

- Increased anion gap (>12 mEq)
  - Increased acid production:
    — Ketoacidosis (e.g., diabetes, alcohol abuse, starvation)
    — Lactic acidosis (e.g., circulatory or respiratory failure, shock, drugs and toxins, enzyme defects); associated with other disorders (e.g, severe anemia, pulmonary disease, neoplasms)

  — Poisoning (e.g., salicylates, ethylene glycol, methanol)
  - Renal failure
- Normal anion gap (due to retention of chloride)
  - Renal tubular dysfunction (e.g., renal tubular acidosis, hypoaldosteronism, potassium-sparing diuretics)
  - Loss of alkali (e.g., diarrhea, ureterosigmoidoscopy, enteric fistula, ileostomy, ileal loop bladder, carbonic anhydrase inhibitors)
  - Excess intake (e.g., ammonium chloride, cationic amino acids)

RESPIRATORY ALKALOSIS

Alveolar hyperventilation leads to decreased arterial P_{CO_2} levels and elevated pH.

- Common causes
  - Anxiety
  - Improper ventilation during anesthesia, mechanical ventilation, or resuscitation

Text continued on page 275

TABLE 8-4. **Some Hematologic Abnormalities**

TERM/ABNORMALITY	DEFINITION
Leukocytosis	Total WBC count >10,000–15,000/mm³
Leukopenia	Total WBC count <4000/mm³
Neutrophilia	Absolute neutrophil count >8000/mm³
Neutropenia	Absolute neutrophil count <1500–2000/mm³, <1000–1500/mm³ in blacks
Lymphocytosis	Lymphocyte count >4000/mm³ in adults, >7200 in adolescents, >9000 in young children and infants
Lymphocytopenia	Lymphocyte count <1500/mm³ in adults, <3000/mm³ in children
Monocytosis	Monocyte count >10% in differential count, or absolute count >500/mm³
Eosinophilia	Eosinophil count >500/mm³, or >10% in differential count
Basophilia	Basophil count >150/mm³, or >3% in differential count
Granulocytosis	Abnormally high count of PMNs (includes neutrophils, eosinophils, and basophils)
Granulocytopenia	Abnormally low count of PMNs
Agranulocytosis	Extremely low count of PMNs (<500/mm³)
Thrombocytosis	Platelet count >500,000/mm³
Thrombocytopenia	Platelet count <100–150 × 10³/mm³
Pancytopenia	Abnormally low counts of RBCs, all WBC types, and platelets
Polycythemia	RBC count >5.1–5.5 × 10⁶/mm³
Reticulocytosis	Reticulocyte (young RBCs) count >2.5–4% of RBCs
Anemia	Any condition in which the RBC count, the Hb level, or the Hct are less than normal:
Aplastic	Failure of bone marrow with pancytopenia
Fanconi's	Congenital aplastic anemia
Hemolytic	Hemolysis of RBCs caused by RBC injury
Iron deficiency	↓ iron for RBC production resulting in ↓ Hb levels
Megaloblastic	↑ Megaloblasts due to ↓ vitamin B_{12} or folate
Macrocytic	With ↑ size of RBCs (↑ MCV)
Microcytic	With ↓ size of RBCs (↓ MCV)
Normocytic	With normal sized RBCs (normal MCV)
Pernicious	Chronic anemia caused by malabsorption
Hemoglobinopathy	Any disorder affecting the structure, function, or production of Hb (e.g., sickle cell syndromes, thalassemia)
Myeloproliferative disorders	Acquired clonal abnormalities of hematopoietic stem cells resulting in changes in myeloid, erythroid, and platelet cells (e.g., polycythemia vera, primary thrombocytopenia)
Myelodysplastic syndromes	A group of disorders characterized by cytopenias of 1–3 cell lines and abnormal cellular morphology in the bone marrow and peripheral blood (e.g., refractory anemia).
Leukemia	Uncontrolled proliferation of a malignant clone of hematopoietic stem cells resulting in marked increase in functionless cells and decreased normal cells
Acute	Characterized by anemia, thrombocytopenia, and granulocytopenia:
ALL	Acute lymphocytic leukemia (↑ number of lymphoid cells)
AML	Acute myelogenous leukemia (↑ number of granulocytes)
ANLL	Acute nonlymphocytic leukemias—all others (myeloid, promyeloid, monocytic, myelomonocytic, erythroleukemia)
Chronic	Proliferative disorders derived from myeloid or lymphoid precursor cells that retain some capacity for differentiation to recognizable mature elements:
CLL	Chronic lymphocytic leukemias (B cell is more common, T cell more aggressive)
CML	Chronic myelocytic/myelogenous leukemia
HCL	Hairy cell leukemia
Leukemoid reaction	A nonleukemic WBC count >50,000/mm³ or differential with >5% metamyelocytes or earlier cells

Hct = hematocrit, Hb = hemoglobin, MVC = mean corpuscular volume, PMN = polymorphonuclear leukocyte, RBC = red blood cell, WBC = white blood cell.

TABLE 8-5. **Normal Reference Values for Coagulation Studies and Common Causes of Abnormalities***

ANALYTE	REFERENCE VALUES	COMMON CAUSES OF ABNORMAL RESULTS
Antithrombin III	80–120% 22–39 mg/dL	Increased: warfarin, post-MI. Decreased: hereditary deficiency, DIC, PE, thrombolytic therapy, cirrhosis, chronic liver failure, postsurgery, late pregnancy, oral contraceptives, sepsis, nephrotic syndrome, IV heparin >3 days.
Bleeding time	2–9.5 min	Increased: thrombocytopenia, capillary wall abnormalities, platelet abnormalities, drugs (aspirin, warfarin, anti-inflammatory drugs, streptokinase, urokinase, dextran, β-lactam antibiotics, moxalactin).
Coagulation factors I (fibrinogen)	0.15–0.35 g/dL	Increased: tissue inflammation or damage, oral contraceptives, pregnancy. Decreased: DIC, hereditary afibrinogenemia, liver disease, fibrinolysis, or abnormal fibrinogen, or abnormal prothrombin; accompanied by prolonged PT and PTT; vitamin K dependent.
II (prothrombin)	60–140%	Accompanied by prolonged PT and PTT.
V (labile factor)	60–140%	
VII (stable factor)	60–140%	Accompanied by prolonged PT but not PTT; vitamin K dependent.
VIII (antihemophilic factor) + (von Willebrand factor)	50–200%	Increased hemophilia A. Decreased: von Willebrand's disease.
IX (Christmas factor)	60–140%	Decreased: Christmas disease.
X (Stuart-Prowe factor)	60–140%	Accompanied by prolonged PT and PTT; vitamin K dependent.
XI (prekallikrein)	60–140%	Accompanied by prolonged PTT.
XII (Hageman factor)	60–140%	Accompanied by prolonged PTT.
XIII (fibrin stabilizing factor)	Negative screen	
Partial thromboplastin time (PTT)	24–37 sec	Prolonged: anticoagulation therapy, coagulation factor deficiencies (hemophilia, ↓ fibrinogen, etc.), liver disease, ↓ vitamin K, DIC, prolonged use of tourniquet before drawing blood sample. Decreased: extensive cancer without liver involvement, immediately after acute hemorrhage, early DIC.
Platelet count	150–350 × 10^3/mm³	See page 268.
Prothrombin time (PT)	8.8–11.6 sec	Prolonged: anticoagulation therapy, DIC, liver disease, ↓ vitamin K, coagulation factor deficiencies, drugs (salicylates, chloral hydrate, diphenylhydantoin, estrogens, antacids, phenylbutazone, quinidine, antibiotics, allopurinol, anabolic steroids), biliary obstruction, prolonged use of tourniquet before drawing blood sample. Decreased: vitamin K supplementation, thrombophlebitis, drugs (gluthetimide, estrogens, giseofulvin, diphenhydramine).
Thrombin time	+/−5 sec of control	Prolonged: heparin therapy, DIC, fibrinogen, streptokinase, urokinase.

*Normal reference values used at Massachusetts General Hospital.[4]
DIC = disseminated intravascular coagulation, IV = intraveneous, MI = myocardial infarction, PE = pulmonary embolism.

TABLE 8–6. Normal Reference Values for Selected Immunologic Analytes and Common Causes of Abnormalities*

ANALYTE	REFERENCE VALUES	COMMON CAUSES OF ABNORMAL VALUES
Autoantibodies Antinuclear (ANA)	Negative at 1:8 dilution	Positive: mixed connective tissue diseases (SLE, RA, scleroderma, dermatomyositis, polyarteritis), drug-induced lupus-like syndromes, chronic active lupoid hepatitis, pulmonary interstitial fibrosis, TB, necrotizing vasculitis, Sjögren's syndrome, idiopathic.
Mitochondrial	Negative at 1:20 dilution	Positive primary biliary cirrhosis, long-standing hepatic obstruction, chronic hepatitis, cryptogenic cirrhosis.
Smooth muscle	Negative at 1:20 dilution	Positive: chronic active hepatitis, lupoid hepatitis, intrinsic asthma, acute viral hepatitis, biliary cirrhosis.
Cold agglutins[2]	<1:32	Increased: Mycoplasma pneumonia, CMV infections, infectious mononucleosis, cirrhosis, acquired hemolytic anemia, frost bite, malaria.
Complement C3	83–177 mg/dL	Increased: inflammatory states as acute-phase response (RA, rheumatic fever, early SLE), neoplasms. Decreased: active SLE, glomerulonephritis, chronic active hepatitis, DIC, hereditary C3 deficiency, celiac disease, anorexia nervosa, SBE, chronic liver disease, Gram-negative sepsis, fungemia, cryoglobulinemia, immune complex disease.
C4	15–45 mg/dL	Increased: neoplasms, juvenile RA, ankylosing spondylitis. Decreased: acute early SLE, early glomerulonephritis, hereditary angioneurotic edema, hereditary C4 deficiency, cryoglobulinemia, immune complex disease.
Immunoglobulins IgA	70–312 mg/dL	Increased: cirrhosis, hepatitis, gamma A myeloma, subacute and chronic infections, RA, SLE, CML, exercise. Decreased: hereditary deficiency, lymphocytic leukemias, ataxia telangiectasia, acquired immunodeficiency states, chronic sinopulmonary disease, protein-losing enteropathy, late pregnancy.
IgG	639–1349 mg/dL	Increased: infections of all types, severe malnutrition, RA, myeloma, hyperimmunization, liver disease. Decreased: hereditary or acquired deficiency, CLL, protein-losing syndromes, pregnancy, IgA myeloma.
IgM	56–352 mg/dL	Increased: liver disease, chronic infections, primary biliary cirrhosis, Waldenström's macroglobulinemia, RA, SLE. Decreased: hereditary deficiency, CLL, protein-losing syndromes, IgG and IgA myelomas, hepatoma, lymphoid aplasia, infancy and early childhood.
IgE	<103 IU/ml	Increased: atopic diseases (exogenous asthma, atopic eczema, hay fever), parasitic diseases, IgE myeloma. Decreased: hereditary deficiency, acquired immunodeficiency, ataxia telangiectasia, non-IgE myelomas.
Rheumatoid factor (fasting)	<30 IU/ml	Increased: RA, SLE, syphilis, chronic inflammation, SBE, cancer, some lung diseases (i.e., TB), sarcoidosis, viral infections.

*Normal reference values used at Massachusetts General Hospital[4] unless otherwise footnoted.
↓ = decreased, ↑ = increased, CLL = chronic lymphocytic leukemia, CML = chronic myelocytic/myelogenous leukemia, CMV = cytomegalovirus, DIC = disseminated intravascular coagulation, RA = rheumatoid arthritis, SBE = subacute bacterial endocarditis, SLE = systemic lupus erythematosus, TB = tuberculosis.

TABLE 8-7. **Normal Arterial Blood Gas Values**

MEASUREMENT	NORMAL VALUES
P_{O_2}	75–100 mm Hg
P_{CO_2}	35–45 mm Hg
pH	7.35–7.45
O_2 saturation	>95%
$[HCO_3^-]$	22-26 mEq/L
Base difference (deficit/ excess)	−2–+2

TABLE 8-8. **Summary of Acid-Base Changes in the Blood**

	PH	PCO₂	[HCO₃]
Acidosis			
Acute respiratory	↓	↑	Nl
Compensated respiratory	Nl	↑	↑
Acute metabolic	↓	Nl	↓
Compensated metabolic	Nl	↓	↓
Alkalosis			
Acute respiratory	↑	↓	Nl
Compensated respiratory	Nl	↓	↓
Acute metabolic	↑	Nl	↑
Chronic metabolic	↑	↑	↑

↓ = decreased, ↑ = increased, Nl = normal.

TABLE 8-9. **Hyperlipidemias**

TYPE	LIPOPROTEIN ABNORMALITY	PLASMA LIPIDS		CAD RISK	PREVALENCE
		CHOLESTEROL	TRIGLYCERIDES		
I	↑↑↑ Chylomicrons	Nl–↑	↑↑↑	Low	Rarest
IIa	↑↑↑ LDL cholesterol	↑↑↑	Nl	Very high	Common
IIb	↑↑ LDL, ↑ VLDL	↑↑	↑	Very high	Probably common
III	Broad band B-lipoprotein	↑↑	↑↑	Very high	Rare
IV	↑ VLDL	Nl–↑	↑↑	High	Most common
V	↑↑ VLDL,↑↑ Chylomicrons	↑	↑↑	Low	Rare

↑ = somewhat increased, ↑↑ = moderately increased, ↑↑↑ = markedly increased, CAD = coronary artery disease, LDL = low-density lipoprotein, Nl = normal, VLDL = very low-density lipoprotein.

TABLE 8-10. Serum Chemistry Values in Acute Myocardial Infarction*

ANALYTE (NORMAL VALUES)	BEGINS TO RISE	REACHES PEAK	RETURNS TO NORMAL
Creatine kinase (CPK) (F: 40–150 U/L) (M: 60–400 U/L)	2–12 hr	12–40 hr	2–6 days
MBs (0–7.5 ng/mL) (<4%)	2–12 hr	12–24 hr	1.5–3 days
Aspartate aminotransferase (AST) (F: 9–25 U/L) (M: 10–40 U/L)	6–24 hr	24–48 hr	3–6 days
Lactate dehydrogenase (LDH) (110–210 U/L)	12–48 hr	2–6 days	7–14 days
LDH-1 (17–27%) (LDH-1 < LDH-2)	12–48 hr	2–6 days	7–14 days

*Normal reference values used at Massachusetts General Hospital.[4]
F = female, M = male.

- Hypoxic stimulation of the peripheral chemoreceptors (e.g., asthma attack, CHF, PE, pneumonia)
- Stimulation of the midbrain respiratory centers (e.g., lesions, cerebrovascular accident, drugs, endotoxins)
- Increased intracranial pressure
- Fever
- Pregnancy
- Ascites

METABOLIC ALKALOSIS

Abnormally high blood pH can also result from metabolic abnormalities:

- Common causes
  - Associated with volume (and chloride) depletion (e.g., vomiting, nasogastric suction, diuretic therapy, abrupt decrease in P_{CO_2} during treatment of chronic respiratory acidosis)
  - Associated with hyperadrenocorticism leading to renal acid excretion (e.g., Cushing's syndrome, hyperaldosteronism)
  - Severe potassium depletion
  - Excessive alkali intake (e.g., bicarbonate or precursors, alkalining salts, milk-alkali syndrome)
- A summary of acid-base changes that are seen with various disorders are shown in Table 8–8.

8.7 ABNORMALITIES SEEN IN SPECIFIC DISEASE STATES

Frequently, disease states produce specific abnormalities in a number of laboratory blood tests. Some of these of particular interest in patients with cardiopulmonary dysfunction are listed below:

- The various types of hyperlipidemias are shown in Table 8–9.
- The serum enzyme abnormalities seen in acute myocardial infarction are listed in Table 8–10. In addition, the changes in these enzyme levels as a function of time are illustrated in Figure 8–2.
- Table 8–11 depicts the characteristic patterns observed in renal impairment and failure.
- Some possible patterns of abnormalities seen in liver disease are shown in Table 8–12.

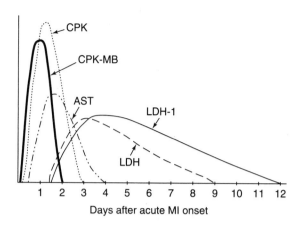

FIGURE 8-2. Changes in cardiac enzyme levels over time in acute myocardial infarction (MI). CPK = creatine phosphokinase, CPK-MB = myocardial band or cardiac isoenyzme, AST = aspartate transaminase, LDH = lactate dehydrogenase, LDH-1 = cardiac isoenzyme.

Days after acute MI onset

TABLE 8-11. **Characteristic Patterns of Renal Impairment and Failure**

ANALYTE (NORMAL VALUES)*	PRERENAL AZOTEMIA	ACUTE TUBULAR INJURY	CHRONIC RENAL FAILURE
Urine osmolality (500–1200 mOsm/L)	>500	<350	<50
Urine/plasma urea	>10	<10	>10
Urine/plasma creatinine	>40	<20	<20
Urine Na⁺ (40–240 mEq/ 24 hr)	<10–20	>40	May be ↑ or may be ↓
Renal failure index	<1	>2	>2
Excreted fraction of filtered Na⁺	<1	>3	>2
Other	No casts in UA, ↑ BUN > ↑ creatinine	Clinical evidence of acute onset, positive casts or cells in UA, ↑ serum WBC, slight ↑ BUN, ↑ serum creatinine, metabolic acidosis; may be ↓ Ca⁺⁺, ↑ K⁺, normal–↓ serum Na⁺	Proteinuria, ↑ BUN, ↑ serum creatinine, ↓ serum Na⁺, ↑ serum K⁺, metabolic acidosis, ↑ serum Ca⁺⁺, ↑ triglycerides, ↑ cholesterol, ↑ VLDL, ↓ Hct (anemia), ↓ serum albumin, ↓ total protein, ↑ phosphate

*Normal reference values used at Massachusetts General Hospital.[4]
↓ = decreased, ↑ = increased, BUN = blood urea nitrogen, Hct = hematocrit, UA = urinalysis, VLDL = very low-density lipoprotein, WBC = white blood cell.

TABLE 8-12. Characteristic Patterns of Liver Function Tests

DISORDER	BILIRUBIN	ALKALINE PHOSPHATASE	AST (SGOT)	ALT (SGPT)	PTT	OTHER
Hepatocellular jaundice	↑	↑–↑↑	↑ AST < ALT	↑	Nl–↑ (poor response to vitamin K)	↓ Serum albumin; ↓↓ Cholesterol (total and esters)
Uncomplicated obstructive jaundice	↑–↑↑↑	↑↑↑	Nl–↑ AST > ALT	Nl–↑	Nl–↑↑ (responds to vitamin K)	↑ Total cholesterol (normal esters); Nl–↓ albumin; ↑ GGT
Acute viral or toxic hepatitis	↑–↑↑↑	↑–↑↑	↑↑↑	↑↑↑	Nl–↑↑↑	↑ IgM if hepatitis B
Chronic active (non-A, non-B) hepatitis	Nl–↑	Nl–↑	↑–↑↑	↑–↑↑	Nl–↑↑ (No response to vitamin K)	Nl–↑ serum albumin; ↑ IgG, IgM
Alcoholic hepatitis	Nl–↑↑	Nl–↑↑	Nl–↑↑↑	Nl–↑↑	Nl–↑↑	Nl–↓ serum albumin; ↑ Gamma globulin; ↑ GGT; ↑ MCV; May be anemia
Cirrhosis	Nl–↑	Nl–↑	Nl–↑↑	Nl–↑	Nl–↑↑	Anemia is common; ↑ Gamma globulin, especially IgM; ↓ Serum albumin; Positive mitochrondrial antibody

↓ = decreased, ↑ = somewhat increased, ↑↑ = moderately increased, ↑↑↑ = markedly increased, GGT = gamma glutamyl transpepidase, Ig = immunoglobulin, MCV = mean corpuscular volume, Nl = normal.

REFERENCES

1. Ferri FE: *Practical Guide to the Care of the Medical Patient.* St. Louis, The C.V. Mosby Co., 1987.
2. Fischbach F: *A Manual of Laboratory & Diagnostic Tests,* 4th Ed. Philadelphia, J.B. Lippincott Co., 1992.
3. Gomella LG (ed.): *Clinician's Pocket Reference,* 6th Ed. Norwalk, CT, Appleton & Lange, 1989.
4. Jordan CD, Flood JG, Laposata M, Lewandrowski KB: Normal reference laboratory values. *New Engl. J. Med.* 327:718–724, 1992.
5. Krupp MA, Tierney LM, Jawetz E, Roe RL, Camrgo CA: *Physician's Handbook,* 21st Ed. Los Altos, CA, Lange Medical Publications, 1985.
6. Pagana KD, Pagana TJ: *Mosby's Diagnostic and Laboratory Test Reference.* St. Louis, The C.V. Mosby Co., 1989.
7. Ravel R: *Clinical Laboratory Medicine: Clinical Application of Laboratory Data,* 5th Ed. Chicago, Year Book Medical Publishers, Inc., 1989.
8. Schroieder SA, Tierney LM, McPhee SJ, Papadakis MA, Krupp MA (eds.): *Current Medical Diagnosis & Treatment.* Norwalk, CT, Appleton & Lange, 1992.
9. Wallach J: *Interpretation of Diagnostic Tests: A Synopsis of Laboratory Medicine,* 5th Ed. Boston, Little, Brown & Co., 1992.

ABBREVIATIONS

AAA Abdominal aortic aneurysm

A & B Apnea and bradycardia

A-a gradient Alveolar-to-arterial gradient

ABE Acute bacterial endocarditis

ABGs Arterial blood gases

ACE Angiotensin converting enzyme

A/C Assist control (on ventilator)

ACB Aortocoronary bypass

AF Aortofemoral, atrial fibrillation

a-fib Atrial fibrillation

AI Aortic insufficiency

AICD Automatic implantable cardiac defibrillator

ALT Serum alanine aminotransferase (= SGPT)

AML Anterior mitral leaflet

AMV Augmented minute ventilation

Ao Aorta

AP Anteroposterior, aortopulmonary

APC Atrial premature complex/contraction (= PAC)

ARDS Adult respiratory distress syndrome

ARF Acute renal failure, acute rheumatic fever

AS Aortic stenosis

ASCAD Atherosclerotic coronary artery disease

ASCVD Atherosclerotic cardiovascular or cerebrovascular disease

ASD Atrial septal defect

ASHD Atherosclerotic heart disease

AST Serum aspartate aminotransferase (= SGOT)

AT Anaerobic threshold

AV Atrioventricular

(a-v)O$_2$ Arteriovenous oxygen difference

AVB Atrioventricular node block

AVR Aortic valve replacement

BE Base excess/deficit

BP Blood pressure

bpm Beats per minute, breaths per minute

BR Breathing reserve

BS Breath sounds, bowel sounds

BSA Body surface area

CABG Coronary artery bypass graft (surgery)

CAD Coronary artery disease

CBF Coronary blood flow

CF Cystic fibrosis

CHD Coronary heart disease, congenital heart disease

CHF Congestive heart failure

CI Cardiac index

CMC Closed mitral commissurotomy

CO Cardiac output, carbon monoxide

COAD Chronic obstructive airway disease

COLD Chronic obstructive lung disease

COPD Chronic obstructive pulmonary disease

cp Chest pain

CPAP Continuous positive airway pressure

CPA Cardiophrenic angle (on chest x-ray [CXR] examination)

CPB Cardiopulmonary bypass

CPK Creatine phosphokinase

CT Computed tomography

Cx Circumflex (coronary artery)

CVP Central venous pressure

CWE Chest wall excursion

CXR Chest x-ray

DBP Diastolic blood pressure

D$_{LCO}$ Diffusion capacity for carbon monoxide

DOE Dyspnea on exertion

ECG Electrocardiogram

EDP End-diastolic pressure

EDV End-diastolic volume

EF Ejection fraction

EPS Electrophysiologic studies

EST Exercise stress test

ESV End-systolic volume

ET Endotracheal

ETT Exercise tolerance test, endotracheal tube

f Respiratory rate

FEF$_{25\%-75\%}$ Forced expiratory flow during midhalf of forced vital capacity

FEV$_1$ Forced expiratory volume in 1 second

FEV$_1$/FVC Percentage of forced vital capacity in 1 second

FIO$_2$ Fraction of inspired oxygen
FRC Functional reserve capacity
FVC Forced vital capacity
FWC Functional work capacity
GBPS Gated blood pool study (= MUGA, RNA)
GXT Graded exercise test
HBP High blood pressure
HCM Hypertrophic cardiomyopathy (formerly IHSS)
HCO$_3^-$ Bicarbonate
HCTZ Hydrochlorothiazide
HCVD Hypertensive cardiovascular disease
HDL High-density lipoproteins
HJR Hepatojugular reflex
HOCM Hypertrophic obstructive cardiomyopathy
HR Heart rate
HR$_{max}$ Maximal heart rate (= MHR)
HRR Heart rate reserve
HTN Hypertension
IABP Intraaortic balloon pump
IC Inspiratory capacity
ICS Intercostal space
IHSS Idiopathic hypertrophic subaortic stenosis (= HOCM)
IMV Intermittent mandatory ventilation
IPPB Intermittent positive pressure breathing
IRBBB Incomplete right bundle-branch block
IRV Inspiratory reserve volume
ISA Intrinsic sympathetic activity
IVCD Intraventricular conduction delay
IVS Interventricular septum
JVD Jugular venous distension
LA Left atrium
LAD Left anterior descending (coronary artery), left axis deviation
LAE Left atrial enlargement
LAH(B) Left anterior hemiblock
LAO Left anterior oblique
LAP Left atrial pressure
LBBB Left bundle-branch block
LDH Lactic dehydrogenase
LDL Low-density lipoproteins
LDL/HDL Ratio of low-density lipoproteins to high-density lipoproteins
LLL Left lower lobe
LM(CA) Left main (coronary artery)
LPH(B) Left posterior hemiblock
LV Left ventricle
LVEDP Left ventricular end-diastolic pressure
LVEDV Left ventricular end-diastolic volume
LVEF Left ventricular ejection fraction

LVESV Left ventricular end-systolic volume
LVET Left ventricular ejection time
LVH Left ventricular hypertrophy
LVOT Left ventricular outflow tract
LVSWI Left ventricular stroke work index
(m) Murmur
MAP Mean aortic pressure
MCL Midclavicular line
MET(s) Metabolic equivalent of energy expenditure
MHR Maximal heart rate (= HR$_{max}$)
MHRR Maximal heart rate reserve
MI Myocardial infarction
MIF Maximal inspiratory flow
MMEF Maximal midexpiratory flow
MR Mitral regurgitation
MRI Magnetic resonance imaging
MS Mitral stenosis
MUGA Multiunit gated acquisition scan (= GBPS, RNA)
MV̇o$_2$ Myocardial oxygen consumption
MVP Mitral valve prolapse
MVR Mitral valve replacement
MVV Maximal voluntary ventilation
NSR Normal sinus rhythm
NT Nasotracheal
NTG Nitroglycerine (= TNG)
O$_2$ Oxygen
O$_2$ sat Oxygen saturation (= SaO$_2$)
OMC Open mitral commissurotomy
PA Pulmonary artery
PA line Pulmonary artery line
PAC Premature atrial complex/contraction (= APC)
P$_{ao}$ Pressure at airway opening
P$_{alv}$ Alveolar pressure
PAP Pulmonary artery pressure
PAT Paroxysmal atrial tachycardia
P$_{aw}$ Pressure at any point along airways
PAW(P) Pulmonary artery wedge pressure (= PCW[P])
P$_{bs}$ Pressure at the body surface
PaCO$_2$, PCO$_2$ Carbon dioxide tension or pressure
PCW(P) Pulmonary capillary wedge (pressure) (= PAW(P))
PD Postural drainage
PDA Patent ductus arteriosus, posterior descending artery
PE Pulmonary embolus, physical examination
PEEP Positive end-expiratory pressure
PEF Peak expiratory flow
PEP Preejection period

P_{es} Esophageal pressure used to estimate P_{pl}

PET Positron emission tomography

PFO Patent foramen ovale

PFT(s) Pulmonary function test(s)

P_L Transpulmonary pressure ($= P_{alv} - P_{pl}$)

PMI Point of maximal impulse

PND Paroxysmal nocturnal dyspnea

PaO_2, PO_2 Oxygen tension or pressure

P_{pl} Pleural pressure

PR Pulmonary regurgitation

PS Pulmonary stenosis

PTCA Percutaneous transluminal coronary angioplasty

PVC Premature ventricular complex/contraction ($= VPC$)

PVR Pulmonary or peripheral vascular resistance

P_w Transthoracic pressure ($= P_{pl} - P_{bs}$)

PWP Pulmonary wedge pressure

$\dot{Q}$ Volume of blood flow, cardiac output

$\dot{Q}s$ Shunt volume

$\dot{Q}s/\dot{Q}t$ Shunt fraction

Qt Total volume

R Respiratory exchange ratio ($= \dot{V}CO_2/\dot{V}O_2$)

RA Right atrium

RAD Right axis deviation

RAE Right atrial enlargement

RAO Right anterior oblique

RAP Right atrial pressure

R_{aw} Airway resistance

RBBB Right bundle-branch block

RCA Right coronary artery

RF Rheumatic fever

RHD Rheumatic heart disease

RHR Resting heart rate

RLL Right lower lobe

RML Right middle lobe

RNA Radionuclide angiography ($= GBPS$, MUGA)

RNV Radionuclide ventriculography ($= GBPS$, RNA)

RPE Rating of perceived exertion

RPP Rate-pressure product

RR Respiratory rate ($= f$)

RUL Right upper lobe

RV Right ventricle, residual volume

RV/TLC Percentage of total lung capacity taken by the residual volume

RVH Right ventricular hypertrophy

S_1 First heart sound

S_2 Second heart sound

S_3 Third heart sound

S_4 Fourth heart sound

SA Sinoatrial

SAM Systolic anterior motion (re: anterior mitral valve leaflet)

SaO_2 Oxygen saturation ($= O_2$ sat)

SBE Subacute bacterial endocarditis

SBP Systolic blood pressure

SEM Systolic ejection murmur

SGOT Serum glutamic-oxaloacetic transaminase ($= AST$)

SGPT Serum glutamic-pyruvic transaminase ($= ALT$)

SIMV Synchronous intermittent mandatory ventilation

SPECT Single-photon emission computed tomography

ST ST segment of the electrocardiogram (ECG)

SV Stroke volume

SVR Systemic vascular resistance

SVT Supraventricular tachycardia

SWI Stroke work index

TGA Transposition of the great arteries

TI Tricuspid insufficiency

TLC Total lung capacity

TMT Treadmill test

TNG Trinitroglycerine ($= NTG$)

TPA Tissue plasminogen activator (or tPA)

TPR Total peripheral resistance

TR Triscuspid regurgitation

TS Triscuspid stenosis

TTI Tension-time index

TVR Tricuspid valve replacement

URI Upper respiratory infection

$\dot{V}A$ Alveolar ventilation

VC Vital capacity

VCG Vectorcardiogram

$\dot{V}CO_2$ Volume of carbon dioxide produced

VD Dead space ventilation

VD/VT Dead space to tidal volume ratio

$\dot{V}E$ Expired ventilation per minute

VEA Ventricular ectopic activity

$\dot{V}O_2$ Oxygen consumption or uptake (total body)

VPB Ventricular premature beat

VPC Ventricular premature complex/contraction ($= PVC$)

$\dot{V}/\dot{Q}$ Ventilation-perfusion ratio

VSD Ventricular septal defect

VT Tidal volume

v-fib, VF Ventricular fibrillation

v-tach, VT Ventricular tachycardia

WPW Wolff-Parkinson-White syndrome

A wave The rise in the atrial pressure curve caused by active contraction of the atria

Acetylcholine A chemical neurotransmitter released from the preganglionic and postganglionic endings of parasympathetic nerve fibers and from the preganglionic endings of sympathetic fibers, which causes cardiac inhibition, vasodilation, gastrointestinal peristalsis, and other parasympathetic effects

Acetylcholinesterase An enzyme that catalyzes the hydrolysis of acetylcholine and thus controls its effect

Acidemia A decrease in the pH of the blood due to an increase in its hydrogen ion concentration

Acidosis A disorder of normal acid-base balance resulting from accumulation of acid (hydrogen ion) and/or reduction of base (bicarbonate) in the blood or tissues

Acinus The portion of the lung distal to the terminal bronchiole comprising respiratory bronchioles, alveolar ducts, alveolar sacs, and alveoli

Adrenergic Related to epinephrine (adrenaline) or substances with similar activity; pertaining to or affecting the sympathetic nervous system

β-Adrenergic blocker A substance that selectively inhibits or blocks β-adrenergic (sympathetic nervous system) stimulation of effector cells

Adventitious breath sounds Abnormal sounds heard on auscultation that are superimposed over normal breath sounds

Aerobic Relating to the use of oxygen to produce energy

Afterload The load or pressure against which the ventricle must exert its contraction force to eject blood

Airway reactivity Alteration of bronchomotor tone in response to noxious stimuli

Airway resistance (R_{aw}) The force opposing the flow of gases during ventilation; results from obstruction or turbulence in the upper and lower airways

Akinesis Lack of movement; in cardiology, lack of movement of an area of myocardium

Aldosterone A steroid hormone produced by the kidneys that effects resorption of sodium and excretion of hydrogen and potassium

Alkalemia An increase in the pH of the blood due to a decrease in its hydrogen ion concentration

Alkalosis A disorder of normal acid-base balance resulting from excessive accumulation of base (bicarbonate) or excessive loss of acid (hydrogen ion)

Alveolar ventilation ($\dot{V}A$) The amount of air that participates in gas exchange

Alveolitis Inflammation of the alveoli

Alveolus One of the smallest terminal air sacs involved in gas exchange

Anaerobic Relating to the production of energy without the use of oxygen

Anaerobic threshold (AT) The onset of blood lactate accumulation that occurs as exercise intensity increases beyond the level that can be met by predominantly aerobic metabolism; also called ventilatory threshold

Anemia An abnormally low number of red cells in the blood

Aneurysm An area of muscular weakness and dilation occurring in an artery or cardiac chamber

Angina pectoris Pain, pressure, or heaviness, occurring usually in the chest or surrounding areas, which is caused by insufficient myocardial oxygen supply

Angiography Radiologic examination of blood vessels injected with contrast medium

Antibody A class of immunoglobulins capable of attacking invading antigens

Antidiuretic hormone (ADH) A hormone secreted by the pituitary gland that causes the kidneys to retain water and in high concentrations causes contraction of vascular smooth muscle; vasopressin

Antigen Any substance capable of causing the production of antibodies

Apgar score A 10-point scoring system used to assess the status of newborns (heart rate, respiratory effort, muscle tone, response to stimulation, and skin color); usually performed at 1 and 5 minutes of age

Apnea A temporary cessation of breathing

Arrhythmogenic Capable of producing arrhythmias

Arteriovenous oxygen difference ([a-v]O$_2$) The difference between arterial and central venous oxygen content

Atelectasis Collapse and airlessness of alveoli

Atherosclerosis Disease process characterized by irregularly distributed lipid deposits in the intima of large and medium-sized arteries

Atrial gallop The presence of a late diastolic (presystolic) fourth heart sound (S$_4$) in addition to the normal first and second heart sounds

Atrioventricular (AV) block Delayed or interrupted conduction of the electrical impulse as it passes from the atria through the atrioventricular node to the ventricles; also called heart block

Automaticity The ability of a cell to initiate its own depolarization

Barotrauma Injury caused by excessively high or low pressure (e.g., of the lungs due to high inspiratory pressures during mechanical ventilation)

Bigeminal Paired extrasystoles, as when atrial or ventricular complexes are coupled to sinus beats

Bleb Coalescent alveolar sacs formed from the destruction of alveolar septa, as in emphysema

Borg scale A numeric scale for rating perceived exertion

Bradycardia A slow heart rate, usually defined as less than 50 beats per minute

Bradypnea An abnormal slowing of respiration

Bronchiectasis Dilation and distortion of the bronchial and bronchiolar walls as the result of chronic inflammation or obstruction

Bronchiolitis Inflammation of the bronchioles

Bronchodilator A medication that relieves bronchoconstriction and thereby increases the luminal diameter of the bronchi

Bronchophony Louder, distinct voice transmission heard over areas of consolidated lung tissue

Bulla A thin-walled, air-filled cavity larger than 1 cm in diameter resulting from destruction of alveolar septa

Capacitance vessels The large venules and veins that form a large, variable-volume, and low-pressure reservoir

Cardiac index Cardiac output divided by body surface area (L/min/m^2)

Cardiac reserve The difference between resting cardiac output and the maximal cardiac output of an individual

Cardiac tamponade See "Pericardial tamponade"

Cardiogenic shock A condition where the heart is unable to pump enough cardiac output to perfuse the body tissues

Cardiomyopathy Any primary disease of the heart muscle

Cardioversion Restoration of the normal rhythm of the heart by electrical countershock

Carina Specifically in the pulmonary system, the ridge separating the openings of the right and left main bronchi at their junction with the trachea

Catecholamine Any of the compounds secreted by the adrenal medulla that affect the sympathetic nervous system

Cholinergic Relating to nerve fibers that secrete acetylcholine; pertaining to or affecting the parasympathetic nervous system

Chordae tendinae Fibrous cords that attach the leaflets of the heart valves to the papillary muscles and myocardium

Chronotropic Affecting the heart rate

Cilia Hairlike projections from respiratory epithelial cells that propel mucus and debris toward the pharynx

Closing volume The lung volume at which small airway closure begins during expiration

Clubbing A proliferative change in the soft tissues of the distal fingers and toes, especially the nailbeds, with broadening, loss of the base angle at the cuticle, and increased curvature, giving a bulbous appearance

Commissurotomy A surgical division of the junction between adjacent cusps of a cardiac valve

Compliance A measure of the distensibility of a tissue (i.e., increase in volume per unit of pressure change); regarding patients, adherence to prescribed medical treatment, lifestyle modifications, etc.

Congestion Excessive accumulation of blood in the vessels of an organ

Consolidation Solidification of a normally aerated portion of a lung resulting from the presence of exudative fluid and cells in the alveolar spaces

Contractility The ability of tissue, especially muscle, to shorten and develop tension; in the heart, the innate rate and intensity of force development during contraction

Cor pulmonale Right-sided heart failure due to pulmonary hypertension resulting from acute or chronic pulmonary disease

Costophrenic Pertaining to the ribs and diaphragm, as in the angle between the rib cage and diaphragm on a chest radiograph

Couplet A pair of atrial or ventricular extrasystoles

Crackles Adventitious breath sounds heard over areas where there is fluid accumulation in the distal airways, or over collapsed alveoli, which partially reopen during inspiration; rales

Croup A condition resulting from acute inflammation of laryngeal structures causing a characteristic barking cough

Cuirass A type of negative pressure mechanical ventilator that covers the anterior chest wall

Cyanosis Bluish or purple discoloration of the skin and mucous membranes as a result of insufficient oxygenation with a high concentration of reduced hemoglobin in the capillaries

Decortication Removal of the cortex or external layer, usually applied to a surgical excision of residual clot and/or newly organized scar tissue that form after a hemothorax or empyema

Decubitus Sidelying position

Defibrillation Electrical shock of sufficient power to cause a fibrillating heart to resume normal rhythm

Dehiscence Splitting open of a surgical wound

Desaturate To produce desaturation, an increase in the percentage of unfilled oxygen-binding sites on the hemoglobin molecule

Dialysis A form of filtration that separates the smaller molecules in a solution from the larger ones through the use of a semipermeable membrane

Diaphoresis Perspiration, sweat

Diastole The period of ventricular relaxation in the cardiac cycle

Diffusion The passive tendency of molecules to move from an area of higher concentration to one of lower concentration, as in the movement of oxygen into and carbon dioxide out of the blood in the pulmonary capillaries

Diuretic Type of medication used to decrease body fluid and thereby decrease blood volume, as in heart failure or hypertension

Dopaminergic Relating to those nerves or receptor sites that employ dopamine as their neurotransmitter

Dyskinesis Difficult or abnormal movement; in cardiology, abnormal paradoxic movement of an area of myocardium

Dysphagia Pain and/or difficulty in swallowing

Dyspnea A subjective difficulty or distress in breathing

Echocardiography (echo) The use of ultrasound to depict the structures of the heart and great vessels

Ectopy Abnormal or aberrant origination of myocardial depolarization

Effusion An accumulation of fluid that has escaped from its natural vessels into a body cavity, as in pleural or pericardial effusion

Egophony Abnormal vocal transmission over areas of pulmonary consolidation characterized by the auscultation of $\bar{a}$ when the vowel sound $\bar{e}$ is spoken

Ejection fraction (EF) The portion of filling volume that is actually ejected from the ventricle during systole (i.e., stroke volume/end-diastolic volume)

Electrocardiogram (ECG) A graphic recording of the electrical activity of the heart versus time

Electrolyte Any substance that ionizes in solution and thus conducts electricity and is decomposed by it

Embolism Occlusion of a blood vessel by matter carried by the blood flow from another site

Embolus Undissolved matter (e.g., thrombus, vegetation, mass of bacteria, tumor) lodged in a vessel

Empyema Accumulation of pus in a body cavity, commonly the pleural space

Endocarditis Inflammation of the endocardium

Endocardium The endothelium and subendothelial connective tissue of the heart

Epicardium The outermost layer of the heart; the visceral part of the pericardium

Epiglottitis Inflammation of the epiglottis, the cartilage that protects the trachea from aspirating foodstuff during the normal swallowing process

Ergometer A device for measuring the amount of work, or exercise, performed

Exacerbation An increase in the severity of the signs and symptoms of a disease

Expectoration The act of coughing up and spitting out materials from the lungs

Extracorporeal membrane oxygenation (ECMO) The use of an artificial membrane outside the body to provide oxygenation of the blood

Exudate Any fluid that gradually oozes out of a body tissue because of abnormal leakage, as in inflammation

Fibrosis The formation of fibrous tissue as a reactive or reparative process

Fibrothorax A chronic pleural disease characterized by formation of thick fibrous tissue and adhesion of the two layers of pleura

Fick method (principle) A method of determining cardiac output (L/min) by dividing the oxygen consumption (mL/min) by the difference between the arterial and mixed-venous blood oxygen content (mL/L)

FIO_2 The fraction of inspired oxygen; the portion of an inhaled mixture of gases that is oxygen

Fissure A clearly discernible division in lung tissue that separates two lobes of the lungs

Foramen ovale In the fetus, the oval opening in the interatrial septum secundum; normally it closes soon after birth

Foramen secundum In the fetus, the opening in the dorsal part of the septum primum that forms before the septum fuses with the endocardial cushions

Fremitus A vibration within the thorax that is felt by palpation

Fulminant Suddenly occurring

Functional capacity The ability or power to perform necessary activities

Glottis The fissure between the vocal cords

Granulation The formation of minute, rounded connective tissue projections that form on the surface of a lesion during healing

Granuloma Nodular inflammatory lesions composed of modified macrophages

Hemidiaphragm One of the two domes of the diaphragm

Hemopneumothorax The presence of blood and air in the pleural cavity

Hemoptysis The expectoration of blood from the lungs because of pulmonary or bronchial hemorrhage

Hemothorax The presence of blood in the pleural cavity

High-density lipoprotein (HDL) The major class of lipoproteins containing approximately 50% protein and lower levels of cholesterol and triglycerides than low-density lipoproteins and very low-density lipoproteins

Hilus The point at which the nerves, vessels, and primary bronchi penetrate the parenchyma of each lung

Honeycombing On chest x-ray film, a course reticular density

Huffing A cough assistance technique where forced expiration is performed with an open glottis to assist in the expectoration of secretions

Hyaline membrane An eosinophilic membrane lining the alveolar ducts of infants suffering from respiratory distress syndrome

Hypercapnia The presence of an abnormally high amount of carbon dioxide in the circulating blood; hypercarbia

Hyperkalemia An abnormally high potassium ion concentration in the circulating blood

Hypernatremia An abnormally high sodium ion concentration in the plasma

Hyperpnea An increase in the depth of respiration

Hypersomnolence A condition of drowsiness approaching coma

Hyperventilation Increased alveolar ventilation relative to metabolic carbon dioxide production so that arterial carbon dioxide levels are lower than normal

Hypocapnia Abnormally reduced arterial carbon dioxide level; hypocarbia

Hypokalemia An abnormally low potassium ion concentration in the circulating blood

Hypokinesis Reduced movement; in cardiology, reduced movement of an area of myocardium

Hyponatremia An abnormally low sodium ion concentration in the plasma

Hypotension Abnormally low arterial blood pressure or a fall in arterial blood pressure with an increase in exertion or heart rate

Hypoventilation Inadequate alveolar ventilation relative to carbon dioxide production so that arterial carbon dioxide levels are increased

Hypoxemia Abnormally low arterial oxygen levels in the blood

Hypoxia Subnormal levels of oxygen in inspired gas, arterial blood, or tissues

Idiopathic Of unknown origin or cause

Idiopathic hypertrophic subaortic stenosis (IHSS) Obstruction of the left ventricular outflow tract due to hypertrophy of the left ventricular septum; hypertrophic obstructive cardiomyopathy

Immunodeficiency A state of defective immune response, either humoral or cellular

Immunoglobulin (Ig) Circulating antibodies that protect the body from foreign substances

Immunosuppressive Any agent that prevents or interferes with the development of an immune response

Infarction Sudden insufficiency of arterial or venous blood supply resulting in a macroscopic area of necrosis

Inotrope An agent that influences the contractility of muscular tissue

Intercurrent Occurring during the course of an existing process

Intermittent claudication An attack of pain or lameness, usually in the calf, caused by muscle ischemia (most commonly because of atherosclerosis)

Interpolated Occurring or inserted between two other things

Interstitial Situated between essential parts or in the interspaces of a tissue

Intima The innermost layer of a vessel; tunica intima

Intubation The insertion of a hollow tube through the nose or mouth into the trachea, usually for the purpose of assisted ventilation

Ischemia Inadequate oxygenation of a tissue relative to its demands

Isocapnia A state in which the arterial carbon dioxide tension remains constant or unchanged, despite changes in ventilation

Jugular venous distention (JVD) Stretching or overfilling of the jugular vein, usually due to elevated venous pressure

Junctional rhythm The rhythm of the heart when the atrioventricular node takes over as the predominant pacemaker; nodal rhythm

Kerley B lines Seen on chest radiography, fine horizontal lines a few centimeters above the costophrenic angle; postulated to result from distention of interlobular lymphatics with edema fluid

Korotkoff sounds Sounds heard over an artery when pressure over it is reduced during the determination of blood pressure by the auscultatory method

Kussmaul breathing Deep, rapid respiration characteristic of diabetes or other causes of acidosis

Laryngospasm Involuntary muscular contraction that results in closure of the glottis

Left-to-right shunt A diversion of blood from the left side of the heart to the right or from the systemic circulation to the pulmonary circulation

Lobectomy Surgical resection of a lobe of the lungs

Low-density lipoprotein (LDL) The major class of lipoproteins having a relatively large molecular weight and containing proportionally less protein and more cholesterol and triglycerides than high-density lipoproteins

Manubrium The upper portion of the sternum

Meconium The first stool passed by a newborn

Mediastinal shift A shifting of the mediastinum to one side as the result of lower pressure in one hemithorax compared with the other (e.g., displacement away from a tension pneumothorax or toward an atelectatic segment)

Mediastinum The area of the thoracic cavity containing the structures between the lungs

Mediate percussion The act of tapping on the surface of the chest using one middle finger over the other to evaluate the resonance of the underlying structures

Melanoptysis Expectoration of black sputum, as in coal workers' pneumoconiosis

MET The abbreviation for metabolic equivalent of energy expenditure; the amount of energy or oxygen required to perform particular tasks relative to that required at rest

Metabolic acidosis A decreased level of arterial bicarbonate and pH as the result of metabolic pathologic conditions

Metabolic alkalosis An elevated level of arterial bicarbonate and pH as the result of metabolic pathologic conditions

Methylxanthines A class of drugs (e.g., aminophylline) that have bronchodilator and cardiac and CNS stimulant properties

Microatelectasis Airlessness of a very small part of the lungs caused by resorption of gas from collapsed or blocked alveoli

Midsystolic click A clicking sound heard on auscultation of the heart that is associated with systolic prolapse of the mitral valve leaflets

Mucociliary transport The process of removal of mucus and debris from the airways by way of the wavelike motion of the cilia

Mucokinetic Relating to an agent capable of enhancing the mobilization of secretions

Mucolytic Capable of dissolving, digesting, or liquifying mucus

Mucopurulent Containing both mucus and pus

MV̇o₂ Myocardial oxygen consumption

Myocardial infarction Necrosis of an area of heart muscle due to sudden insufficient or interrupted blood flow

Myocarditis Inflammation of the myocardium

Myocardium The muscular middle layer of tissue in the heart; also used in general reference to the heart

Myocytes muscle cells

Myxoma A benign neoplasm derived from connective tissue

Nares Nostrils

Natriuresis The urinary excretion of sodium; commonly designates enhanced sodium excretion, as in certain diseases or resulting from diuretic therapy

Nitroglycerin (NTG) A drug used as a vasodilator, especially in angina pectoris

Norepinephrine A catecholamine hormone that possesses the excitatory actions of epinephrine but has minimal inhibitory effects

Obesity hypoventilation syndrome A syndrome characterized by hypercapnia and acidemia associated with reduced alveolar ventilation due to massive obesity

Obstructive (airways/lung) disease Lung disease characterized by chronic airflow limitation, or increased airway resistance, which is particularly noticeable on expiration

Opening snap A diastolic sound heard on auscultation of the heart that is associated with the opening of stenotic atrioventricular valves

Opportunistic infection Infection with microorganisms that do not ordinarily cause disease, occurring in individuals whose immune systems are compromised

Orthopnea Discomfort in breathing that develops when lying flat and is relieved by a more upright position

Orthostatic hypotension A fall in blood pressure because of rapid changes to more upright positions

Orthotopic In the normal or usual position, as in heart transplantation where the native heart is removed and the donor heart is positioned in its place

Osteoarthropathy Joint swelling and pain caused by numerous chronic pulmonary infections and other disorders

Oximeter An instrument that measures oxygen saturation

Oxygen pulse The volume of oxygen consumed per heart beat

Oxygen saturation The percentage of hemoglobin bound with oxygen

Oxygen toxicity An inflammatory response of various tissues (e.g., eyes, lungs, central nervous system) to prolonged exposure to exceedingly high concentrations of inspired oxygen

Palliative Mitigating; reducing the severity of

Pallor Paleness of the skin

Palpitation A pulsation of the heart perceived by an individual

Panacinar or panlobular Involving the entire acinus or lobule of the lung, as in panlobular emphysema

Pancarditis Inflammation of all the structures of the heart

Papillary muscles Projections of cardiac muscle that terminate in the chordae tendinae and anchor the valves

Paradoxic Occurring contrary to the normal rule

Parasympatholytic Relating to an agent that inhibits the cholinergic receptors of the autonomic nervous system

Parasympathomimetic Relating to an agent that stimulates the cholinergic receptors of the autonomic nervous system

Parenchyma The essential functioning cells of an organ

Parietal pleura The layer of the pleural sac that is adjacent to the chest wall

Paroxysmal Occurring with a sudden onset and cessation

Partial thromboplastin time (PTT) The time it takes for a fibrin clot to form after calcium and a phospholipid have been added to a blood sample; activated partial thromboplastin time; evaluates intrinsic clotting mechanism

Pathophysiology The science of disordered function in disease

Pectoriloquy The transmission of whispered voice sounds to the chest wall

Pectus carinatum Excessive prominence of the sternum; pigeon breast

Pectus excavatum Excessive depression of the sternum; funnel breast

Perfusion Blood flow per unit volume of tissue; in the lungs the blood flow through the pulmonary circulation that is available for gas exchange

Pericardial tamponade Compression of the heart with restriction of ventricular filling due to accumulation of fluid within the pericardial sac; cardiac tamponade

Pericardiectomy Surgical resection of part of the pericardium

Pericardiocentesis The removal of fluid from the pericardial sac using a needle

Pericarditis Inflammation of the pericardium

Pericardium The fibroserous membrane surrounding the heart and the origins of the great vessels

Periodic respiration Alternating periods of hyperpnea and apnea

Pertussis Inflammation of the larynx, trachea, and bronchi; whooping cough

Petechiae Pinpoint purplish discolorations of skin or mucous membrane caused by intradermal bleeding

Physiologic dead space Areas of the lungs that are ventilated but not perfused so there is no gas exchange

Pleura The serous membrane enveloping the lungs and lining the chest wall

Pleural rub Inspiratory and expiratory grating, creaking sounds heard on auscultation that result from pleural inflammation

Pleurectomy Surgical resection of the pleura, usually the parietal pleura

Pleurisy Inflammation of the pleura; pleuritis

Pleurodesis Creation of an adhesion between the parietal and visceral pleurae by surgical or medical means

Plethysmograph An airtight chamber into which an individual is placed to measure various pulmonary function values

Pneumatocele A thin-walled cavity within the lung; characteristic of staphylococcal pneumonia

Pneumoconiosis An inflammatory fibrosis of the lungs due to the inhalation of dust particles, usually from occupational exposure

Pneumomediastinum Air within the mediastinal space

Pneumonectomy Surgical resection of an entire lung

Pneumonia Inflammation of the lungs, particularly due to infection

Pneumonitis Any inflammation of the lungs

Pneumothorax Air within the pleural space

Polycythemia An abnormally high number of red cells in the blood

Postperfusion syndrome A condition of decreased cardiac output in conjunction with other cardiovascular symptoms that arise following cardiopulmonary bypass during cardiac surgery

Postpericardiotomy syndrome The occurrence, often repeatedly, of the symptoms of pericarditis, with or without febrile episodes, weeks or months after cardiac surgery

Postural drainage The use of gravity and positioning to facilitate the removal of secretions from the airways

Postural hypotension Low blood pressure that develops on assumption of upright postures; orthostatic hypotension

Preload The volume of blood in the ventricle just before systole; the end-diastolic volume

Preprandial Before a meal

Pressor An agent that enhances vasomotor tone and increases blood pressure

Prinzmetal's angina See "Variant angina"

Prothrombin time (PT) The time it takes plasma to form a fibrin clot after the addition of calcium and thromboplastin are added; evaluates extrinsic clotting mechanism

Pulsus alternans The mechanical alteration of the pulse characterized by a regular rhythm and alternating strong and weak pulses; seen with serious myocardial disease

Pulsus paradoxus A marked variation in cardiac stroke volume with respiration characterized by a stronger pulse during expiration and a weaker pulse during inspiration; seen in pericardial effusion or restrictive pericarditis

Purulent Consisting of, containing, or discharging pus

Pyogenic Producing or able to produce pus

R-on-T phenomenon The occurrence of a premature ventricular complex (R wave) during the relative refractory period (during or on the T wave) of the preceding beat

Rales Discontinuous adventitious breath sounds of a crackling nature heard throughout inspiration and the first third of expiration; crackles

Rate-pressure product The product of heart rate times systolic blood pressure; an indirect indicator of myocardial oxygen demand

Respiratory failure The inability of the respiratory system to adequately ventilate the alveoli

Restrictive lung dysfunction (RLD) An abnormal reduction in pulmonary ventilation due to restriction of expansion by the lungs or chest wall

Retinopathy Noninflammatory degenerative disease of the retina

Rhonchi Continuous, "snoring" adventitious sounds heard on auscultation during both inspiration and expiration; caused by air passing through larger airways with secretions; low-pitched wheezes

Right-to-left shunt A diversion of blood from the right side of the heart to the left without participating in gas exchange; intrapulmonary shunt

Scintigraphy A diagnostic procedure involving the intravenous injection of a radionuclide and radiologic imaging

Sensitivity The probability that, given the presence of a disease, an abnormal test result indicates the presence of the disease

Shock A state of profound physical depression due to severe physical injury or illness

Sick sinus syndrome A condition characterized by alternating episodes of bradycardia and recurrent extrasystoles and supraventricular tachycardia

Silent ischemia A condition of inadequate myocardial circulation without the typical symptoms of ischemia

Silicosis A type of pneumoconiosis that results from occupational exposure over years to silica dust

Sinus block Failure of an impulse to be transmitted from the sinoatrial node

Sleep apnea Episodes of breathing cessation caused by an upper airway obstruction during sleep

Specificity The probability that, given the absence of disease, a normal test result excludes the presence of the disease

Spirometry Measurement of the various lung volumes using a spirometer (a counterbalanced cylindric bell sealed via a water trough)

Status asthmaticus Severe, intractable asthma

Sternotomy A surgical incision through the sternum

Stridor A high-pitched inspiratory and expiratory sound created by obstruction of the larynx or trachea to airflow

Stroke volume The volume of blood (mL) ejected with each heart beat

Subcutaneous emphysema The presence of free air in the subcutaneous tissue, due to air leak from the lungs

Sudden cardiac death Death within 1 hour of the onset of cardiac symptoms

Summation gallop The presence of third and fourth heart sounds, which are fused, in addition to the normal first and second heart sounds

Suppuration The formation of pus

Surfactant A surface-active agent lining the alveolar surfaces that reduces surface tension and retards the tendency of the alveoli to collapse

Sympatholytic Denoting an agent that inhibits adrenergic receptors of the autonomic nervous system

Sympathomimetic Denoting an agent that produces effects similar to those produced by stimulation of the sympathetic nervous system

Syncope Sudden, transient loss of consciousness due to inadequate cerebral perfusion

Systole The period of ventricular contraction

Tachycardia An abnormally fast heart rate, usually considered greater than 100 beats per minute

Tachypnea An abnormally fast respiratory rate; polypnea

Tamponade Compression of the heart as a result of fluid accumulation within the pericardial sac

Tension pneumothorax The accumulation of air in the pleural space due to a valve effect where air leaks on inspiration but is trapped on expiration

Thermodilution method A method of measuring cardiac output where a bolus of cold saline is injected into the right atrium and the resultant temperature change is measured in the pulmonary artery

Thoracentesis The removal of fluid from the pleural space using a needle

Thoracoplasty The surgical resection of ribs to allow inward retraction of the chest wall, to reduce the size of the pleural space

Thoracotomy Surgical opening of the thoracic cavity

Thrombocytopenia An abnormally low number of platelets in the blood

Thrombolysis The dissolving of a thrombus

Tissue plasminogen activator (TPA, tPA) A genetically engineered thrombolytic agent used in conjunction with heparin to limit the size of a myocardial infarction

Torsade de pointes A 5- to 20-beat salvo of paroxysmal ventricular tachycardia with an undulating QRS axis that progressively changes direction

Total peripheral resistance (TPR) The force opposing the flow of blood in the systemic circulation; derived from dividing the mean arterial pressure by the cardiac output

Tracheitis Inflammation of the mucosal lining of the trachea

Tracheoesophageal fistula An abnormal communication between the esophagus and the trachea

Tracheomalacia An erosion of the trachea, usually because of excessive pressure from a cuffed endotracheal tube

Transudate Any liquid that passes through a membrane as a result of an imbalance between the hydrostatic and osmotic forces on the two sides of the membrane

Triplet Three consecutive atrial or ventricular extrasystoles

Tympany A low-pitched, resonant, drumlike sound obtained by percussing the chest wall or other hollow organ

Unstable angina (pectoralis) Preinfarction chest pain characterized by discomfort occurring at rest and low levels of activity

V **wave** The rise in the atrial pressure curve near the end of ventricular systole caused by gradual passive filling of the atria with the atrioventricular valves closed

Valsalva maneuver Contraction of the muscles of the abdomen, chest wall, and diaphragm in a forced expiratory effort against a closed glottis

Valvular insufficiency Inadequate closure of one of the cardiac valves so that blood regurgitates through the closed valve

Valvular stenosis Narrowing of a valve orifice

Valvuloplasty The surgical reconstruction of a defective valve to relieve incompetence or stenosis

Valvulotomy A surgical incision through a stenosed valve or valve leaflet to relieve an obstruction

Variant angina Atypical angina; angina that is not precipitated by increased myocardial demand, is often of longer duration and more severe, and is associated with ST elevation; Prinzmetal's angina

Vasopressor An agent that produces vasoconstriction or an increase in blood pressure

Ventilation Movement of gas into and out of the alveoli

Ventilation-perfusion ($\dot{V}/Q$) matching/ratio The degree of physical correspondence between ventilated and perfused areas of the lungs

Ventilatory failure Inability of the lungs to adequately perform gas exchange; specifically because of impairment of the ventilatory pump

Ventilatory reserve The difference between normal pulmonary ventilation and the maximal breathing capacity of an individual

Ventricular fibrillation (VF, v-fib) An erratic quivering of the ventricular myofibrils that produces no cardiac output and clinical death if untreated

Ventricular gallop The presence of an early diastolic, third heart sound (S_3) in addition to the normal first and second heart sounds

Ventriculography The radiologic visualization of the ventricles using injection of a radiopaque material

Venturi mask A supplemental oxygen delivery device that can be adjusted to deliver a specific fraction of inspired oxygen at relatively high flow rates

Very low-density lipoproteins (VLDL) The major class of lipoproteins containing a high concentration of triglycerides and a moderate concentration of cholesterol and phospholipids

Visceral pleura The serous membrane covering the surface of each lung

Wandering pacemaker An abnormal cardiac rhythm in which the site of the controlling pacemaker shifts from beat to beat, usually between the sinus and atrioventricular nodes

Wheezes Continuous, musical sounds of variable pitch and duration heard on auscultation of the lungs, caused by airway narrowing

Whispered pectoriloquy Distinct transmission of whispered words over an area of consolidated lung tissue

INDEX

Note: Page numbers in *italics* refer to illustrations; page numbers followed by t refer to tables.

Children *(Continued)*
  oxygen saturation in, 249t
  patent ductus arteriosus in, 232–233, *232*
  pericarditis in, 238–239
  physical therapy for, 239–240, 244, 247–248, 251–256
    bronchial drainage in, 251, *252*, 253t
      contraindications to, 253t
      precautions with, 253t
    bronchial hygiene techniques in, 251, *252*, 253t, 254t, *255*, 256t
    chest percussion in, 251, *254*, 254t, *255*, 256t
      contraindications to, 254t
      precautions with, 254t
    chest vibration in, 251, 254t, *255*, 256t
      contraindications to, 254t
      precautions with, 254t
    endurance exercise training in, 254
    patient position in, 244, 251
    physiologic monitoring in, 244
    suctioning in, 251, 256t
  pulmonary stenosis in, 234
  respiratory distress in, 242–243, *242*, 249t
  respiratory rate in, 250t
  rheumatic fever in, 238
  skeletal system of, 249t
  skin color in, 249t
  tetralogy of Fallot in, 235–237, *236*
  transposition of great arteries in, 237–238, *237*
  trisomy 21 syndrome in, 247
  ventricular septal defect in, 231–232, *231*
  vital signs in, 250t
Chlorambucil, pulmonary toxicity of, 108
Chloride, reference values for, 263t
  sweat, reference values for, 266t
Chlorothiazide (Diuril), as antihypertensive agent, 113–114, 114t, 115t
Chlorpropamide (Diabinese), 144, 144t
Chlorthalidone (Hygroton; Thalitone), as antihypertensive agent, 113–114, 114t, 115t
Cholesterol, drug reduction of, 133, 134t
  reference values for, 263t, 264t, 274t
Cholestyramine (Cholybar; Questran), as hyperlipidemic agent, 133, 134t
Choloxin (dextrothyroxine), as hyperlipidemic agent, 133, 134t
  cardiac effects of, 136t
Cholybar (cholestyramine), as hyperlipidemic agent, 133, 134t
Christmas factor (factor IX), reference values for, 272t
Chronic obstructive pulmonary disease (COPD), 88–89
  adventitious sounds in, 193t
  breath sounds in, 193t
  chest examination in, 150t
  chest x-ray in, 151t
  cor pulmonale with, 99
  diaphragmatic excursion in, 170

Chronic obstructive pulmonary disease (COPD) *(Continued)*
  diaphragmatic motion in, 168
  dyspnea in, positioning for, *220*, 221
  expiration in, 158t
  expiratory flow-volume curve in, 51
  flow-volume loop in, *51*
  in peripheral vascular disease, 101t
  inspection in, 193t
  lung capacities in, 47
  lung sounds in, 161t
  lung volumes in, 47
  percussion in, 193t
  physical signs in, 193t
  pulmonary function tests in, 151t
  pursed-lip breathing in, 211–212, *211*
  respiratory muscle training in, 206
  tactile fremitus in, 193t
  ventilatory muscle training in, 206–207
  voice sounds in, 193t
Chylomicrons, laboratory values for, 274t
Cirrhosis, liver function tests in, 277t
Claudication, intermittent, 8t, 105, 106, 106t, 154t
Clicks, midsystolic, 164t
Clofibrate (Atromid-S), as hyperlipidemic agent, 133, 134t
  cardiac effects of, 136t
Clonidine (Catapres), 118t
Closing volume (CV), in pulmonary function testing, 49t
Clubbing, digital, 8t, 41t
  in physical therapy examination, *157*, 158
Cluster breathing, 158t
Coagulation, laboratory studies of, 259–260, 272t
Coagulation factors, reference values for, 272t
Coagulation necrosis, in myocardial infarction, 71
Coarctation of the aorta, 229t, 233–234, *233*
Cocaine, in coronary disease, 148
Coffee, atrial dysrrhythmias with, 180
  paroxysmal atrial tachycardia with, 181
  paroxysmal supraventricular tachycardia with, 181
  premature ventricular complexes with, 185
Cold agglutins, reference values for, 273t
Colestipol (Colestid), as hyperlipidemic agent, 133, 134t
Collagen vascular disease, cardiopulmonary complications of, 100t, 101t, 106
Coma, 41t
Commissurotomy, valvular, 29
Complement, reference values for, 273t
Compliance, patient. See *Patient compliance.*
Compliance (C), pulmonary, 38t, 50t
  in infant respiratory distress syndrome, 242
  ventricular, 5
Computed tomography, 17–18, *18*, 44
Confusion, in pulmonary disease, 41t
Congenital heart disease, 227, 229–238, 229t
  acyanotic, 229–234, *231–233*
  aortic stenosis as, 234
  atrial septal defect as, 230–231, *231*

ISBN 0-7216-6709-0

90016

9 780721 667096